hairdressing

Withdrawn

with barbering

for the 2003 Standards

S/NVQ level 2

hairdressing

with barbering

Leah Palmer
Nicci Moorman

www.heinemann.co.uk
✓ Free online support
✓ Useful weblinks
✓ 24 hour online ordering

01865 888058

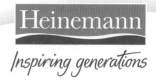

Heinemann
Inspiring generations

Heinemann Educational Publishers
Halley Court, Jordan Hill, Oxford OX2 8EJ
Part of Harcourt Education

Heinemann is the registered trademark of
Harcourt Education Limited

© Fareham College, 2003

First published 2003

08 07 06 05 04
10 9 8 7 6 5 4 3 2

British Library Cataloguing in Publication Data is available
from the British Library on request.

ISBN 0 435 45155 3

Copyright notice

Page layout and illustrations by Hardlines Ltd, Charlbury, Oxon
Original illustrations © Harcourt Education Limited, 2002

Cover design by bigtop, Bicester, UK

Printed in the UK by Bath Press Ltd

Cover photo: © PR: Harriet Evans, Hair by Annakarin Sjoberg
for Headmasters, photography by Simon Coates, make-up by
Annakarin Sjoberg, stylist: Annakarin Sjoberg and products by
L'Oreal Professionnel

Headmasters website: www.hmhair.co.uk

Websites

Please note that the examples of websites suggested in this book
were up to date at the time of writing. It is essential for tutors to
preview each site before using it to ensure that the URL is still
accurate and the content is appropriate. We suggest that tutors
bookmark useful sites and consider enabling students to access
them through the school or college intranet.

Tel: 01865 888058 www.heinemann.co.uk

Contents

Acknowledgements

We would like to thank our respective families (in particular Leah would like to thank her husband and children and Nicci would like to thank her partner) for your devotedness during the long and often bumpy journey along the route to being authors. Your steadfastness and huge support during this project has made this tremendous achievement possible. Thank you for giving us the time when we needed it.

We would also like to thank:

All our models, without whom this book would not be so beautiful. Thanks for all your time and patience during the photo shoots.

All our colleagues at Fareham College. In particular, thank you to the management team, Mary Mussell and Joan Champion for all your support over the last two-and-a-half years and to our fellow lecturers, past and present, for your valuable contributions to the content of this book and for your understanding during its birth.

Our fantastic photographers, Gareth and Tony, for making our first-ever photo shoot such a pleasure. Thanks guys!

Sally Smith, our photo researcher, who learnt some vital hairdressing skills whilst working with us and Chris Honeywell for the final photo shoot.

Tina Lawton and Sue Williams from Warrington College for their hard work on the Key Skills development and to their colleagues for sharing good practice.

Pen, Gillian and Maggie at Heinemann.

Finally, we would like to thank our good friends. Without your unquestionable support and friendship, you would not be reading this now.

Leah Palmer and Nicci Moorman

The authors and publisher would also like to thank Judith Hughes, Sylvia Stephenson, Byron Calame, Wesley Ricketts, Emma Fairfield and Jenny Sealey for their input into the African Caribbean units. We would also like to thank Dr Ali N Syed, Master Chemist and President of Avlon Inc, for his help and advice with the African Caribbean units. Thanks must also go to Susan Ross for all her hard work on the original manuscript.

Use of HABIA unit titles and element headings by kind permission of HABIA, Fraser House, Nether Hall Road, Doncaster, South Yorkshire, DN1 2PH, Tel: 01302 380000, Fax: 01302 380028, Email: enquiries@habia.org.uk, Website: www.habia.org.uk.

Photo acknowledgements

Gareth Boden: page 89
John Carne Hairdressing Group: pages 1 (centre and right), 48, 53
Lakmé: page 95
Daniel Lee: page 45, 286
Lido's: pages 1, 47 (left)
Photodisc: page 7
Science Photo Library: pages 94 (top left, top right, bottom left, bottom right), 317

All other photos © Gareth Boden and Chris Honeywell

Every effort has been made to contact copyright holders of material published in this book. We would be glad to hear from unacknowledged sources at the first opportunity.

INTRODUCTION

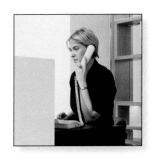 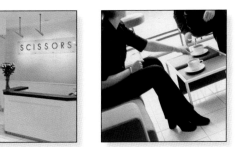 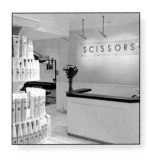

How to use this book

This book has been designed with a dual purpose:

To lead you through the Hairdressing Level 2 NVQ qualification, providing you with background and technical guidance, suggested evidence collection and key skills information.

To provide a reference book that, hopefully, you will find useful to dip into long after you have gained your qualification. The comprehensive cross mapping within the individual units will guide you through the NVQ units and indicate how the information applies, and should prevent repetition!

Important information about the hair and skin is included in the section 'Facts about hair and skin'. Read this thoroughly before you do anything else. The information it gives applies to many of the units throughout the book, so if you learn and understand this first, all the other areas should make sense. Remember that you only have to learn the information once and then apply your knowledge to the practical skills unit you are working through.

Some helpful features

To reinforce your learning process and get you thinking, there are several features included throughout the book to help you:

 In the salon – these are case studies based on real-life events that you may face in an actual salon! They are designed to allow you to consider situations which may actually arise and circumstances that need to be dealt with, for example, a customer complaint which may require you to relate to your knowledge of legislation and inter-personal skills. Case studies help you to think ahead and give an indication of what may happen in a commercial salon.

 Reality check! – offers a guide to good practice and to help you anticipate any problems that may arise. They cover health and safety aspects as well as good working professional practice.

 Check it out – provides activities that apply the theory in a practical situation and can be used to provide portfolio evidence, key skills evidence or customer service evidence.

 Remember – highlight specific areas you need to pay particular attention to.

 Contraindication – indicates when you should be aware that a treatment might be inappropriate or needs adapting.

These features appear in the practical skills units only:

- **Prompt** – you will find this at the end of each element. It will provide you with the key points for revision.
- **Your questions answered** – you will find this at the end of each unit. It offers a quick problem-solving page, answering the 'What if?' questions you might think of as you work through a unit.
- **Test your knowledge** – you will find this after 'Your questions answered'. It will test your knowledge and understanding acquired during the unit. 'Test your knowledge' will not be valid as evidence for your portfolio unless it is carried out under assessment conditions, but it is very good revision!

NVQ guidance – back to basics

If you are familiar with the NVQ system and are confident about the background to this method of gaining a qualification, then skip this part, and move on! If, however, you are new to the NVQ system, read on!

What is an NVQ?

NVQ stands for **National Vocational Qualification**. You may not be familiar with the way this qualification is gained, particularly if you have come from school via the GCSE route, or if you have not been in a training situation for some time.

NVQ is a highly successful method of gaining a qualification. It does not involve an exam with a pass or fail outcome. There is no one-off, scary day of reckoning! NVQ uses continual **assessments** in each unit, building up to a qualification – another option for those of us who panic at the thought of an exam room! However, you will still need to sit written assessments set by your Awarding Body.

There are several hairdressing Awarding Bodies offering NVQs. The qualification can be taken at different levels – 1, 2 or 3. Your college or training institution will be able to guide you through the requirements of the particular Awarding Body it uses, but the standards do not vary much and the information within this book should cover all eventualities!

How to gain an NVQ

To gain an NVQ, you will need to show plenty of **evidence** that you have undertaken each NVQ unit. It is a practical qualification, so each student gets a very good grounding in all the skill areas. This means that when you go into a salon, you will have dealt with most client requests and have lots of confidence to perform the service.

How do I get my evidence?

Many forms of evidence are acceptable – your lecturer or trainer will be able to guide you through the best options for your individual learning programme. Each of the following types of evidence is valid:

- observed work
- witness statements
- assessment of prior learning and experience (APL)
- oral questions
- written questions and/or assignments
- other – for example photographs, project work, videotape, client record cards.

You should record your evidence on the **evidence sheets** provided and these will form your **portfolio**, which is simply a collection of all your evidence.

Organising your portfolio

It is essential to present your work in a clear format so that it can be assessed easily. For this reason, you should produce an **index** listing of what is in your portfolio.

An **assessor** will observe or guide you through the types of evidence listed previously. He or she will have had special training and will hold a specific qualification designed to help you present your evidence in a format suitable for your Awarding Body.

For quality control and fairness across the subject areas, an **internal verifier** will check the assessor and the portfolio instruction. This will be performed at your place of training and should take place regularly.

The Awarding Body also has an **external verifier** who will visit your college or training institution regularly and check that both assessors and internal verifiers are giving the correct information to you, the candidate. Then your portfolio can be accredited with a certificate. This can be achieved a unit at a time or applied for all at once. So, a clear and well-organised portfolio is vital!

What evidence do I need?

Ask your assessor the most suitable method for the work you are doing. Most portfolios contain a mixture of evidence.

If you have external previous experience (APL) or recent qualifications, this can be counted as evidence. For example, if you work part time in a shop (not necessarily a salon) and have experience using the till, dealing with customers and complaints, then a **witness statement** from your employer that is current, valid, signed and dated (such as the one shown here) is acceptable evidence.

Ali's Grocery Store
12 Arcadia Avenue
No Man's Land
Surrey

12 January 2003

To whom it may concern:

Angela Smith has been working for me for two years and is a trustworthy and honest employee. In the course of her duties she works the till, deals with cheques, credit cards and cash, and regularly cashes up. Angela has dealt with returned faulty goods, difficult customers and the odd complaint. I find her helpful, courteous and she works well with colleagues. She follows instructions and works well on her own.

Yours faithfully

Ali Shubvala

(Owner)

The evidence shown in the sample letter would cover some of the reception units, as well as some communication units and the interpersonal skills required. It also covers some of the **ranges** required in your **assessment book** (see below).

What do I have to achieve?

Now let's take an overall look at what you are going to need to do to gain your NVQ qualification.

Your college or training institution will register you with its Awarding Body. The Awarding Body will then issue you, the candidate, with your assessment book. Take care of it; treat it like gold, as it is very precious. This together with your portfolio are your sources of evidence of your hard work.

The assessment book contains guidance on how to achieve each NVQ unit. Each unit is divided into elements. You will need to complete the following for each element:

- **Performance criteria** – you must perform these in the course of your assessed service treatment. They are numbered and your assessor will tick them off as they are observed, for example, 'Identify what clients want' (Unit G7, Outcome 1). You will need to show that you have met all the performance criteria to be considered competent.
- **Range statements** – you need to demonstrate your competence in a variety of different situations and these are described in the range statements of each Element. They must be covered through the various methods of assessment described above – observed performance, oral question or simulation, written question, project or through APL. For example, the range statements for Unit H7, Outcome 2 include 'Creating neckline shapes as tapered, squared and rounded'.
- **Essential knowledge** – each Element identifies the knowledge and understanding supporting the practical application:
- 'Need to know' may not be directly assessable but supports the essential knowledge. This may be in the form of an oral question. For example, using a steamer is not a range to be assessed within Unit H9, but you need to know about it and the effects it has in relation to a conditioning treatment. You may be shown a demonstration of how to use one, without being assessed upon it. You may be asked a question on it.
- 'Need to understand' provides the evidence and is directly assessable.

Why hairdressing?

NVQ Level 2 is the beginning of a career in hairdressing, an industry that is ever changing and has no boundaries to success or the avenues that may be followed. Your NVQ will give you the basic elements that you need to help you become a qualified hair stylist. However, it is important to make sure that you gain your NVQ qualification either through a reputable salon or college/training institution. Once completed, your qualification will open up a world full of opportunities within the fashion and media industries, such as:

- salon stylist/colour technician
- photographic work for magazines
- television work
- fashion shows
- films/theatre work
- salon owner (and that can also be home based)
- hairdressing shows and seminars
- working on cruise ships.

The hairdressing industry has a very flexible employment pattern. As well as working in a salon as a stylist or a technician, many people working in hairdressing are self-employed and enjoy the range of contacts that this brings.

Earning possibilities have improved immensely in recent years. Hairdressing is now classed as very much a fashion accessory. Clients buy designer clothes and they now look to buy designer hairstyles and will pay the appropriate price for a top stylist to create their image. This has led to hairdressers being paid the right salary for their job.

After completing your NVQ, you will take the role of a junior stylist. Here you will put into practice the basic elements that you have learnt and find out what fun the hairdressing industry can be. You will gain excellent customer service skills in monitoring and looking after your clientele as well as creating your own artistic flair and style in hairdressing.

When you start work, you will find that you need to develop the skills you began to acquire as you trained, including:

- customer service
- reception
- communication
- teaching
- management

- accountancy
- presentation
- artistic talent
- marketing
- advertising

Hairdressing is a 'people profession' as well as being creative and innovative. It is fun and rewarding, as well as hard work! There are many avenues open to you in terms of careers. Below are four very different career paths that individuals have followed. A profile of each of these people may show you the range of options available.

A salon manager with a specialist interest in colour

John Carne started his career at the age of 16 in a small barber shop in Surrey. This was his first experience in hairdressing and it was here that he started reading the *Hairdressers Journal*, which opened his eyes to the exciting world of the hairdressing industry. He completed a City and Guilds apprenticeship and opted for an in-house training scheme at a well-known London salon. All the shampooing, coffee making and floor sweeping was a bit of a shock. Gradually it all fell into place and he realised that all the training was worthwhile. He took full advantage of the opportunities to assist in shows and seminars as well as mastering all the essential skills in the basic training.

Before he started his own business in Guildford, John had travelled around the globe for four years, working in Japan, America and Switzerland, performing shows and seminars. He had also been involved in producing photographic work for magazines which immediately gave him international recognition.

He opened the Guildford salon in 1981 and his first priority was to build a strong team of technicians and stylists. He had always been interested in colour as a specialist aspect of styling. Another interest was in establishing salons with a calm, spacious and comfortable feel. He believes that managing a salon gives a unique opportunity for a stylist to express his or her own personality and interests in a very particular way.

Opening your own salon

I'm Lucia Fabrizio. I left school after my GCSEs when I was 16 and went straight to college. I had worked as a Saturday girl in a salon in our town and had loved it even though I had to get up really early on Saturday morning. I enjoyed meeting different clients and came to know some of them well in the year and a half I worked at Cuts 4 U.

I found the work for NVQ Level 2 quite hard because there was so much to learn and get right, but all my friends enjoyed the course and we had lots of practical experience. I did find it quite tiring: it can be, standing up all day! It's especially difficult when you don't really feel well or have been out clubbing the night before!

But I passed the course and was offered a job back at my old salon. However, I decided to return to college to join the part-time Level 3 course and also broaden my experience a bit. I wanted to concentrate on cutting techniques, but I also wanted to own my own salon one day – the Level 3 course gave me both. I really enjoyed the course. It gave me the opportunity to expand on my strengths and overcome my weaknesses. By the end, I felt ready to stand on my own two feet – it was like when I passed my driving test but hadn't gained the confidence to 'go it alone'.

I spent the next couple of years in the salon developing the skills I had learnt, then last week I finally took the step I had been waiting for and opened my own salon.

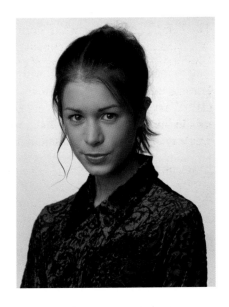

Working in television and films

You may find that your forte is to become a session stylist working all over the world doing hair for television and films. Hanna Coles describes her path into this exciting world.

'I'm Hanna Coles and my first introduction to hairdressing was as a Saturday girl in a London salon. I continued my apprenticeship there, built up a clientele and worked as a stylist for five years – particularly enjoying my involvement in the salon shows and session work.

It was this type of work that I decided to pursue, so after a year at sea, hairdressing on cruise liners (a fantastic and fun way to see the world), I set about making my goal a reality. It took time and determination – endless calls to people in the media industries, gathering lots of advice and information, assisting established session stylists and show designers, often working for free.

It was also suggested that I broaden my knowledge, and therefore increase my work potential, by studying wig-making and make-up. This I did and with my new skills was soon working in the wig department of a West End musical, where I discovered the importance of being able to work quickly and intuitively, because theatre is "live" and anything can happen.

Meanwhile I got a fashion portfolio together by "testing" with up and coming models and photographers and began to have my work published in the fashion pages of magazines such as *Tatler* and *Arena Homme*. Working in this medium taught me that attention to detail and being aware of forthcoming trends is vital.

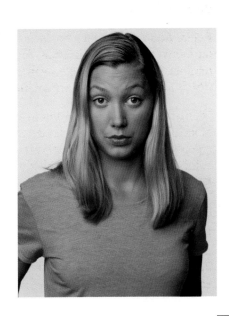

Each job presented an opportunity to make new contacts, learn new things and experiment with new ideas. If people like your efficiency and style of work they use you again and eventually I found myself being booked for pop promos, commercials and television. Then came my first feature film, A *Passion for Life*, shot in beautiful locations in Paris and the south of France.

Now my work is incredibly varied – one day I could be backstage at "Fashion Week" creating contemporary looks on a model, the next, fitting an actor's wig for a seventeenth-century drama, or working with a band on *Top of the Pops*!

It's definitely fulfilling to see your work come to life 40 ft wide at the cinema – or on a billboard or the cover of a book – it can even be a bit scary! But the most important things for me are the fun I have, the colourful and eclectic people I meet and the extraordinary places this work can take me to.

It is hard work and a very competitive industry; I would not like anyone to believe that it's all glamour and going to wonderful parties. Sometimes I am so tired, I can scarcely crawl up the stairs to bed. But if you have the determination and you really want to make it happen – then why not?'

Working as a PA within the hairdressing industry

Amanda West started with John Carne as a Saturday girl and went on to complete her NVQ through the in-salon training system. Unfortunately, Amanda developed dermatitis. This was an allergy to hair products and meant that she could no longer work with hair.

Disappointing though this was, Amanda still wanted to be involved with the hairdressing industry, so she moved on to become a PA. This involves all the other skills needed in hairdressing, for example people management and public relations, so the basic skills learnt in her NVQ were to hold her in good stead when liaising with newspapers and magazines about beauty tips. As in any industry, the people working in the marketing end of a business need to have done their groundwork.

A typical day for Amanda now involves using the following skills:

- customer service in day-to-day personal interaction
- working with beauty editors from fashion magazines if the salon is doing a photo shoot or a show
- organising personnel within the salon
- arranging shows
- talking to model agencies
- liaising with international companies
- writing press/advertising features
- stock controlling to ensure nothing runs out!

How the NVQ qualifications work

Hairdressing Level 2 NVQ is made up of nine units

Each unit is a brick in the wall

When the nine units are completed the wall is finished and your certificate can be applied for

Each unit has performance criteria that you must complete

Range statements that you must cover

Essential knowledge that you must learn to support your practical skills

An assessor will help you to put together your evidence

This is a file called a portfolio

The assessor is helped by an internal verifier

They will make sure the portfolio has all the right information

An external verifier comes to your college or training institution to oversee the whole process and give information from the Awarding Body. The application forms for your qualification can then be signed and your certificate will arrive

hair
FACTS

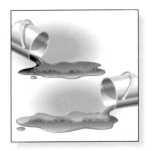  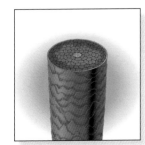

Facts about hair and skin

This section contains some important facts about hair and skin. As you work with hair, you need to know about its structure and how it grows. This will help you understand what effects styling and the use of chemicals such as perm lotion will have on it. Chemicals can badly damage the hair and skin so you should not use these until you fully understand the structure of hair and skin.

The activities in this section will help you to learn these important facts in a practical way.

What you will learn	
• The structure of hair • The structure of skin • Bones of the face and skull	• The growth cycle of hair • The chemical structure of hair • The pH scale

The structure of hair

A single hair is called a hair shaft. It is made up of:

- the cuticle
- the cortex
- the medulla.

Look at the diagram of a hair shaft. It has been magnified many times to show this much detail.

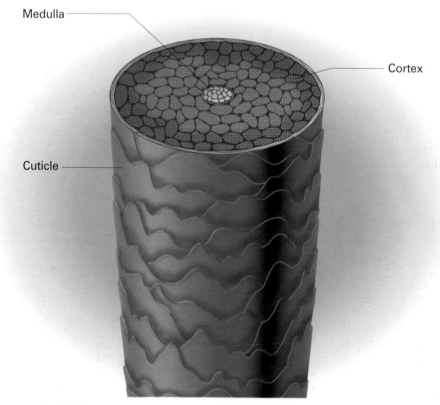

The hair shaft

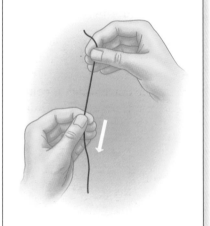

Check it out

ELASTICITY TEST

Take a single strand of your hair and hold each end tightly between the thumb and forefinger of each hand. Now gently pull. The hair should stretch slightly and then return to its original length. If the hair stretches and does not return to its original length, or if the hair snaps, this means the hair is in poor condition. You have just carried out an elasticity test.

The elasticity test

The cuticle

The cuticle is the outside layer of the hair shaft. Its main function or purpose is to protect everything underneath it. It is very tough and holds the insides of the hair shaft together. The diagram shows that the cuticle is made up of many layers of overlapping scales. The number of layers varies but there is an average for each of the different types of hair:

- European/Caucasian hair has 4–7 layers of cuticle scales.
- African Caribbean hair has 7–11 layers of cuticle scales.
- Oriental/Asian hair has more than 11 layers of cuticle scales.

Cuticle scales look like the overlapping scales of a fish or tiles on a roof. The scales are translucent, rather like frosted glass, so the hair's natural colour can be seen through them. The edges of the scales lie away from the scalp.

Although the cuticle layers are tough they can be damaged permanently by the use of strong chemicals such as perms, bleaches and relaxers. However, if the correct treatment procedures are followed the hair will not be damaged. Harsh physical treatment such as over backcombing or the use of elastic bands can also permanently damage cuticle scales.

Healthy cuticle scales lie flat and are closed tightly round the shaft. The hair will appear lustrous and shiny. Damaged cuticle scales lift away from their closest partner. When this happens the hair's appearance will be dull and the hair will feel rough. In this state any chemicals put on to the hair will be absorbed too quickly through the cuticle and into the next layer of the hair shaft – the cortex region.

The cortex

The cortex lies underneath the cuticle and is a very important part of the hair shaft. All the changes take place within the cortex when hair is blow-dried, set, permed, coloured, bleached and relaxed.

The cortex is made up of many strands that are twisted together, like knitting wool. These can stretch, and then return to their original length. However, only hair in good condition will be able to do this.

In European/Caucasian hair the cortex runs evenly through the hair shaft. Naturally curly African Caribbean hair has two different types of cortex due to the curl. The cortex on the outside of the curve has a less dense structure than the cortex on the inside of the curve which is compacted and, therefore, more dense. The flatter shape of the cortex of European/Caucasian hair means that chemicals will process more quickly.

Check it out

POROSITY TEST

Take one strand of hair from your head. Hold it firmly by the root between the thumb and forefinger of one hand. With the thumb and forefinger of the other hand, slide from the root to the end of the hair. If the hair feels rough in places that means the cuticle scales are open or raised and the condition of the cuticle is poor. If the hair feels smooth all the way along, the cuticle scales will be closed and flat and the hair will be in good condition and look smooth and shiny. You have just carried out a porosity test to check the condition of the cuticle scales.

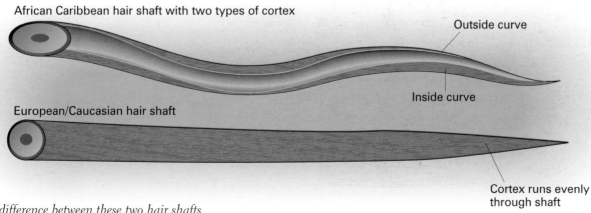

African Caribbean hair shaft with two types of cortex

Outside curve

Inside curve

European/Caucasian hair shaft

Cortex runs evenly through shaft

Notice the difference between these two hair shafts

The cortex contains all the colour pigments in the hair. These are called **melanin**. Melanin is broken down into two types of colour pigments:

- eumelanin – natural black/brown
- pheomelanin – natural red/yellow.

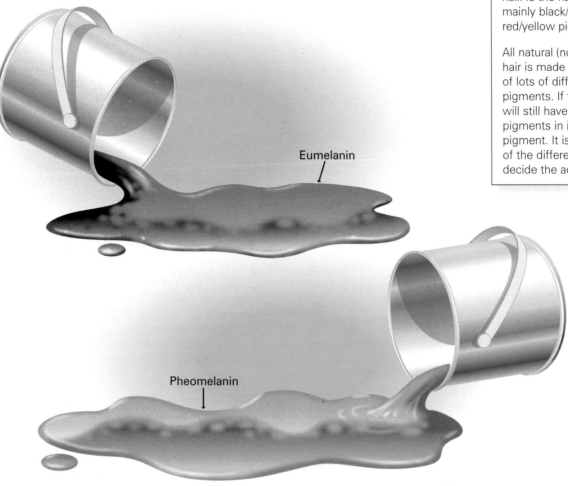

Eumelanin

Pheomelanin

Natural hair colour pigments

The medulla

The medulla is found in the centre of the hair shaft. It is not always present (there is no known reason for this), particularly in fine hair, and scientists have found that it does not have any real function.

The structure of skin

The skin is made up of several parts:

The **epidermis** is the outer layer of the skin. It consists of five layers:

- horny layer
- clear layer
- granular layer
- prickle layer
- basal layer.

The **dermis** is the inner layer of the skin. It lies under the epidermis. Within this region all the following are found:

- **hair shaft** – the part of the hair above the skin or scalp
- **follicle** – the pocket in which the hair grows
- **sebaceous gland** – the gland that produces sebum, the hair's natural oil, which is secreted into the follicle where it lubricates the hair and the skin of the scalp
- **arrector pili muscle** – if you are cold or frightened, this muscle contracts (pulls tight) and the hair stands on end creating 'goose pimples' on the skin
- **sweat gland** – the gland that produces sweat to cool the body
- **blood supply** – tiny blood vessels that bring food, oxygen and nutrients to feed the hair and skin
- **dermal papilla** – promotes cellular activity with nutrients from the nerve and blood vessels
- **hair bulb** – created as new hair cells form.

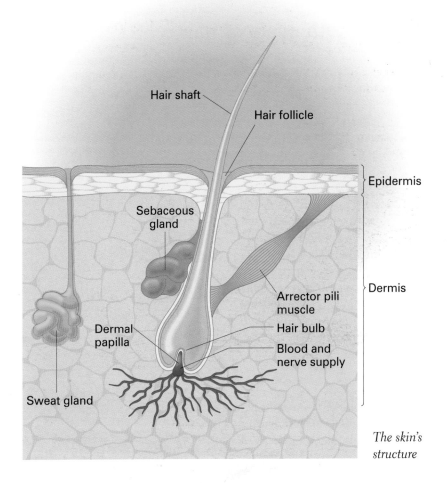

The skin's structure

Bones of the face and skull

The part of the body that protects the brain and forms the framework for the face is called the skull. It is made up of several different bones fused together. The joins are known as sutures. The skull is attached to the body by the vertebral column, which enables the head to turn and tilt. The weight of the head is supported by the neck, the shoulder girdle bones and muscles.

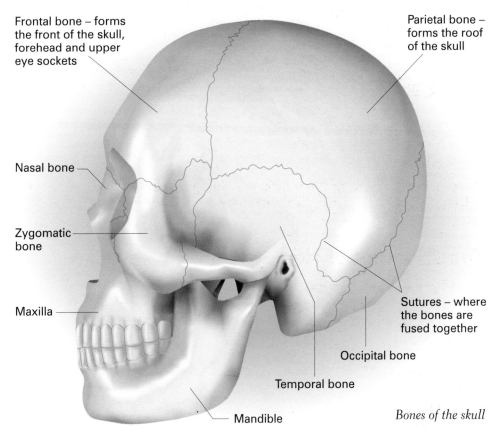

Bones of the skull

The growth cycle of hair

A single strand of hair does not grow continuously throughout its life. Hair follicles (where the hair grows from) undergo alternate periods of activity, when the hair is growing. The stages in the life cycle of hair are known as:

- **anagen**
- **catagen**
- **telogen.**

Anagen

When a hair follicle is active and the hair is growing, this is known as anagen. The period of active growth for scalp hair is from 1.25 years to 7 years. New hairs in early anagen grow faster than old hairs, the average growth being 12.5 mm per month. Between 80 and 90 per cent of scalp hairs are in the anagen state at any one time.

Catagen

Anagen is followed by a short period of change called catagen. During this time, hair follicles undergo a period of change and do not grow. Catagen lasts for about two weeks during which activity (growing) stops and new cells are formed. At any one time only about 1 per cent of follicles are in the catagen state.

Telogen

Finally, the follicle enters a period of rest (dormant like a squirrel in winter hibernation – but still alive) known as telogen. This stage lasts for about three to four months. About 13 per cent of follicles are in the telogen state at any one time.

When the resting phase is complete the follicle begins to lengthen. When the follicle reaches full length a new hair begins to grow. If the old hair is still in the follicle the new hair pushes it out.

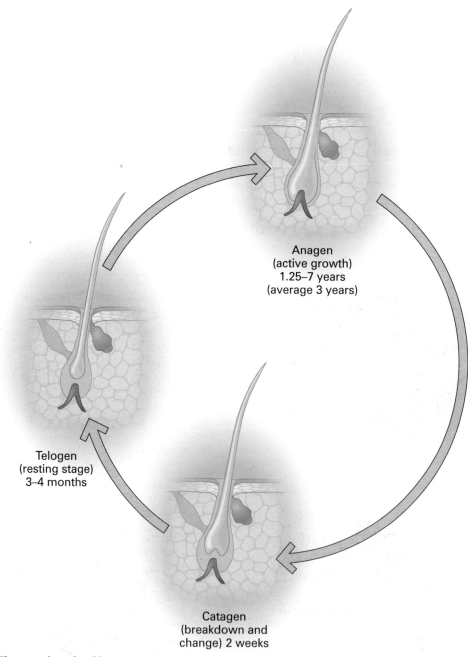

The growth cycle of hair

Anagen
(active growth)
1.25–7 years
(average 3 years)

Telogen
(resting stage)
3–4 months

Catagen
(breakdown and
change) 2 weeks

Changes in the growth cycle

The growth cycle of hair can change. For example, during pregnancy massive cell division is happening throughout the body as the baby grows. This can cause the hair's growth cycle to change and may mean that many hairs change into the anagen (active growth) phase that would, under normal circumstances, not be in anagen. When the abnormally excessive cell division stops, after the baby is born, the hairs that would not normally have been in anagen will return to their previous state and stop their active growth.

This explains why some clients loose excessive amounts of hair after their baby is born. You can, therefore, explain the reasons for this unusual amount of hair loss as hair that your client would not 'normally' have had anyway. You should try to ease your client's fears as hair loss can be very worrying.

Types of hair

There are three main types of hair:

- Asian/Oriental hair – usually very straight with lots of cuticle scales as protection
- Caucasian/European hair – usually wavy but can be straight or tightly curled.
- African Caribbean hair – usually very tightly curled and can be damaged easily by chemical treatments due to the way the cortex and cuticle regions are formed

There are many variations on these hair groups.

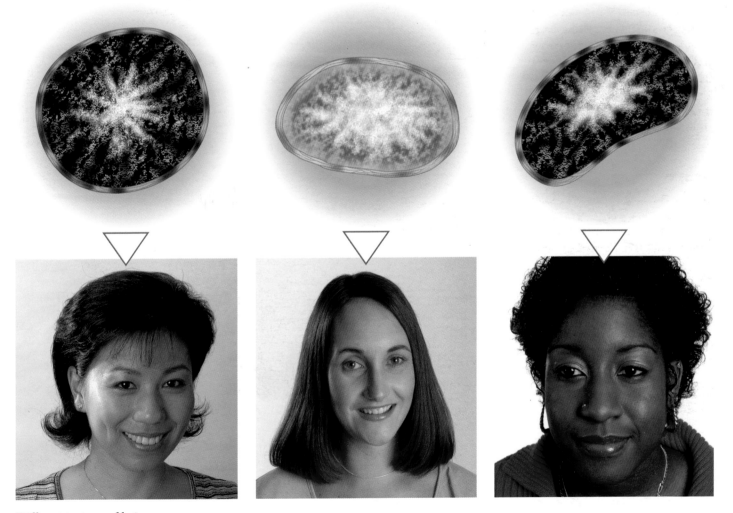

Different textures of hair

There are three kinds of hair on the body:

- Fine vellus hair grows on the body.
- Stronger terminal hair grows on the scalp.
- Lunugo hair is only found on unborn or premature babies but this type of hair usually falls out before the ninth month of pregnancy. You can sometimes see this type of hair on the heads of balding men.

The average person loses up to 100 hairs a day.

In the salon

One of your clients has had hair extensions for some time and is concerned that a lot of hair falls out when the hair extensions are changed. How do you explain this to her?

Hair normally lost each day is held in by the hair extensions and only falls out when the extensions are removed. You need to work out how much hair your client would have lost while wearing the extensions.

For example, if your client has had hair extensions for two weeks, you would calculate the average hair loss by multiplying the number of days (14) by the average number of hairs lost per day (say 75 hairs):

14 days × 75 hairs lost per day = 1050 hairs lost.

Reassure your client that her hair loss is normal.

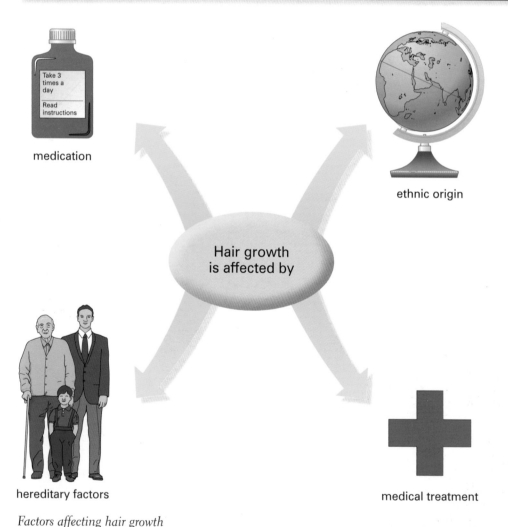

medication

ethnic origin

Hair growth is affected by

hereditary factors

medical treatment

Factors affecting hair growth

Factors affecting the growth cycle

The following can affect a person's hair growth cycle:

- Ethnic origin.
- Hereditary factors – your hair growth cycle is programmed into your genes. For example, if everyone in your family has curly hair, you will probably have curly hair too.
- Medication – this can affect the hair growth and may have long-term effects.
- Medical treatment – this can significantly change many original factors of hair growth. For example, chemotherapy will cause the hair to fall out and regrowth may have a different colour or texture.

In the salon

A client is worried that more of her hair than usual seems to be falling out. You need to find out the answers to the following questions to help your client understand why this is happening:

- Is your client taking any medication? The medication may have an effect on the normal growth of the hair.
- Has she recently had a baby? The change in hormone levels will have an effect on the normal growth of the hair and the client may lose an excessive amount of hair after the baby is born as hormone levels begin to return to normal.
- Is she suffering from stress or worry? Severe stress has been proven as a reason for hair loss. You may need to advise your client to seek medical advice.
- Has she recently had a major shock? Shock can have an effect on hair growth and can, in severe cases, cause all the hair to fall out. Medical advice would be necessary in this instance.
- Has she just had hair extensions removed?

The chemical structure of hair

Hair consists of a hardened protein called **keratin**. Its function is to make the hair elastic and flexible. Keratin is also found in the skin and the finger and toe nails. It is made up of amino acids and peptide bonds. Together they form **polypeptide chains** or links. These chains are found in the cortex of the hair and look like a spiral staircase.

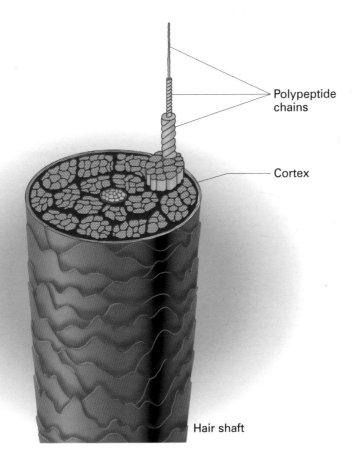

Polypeptide chains

Cortex

Hair shaft

Polypeptide chains

To prevent this spiral from falling down, the polypeptide chains are supported by cross links of hydrogen bonds and disulphide bonds acting like scaffolding poles.

Hydrogen bonds are weak and can be easily broken by water. Therefore, the shape of the hair can be changed temporarily by shampooing and then blow-drying or setting.

Disulphide bonds are very strong and only another chemical can break this stronger link. This change will be permanent and takes place when you perm or relax hair.

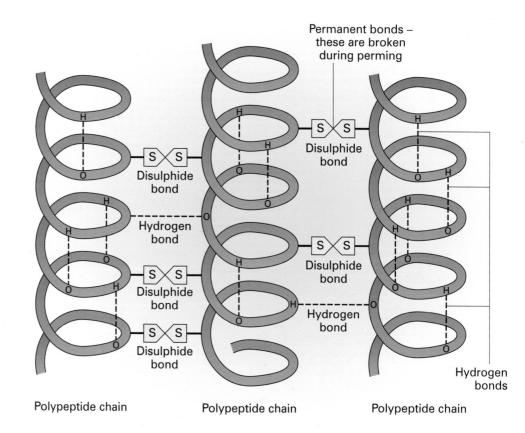

The structure of keratin

Alpha keratin and beta keratin

Hair that has been shampooed and left to dry naturally is described as alpha keratin. This is your natural hair state.

If you shampoo and then set or blow-dry hair into a stretched or unnatural state, this is called beta keratin. This shape changes back easily to alpha keratin by either wetting or being in a damp atmosphere.

Naturally straight hair becomes curly, changing alpha to beta keratin

Naturally curly hair becomes straight, changing alpha to beta keratin

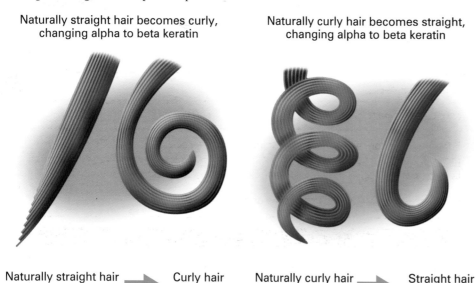

Naturally straight hair (alpha keratin) ➔ Curly hair (beta keratin)

Naturally curly hair (alpha keratin) ➔ Straight hair (beta keratin)

Moving from alpha to beta keratin

The pH scale

It is very important that you understand the pH scale because it will help you appreciate how different products affect the hair and skin.

The scale measures whether a product is acidic or alkaline, with 1 on the scale being the most acidic and 14 the most alkaline. The more alkaline a product, the more damage it can do to the hair and skin. The halfway point on the scale, 7, is classified as neutral so pH 7.1–14 is alkaline and pH1–6.9 is acid. Pure water has a pH of 7.

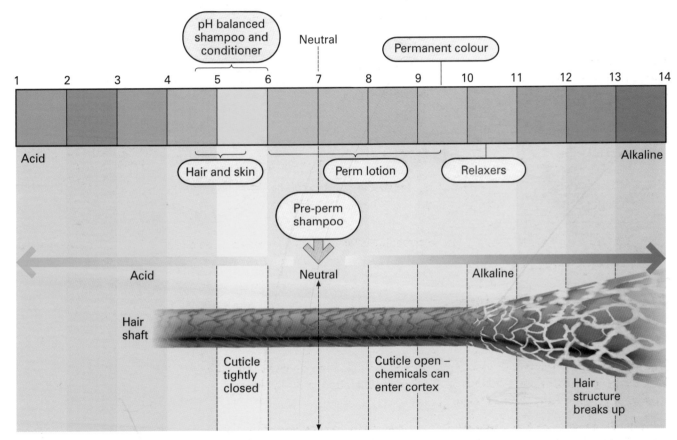

The pH scale. Notice how the hair shaft is damaged by a high level of alkalinity

Generally, an acid-based product will close the cuticle scales to make the hair smooth and shiny (for example conditioner). The exception to this rule is an acid perm which needs heat to open the cuticle scales in order to penetrate the cortex, whereas an alkaline perm will automatically open the cuticle scales. Therefore, an acid perm has a gentler, more conditioning action on the hair but will not improve the condition of the hair as a conditioning treatment would.

Check it out

PRODUCT RESEARCH

Either in the salon, at home or at your local shopping centre, look at different hair products, for example shampoos, conditioners, perm lotions, hair colours, and so on. Look at the packaging to see if you can find the pH value of any of these products.

Draw up and complete a chart like the one below.

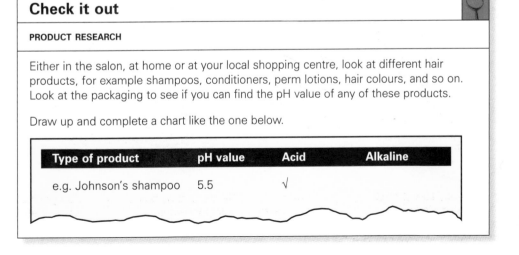

Type of product	pH value	Acid	Alkaline
e.g. Johnson's shampoo	5.5	√	

the workplace
ENVIRONMENT

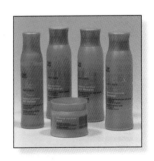 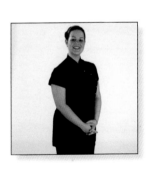 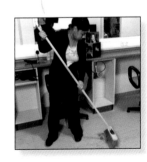

Ensure your own actions reduce risks to health and safety

Unit G1

This unit is *very* important for your working day and focuses on the wellbeing of the stylist, clients, colleagues and all other visitors to the salon. It is about how you can help to make your workplace a safe, secure and healthy place for everyone.

You must consider the health and safety of the client *every* time you carry out a treatment in whichever unit you are being assessed. Whether in the workplace or college/training institution, you have a responsibility to follow health and safety legislation. To help you, the most important aspects of health and safety laws are explained in this unit. If you ignore health and safety procedures when carrying out an assessment or treatment, at best the assessment cannot be competent, at worst your actions could result in injury or damage, for which you may be legally responsible.

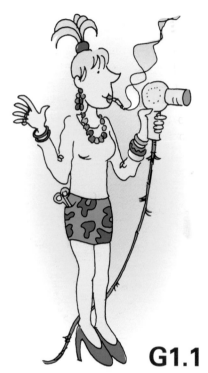

What you will learn

- Identify the hazards and evaluate the risks in your workplace G1.1
- Reduce the risks to health and safety in your workplace G1.2

Identify the hazards and evaluate the risks in your workplace

G1.1

In this element you will learn about your responsibilities in relation to potential hazards in the salon and how you should deal with them. In some cases you will be able to deal with a hazard yourself, but in others you may need to ask the advice of a more qualified member of staff. In these instances you need to know 'who' to approach. You will also need to know your responsibilities for implementing the health and safety policies used in your salon – if you do not know what they are, how can you make sure you stick to them?

It may be helpful to give you the definition of a hazard and a risk:

Hazard = A hazard is something with *potential* to cause harm (something which *may* cause harm).
Risk = A risk is the likelihood of the hazard's potential being realised (the risk of the hazard actually happening).

Almost everything may be a hazard, but it may or may not become a risk. For example, a trailing lead from a hairdryer is a hazard. If it is trailing across the passageway of a client, it has a high risk of someone tripping over it: if it is safely out of the path of the client, the risk is much less.

Hairdressing products, such as hydrogen peroxide, stored in the salon are hazards and because they are toxic and flammable may present a high risk. However, if they are kept in a properly designed secure storage area and handled by trained stylists, the risk is much less than if they are left out in a busy workshop for anyone to use – or misuse.

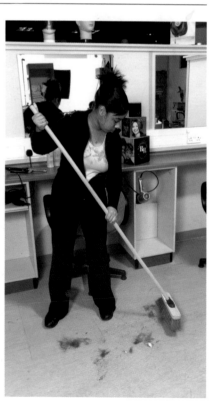

What you will learn

- Responsibilities – who does what
- Policies in your workplace
- Identifying risks
- Reporting and dealing with hazards

Responsibilities – who does what

It is very important to know whom to approach with a salon problem or potential health and safety issue. All salons will have members of staff with different strengths. Some staff will be trained in first aid whilst others may faint at the sight of blood! As a salon trainee, you need to know who to call if your client requires a first aider, how to fill out the accident report book, and where to find the first aider and the accident report book!

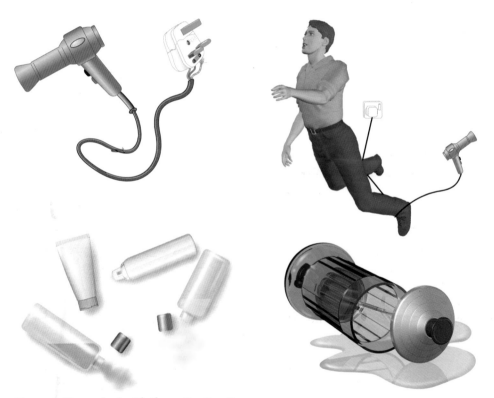

How would you deal with these situations?

Check it out

Find out who you would report health and safety issues to in your salon for:

- faulty machinery or equipment
- accidental breakages and spillages
- accidents resulting in injury to a client
- environmental factors.

Policies in your workplace

Every salon should have a set of rules and procedures for everyone to follow. These should be common knowledge for the safety and protection of all within the salon. By law, a salon has to:

- display health and safety rules and regulations on the wall in a prominent position
- display the fire evacuation procedures.

The salon owner is legally obliged to put into place the rules covering the health and safety of all employees and clients, and to ensure that safe practice is followed by all staff. The employee must follow these rules.

Professionally, the salon will have certain standards to maintain for insurance cover to be valid. Ensuring effective health and safety in the workplace involves:

- regular training, with staff meetings to update on safety issues
- giving future employees a clear outline at their initial interview as to what is expected of them
- maintaining records of injuries or first aid treatment given
- monitoring and evaluating health and safety arrangements regularly
- providing a written health and safety booklet
- consulting the experts and being knowledgeable – ignorance is not an excuse.

Check it out

Does your salon provide a written health and safety booklet? Do you know where to find it?

In the salon

Shelley has just started work at The Cutting Edge. At her interview she was told she would have to attend health and safety training during the first week of her job as junior stylist. She has just completed her second health and safety induction session with the salon owner and has read the salon's health and safety booklet. She has also been told her responsibilities under the following:

- the salon's fire evacuation procedure – including specific action that should be taken as she is responsible for her client's safety
- the Health and Safety at Work Act – she must ensure her own health and safety and that of anyone who may be affected by her work. This involves:
  - being aware of the potential for accidents and having the foresight to prevent them
  - knowing how to phone the emergency services for assistance
  - understanding how to use the different types of fire extinguishers
  - knowing the whereabouts of the water stopcock (turns off the water supply at the mains) and main electricity switch
  - having some knowledge of first aid
  - not misusing any items provided in the interest of health and safety
- Personal Protective Equipment at Work Regulations – where to find the equipment that she has a responsibility to wear when using hairdressing products and chemicals
- the salon's accident procedures including where to find the accident book and how to complete it fully in the event of an accident occurring
- first aid – she has been instructed on basic first aid skills and has been offered a two-day first aid course, which will lead to her holding a recognised first aid certificate
- Manual Handling Regulations – how to properly lift and handle objects within the salon
- where she can safely store her personal belongings – she will need to have money at work for snacks and lunch and this needs to be placed securely out of the main client area.

- What is your salon's fire evacuation procedure?
- Who is trained as a first aider in your salon?
- Where is your salon's first aid kit kept?

Check it out

How would you find out if you should wear gloves or an apron during a chemical process?

Check it out

Find out your salon's accident procedures including where to find the accident book and how to complete it fully in the event of an accident occurring. If you actually fill out the accident book, make sure you put a copy in your portfolio of evidence.

Identifying risks

Can you remember what risk means? If not, look back at page 22 for the definition of a risk.

All hairdressers work very hard, long hours, and are often on the go all day. They are in a busy salon environment, with other people present all the time – own clients, other clients, other staff, outside representatives, management, receptionists and cleaners. Whilst these 'other people' are in your salon you are responsible for making sure you do not endanger their health and safety.

Reporting and dealing with hazards

Hazards can and do happen, and everyone should be aware of the safety implications. As part of personal responsibility, the stylist needs to be able to recognise when the hazard needs to be dealt with immediately, or when help may be needed, and if it needs to be reported to a supervisor, lecturer, technician or manageress.

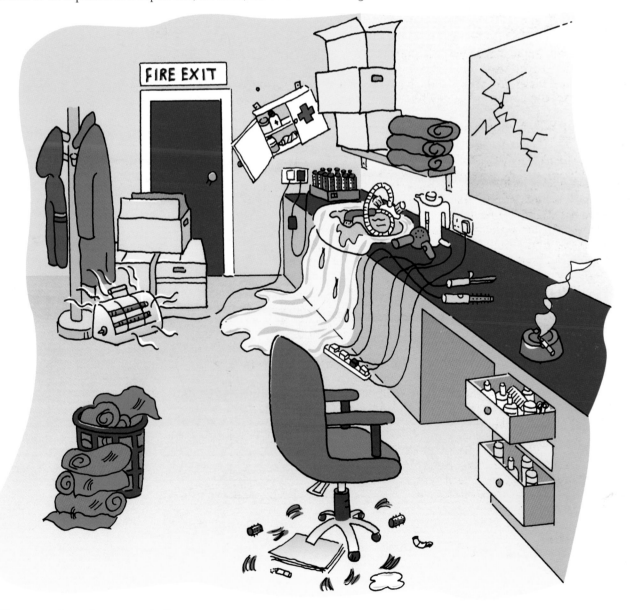

How many hazards can you spot?

It is important to be able to identify hazards before they become risks. Should they become risks it is essential to know how to deal with them.

- **RISK:** Hazards from machinery or equipment (when using or maintaining)
  How to avoid: Make sure machinery and equipment are in good working order, electrical equipment is tested for safety every six months and that all staff are adequately trained to use it.
  When referral may be necessary: When a hazard is identified, you must make sure all staff are aware of it (each salon will have its own procedure for reporting faulty equipment or machinery). You will need to refer to a manager if the machinery or equipment is vital to the smooth running of the salon as he or she will need to authorise its repair or the purchase of a replacement.

- **RISK:** A spillage
  How to avoid: Take care when mixing, pouring and filling.
  When referral may be necessary: When spillage material is corrosive or an irritant.

- **RISK:** Slippery floors resulting from staff not following salon rules for tidying salon
  How to avoid: Make others aware by blocking the area with a chair to prevent an accident. Sweep up powder spills, mop up spills of liquid, refer to COSHH sheets for correct method (COSHH deals with how to handle, store and dispose of chemicals and products – see Element G1.2).
  When referral may be necessary: When acid, grease or polish are spilt.

- **RISK:** Environmental factors
  How to avoid: Make sure all staff follow COSHH sheets and manufacturer's instructions when disposing of chemical products, sharps and infected waste (for example, cut hair infected with head lice).
  When referral may be necessary: When staff are not following specific guidelines; when the skin is pierced by used sharps; when infected waste is left causing a hazard to salon staff and clients.

Check it out

- What would you class as a low risk hazard in your salon?
- Find out your salon's rules for dealing with this type of hazard.
- What would you class as a high risk hazard? Write down how you would deal with this type of hazard and keep it safe in your portfolio of evidence.

Reduce the risks to health and safety in your workplace

G1.2

This element covers health and safety risks and outlines how to reduce the risks that you may come into contact with in the salon. You need to know how to carry out tasks safely following instructions and workplace requirements. You must also have a good understanding of the health and safety policies within your salon that affect your working day. This includes following manufacturer's and supplier's instructions when using products, materials and equipment. You also have to prove your personal presentation and conduct ensures the health and safety of yourself, your clients and colleagues.

What you will learn

- Legal requirements (health and safety legislation)
- Health and safety rules
- Salon/workplace policies
- Rectifying health and safety risks
- Health and safety suggestions
- Personal presentation
- Personal conduct
- Salon security and reducing workplace risks

Legal requirements (health and safety legislation)

This covers all the Acts of Parliament that relate to a business as set down by our government. These Acts of Parliament are being updated continually to fit into modern society, so you will find that Acts have dates after their title stating when they were updated, for example, the Trades Description Act 1968 (amended 1987). This means that these Acts are the law of the land and to break them or to ignore them is an offence and you will be punished. The consequences may be payment of a fine, closure of the business or imprisonment.

As well as following British law we have to follow European law.

Local government bylaws are the ones decided by the Local Authority and can differ from region to region, for example, London has different local bylaws to Birmingham.

To be fully competent in employment, it is essential that you have a sound knowledge of consumer protection and health and safety legislation. Do not worry too much about the years attached to the laws, concentrate more on the Acts themselves and how they protect both the stylist and the consumer, that is, the client.

Health and Safety at Work Act 1974

This requires all employers to provide systems of work that are, as is reasonably practicable, safe and without risk to health.

The employer's duty is to provide:

- premises – a safe place to work
- systems and equipment
- strorage and transport of substances and material
- access to the workplace exits
- good practices in the workplace.

The employer also has a responsibility to other persons not in employment including contractors and self-employed people.

> ### Reality check!
>
> Each of us must take responsibly for our deeds and actions, and we are liable if we do not. Insurance cover will be null and void if it is proven that legislation or establishment rules have been broken and an accident or damage has occurred.

Employers' responsibilities	Shared responsibilities	Employees' responsibilities
Planning safety and security	Safety of the working environment	Correct use of the systems and procedures
Providing information about safety and security	Employees have responsibilities to take reasonable care of themselves and other people affected by their work and to co-operate with their employers to follow the law	Reporting flaws or gaps within the system or procedure when in use
Updating systems and procedures, in workplaces with five or more employees		
Safety of individuals being cared for		

Health and safety responsibilities

Employees have responsibilities to take reasonable care of themselves and other people affected by their work and to co-operate with their employers to follow the law.

The **employee** has a responsibility to:

- take care during time at work to avoid personal injury
- assist the employer in meeting requirements under the Health and Safety at Work Act
- not misuse or change anything that has been provided for safety.

The Act allows various regulations to be made, which control the workplace. The Act also covers self-employed persons who work alone, away from the employer's premises.

In 1992, EU directives updated legislation on health and safety management and widened the existing Acts. These came into being in 1993. There are six main areas:

- provision and use of work equipment
- manual handling operations
- workplace health, safety and welfare
- personal protective equipment at work
- health and safety (display screen equipment)
- management of health and safety at work.

Some of the new provisions of the EU directives are the protection of non-smokers from tobacco smoke, the provision of rest facilities for pregnant and nursing mothers, and safe cleaning of windows.

Manual Handling Operations Regulations 1992

The Health and Safety Executive (HSE) has drawn attention to skeletal and muscular disorders caused by manual handling and lifting, repetitive strain disorders and unsuitable posture causing low back pain. The regulations require that certain measures be taken to avoid these types of injuries occurring.

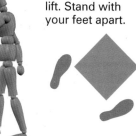
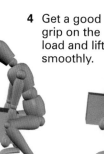
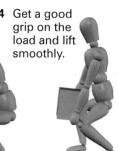
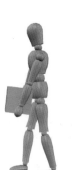
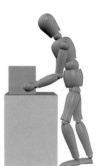

1 Think about the lift. Where is the load to be placed? Do you need help? Are handling aids available?

2 Get ready to lift. Stand with your feet apart.

3 Bend the knees. Keep the back straight. Tuck in your chin. Lean slightly forward over the load to get a good grip.

4 Get a good grip on the load and lift smoothly.

Safe lifting procedures must be observed

Think of all the situations that may apply in the salon:

- stock unpacking and storage – lifting heavy objects
- moving chairs or cutting stools used in the salon
- adjusting trolley height.

It is worth considering all of these factors when purchasing your equipment, as you then have to work with the consequences!

> ## Remember
>
> The employee has a responsibility to:
>
> - her/himself
> - to other employees
> - to the public.

> ## Remember
>
> Follow the golden rule: always lift with the back straight and the knees bent. If in doubt – do not lift at all!

Heat stress

The HSE draws attention to heat stress at work. The best working temperature in hairdressing salons is between 15.5 and 20°C.

Humidity (the amount of moisture in the air) should be within the range of 30–70 per cent, although this will vary if your salon has a sauna and steam area. They should be in a well-ventilated area away from the main workrooms, whilst still being accessible to clients. There should also be sufficient air exchange and air movement, which must be increased in special circumstances, such as chemical mixing and usage. There are different types of ventilation that may be used within the salon.

Mechanical ventilation: extractor fans, which can be adjusted at various speeds.

Natural ventilation: open windows are fine, but be careful of a draught on the client.

Air-conditioned ventilation: passing air over filters and coolers brings about the desired condition, but of course, this is the most expensive method!

A build-up of fumes, or strong smells from chemical preparations such as perm lotion, bleach and tint, may cause both physical and psychological problems, which affect not only clients but staff, too!

Physical effects	Psychological effects
Headaches	Irritability
Sweating	Aggressive behaviour
Palpitations	Nervous fatigue, which may result in mistakes being made
Dizziness	
Nausea or fainting	Lethargy

The effects of heat stress

Protective clothing and equipment

This covers both equipment and protective clothing provisions to ensure safety for all those in the workplace. The regulations also provide that workplace personnel must have appropriate training in equipment use. Protective clothing ensures cleanliness, freshness, and professionalism. For certain treatments it may be advisable to wear extra disposable coverings. The client's clothing must also be protected.

Protection against infectious diseases

Caution: It is important to protect against all diseases, which are carried in the blood or tissue fluids. Protective gloves should be worn whenever there is a possibility of blood or tissue fluid being passed from one person to another, i.e. through an open cut or broken skin. Two specific diseases to mention are:

- AIDS

  Acquired Immune Deficiency Syndrome (AIDS) is a disease caused by the Human Immuno-deficiency Virus (HIV). The virus is transmitted through body tissue. Most people are aware of AIDS because of media coverage. The virus attacks the natural immune system, and therefore carries a strong risk of secondary infection, such as pneumonia, which could be life threatening. As there is no known cure, prevention through protection is vital.

Remember

It is very good practice to investigate what your professional body states about protective clothing. It may make your insurance null and void if you do not follow their directives.

- Hepatitis variants (A, B and C)

  This is an inflammation of the liver. It is caused by a very strong virus also transmitted through blood and tissue fluids. This can survive outside the body and can make a person very ill indeed; it can even be fatal. The most serious form is Hepatitis B and you can be immunised against it by a GP. If a person can prove that he or she needs this protection for employment purposes, there is no cost involved. Most training establishments will recommend this.

Control of Substances Hazardous to Health Regulations 2003 (COSHH)

This law requires employers to control exposure to hazardous substances in the workplace. Most of the products used in the salon are perfectly safe, but some products could become hazardous under certain conditions or if used inappropriately. All salons should be aware of how to use and store these products.

Employers are responsible for assessing the risks from hazardous substances and must decide upon an action to reduce those risks. Proper training should be given and employees should always follow safety guidelines and take the precautions identified by the employer.

On the right are the symbols that show types of hazardous substances. COSHH requires that they are found on packaging and containers in health, beauty and hairdressing salons.

Here are some examples of potential hazards:

- **highly flammable substances**, such as hairspray or alcohol steriliser are hazardous because their fumes will ignite if exposed to a naked flame.
- **explosive materials**, such as hairspray, air freshener or other pressurised cans will explode with force if placed in heat, such as an open fire, direct sunlight, or even on top of a hot radiator.
- **chemicals** can cause severe reactions and skin damage. Vomiting, respiratory problems and burning could be the result if chemicals are misused.

COSHH precautions

Employers must, by law, identify, list and assess in writing any substance in the workplace. This applies not only to products used in the salon, but also to products that are used in cleaning, e.g. bleach or polish. These substances must be given a hazard rating, or risk assessment, even if it is zero.

Finally, you should read all the COSHH sheets used in the salon and be safe: abide by what they say, never abuse manufacturer's instructions, and attend regular staff training for product use – you never know when you might need it!

Electricity at Work Regulations 1989

The Electricity at Work Regulations are concerned with general safety of the use of electricity. They cover the use and maintenance of electrical equipment in the salon.

Q: How do the Electricity at Work Regulations affect the use of electrical equipment in the salon?

A: Regulation 4 of the Act states:

'All electrical equipment must be regularly checked for electrical safety. In a busy salon this may be every six months. The check must be carried out by a

Dust

Toxic

Flammable

Irritant

Corrosive

Oxidising agent

Symbols showing types of hazardous substances

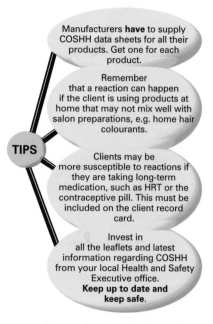

Manufacturers **have** to supply COSHH data sheets for all their products. Get one for each product.

Remember that a reaction can happen if the client is using products at home that may not mix well with salon preparations, e.g. home hair colourants.

TIPS

Clients may be more susceptible to reactions if they are taking long-term medication, such as HRT or the contraceptive pill. This must be included on the client record card.

Invest in all the leaflets and latest information regarding COSHH from your local Health and Safety Executive office. **Keep up to date and keep safe.**

Remember these COSHH tips

"competent person", preferably a qualified electrician and is called PAT testing. All checks must be recorded in a book kept for this purpose only.'

Q: Who is a 'competent person' and what checks must be done?

A: A 'competent person' doesn't need to be a qualified electrician, but he or she must be capable of attending to basic safety checks. The manufacturer may supply its own technical staff to attend to safety checks, as they will be trained in areas of expertise.

Q: If electrical apparatus is found to be faulty, what action must be taken?

A: The equipment must be withdrawn from service and repaired.

Q: What is the purpose of an electrical safety record book?

A: The safety record book should state the dates, the nature of the repair and who carried it out. It should also contain a list of tests carried out on the equipment under inspection, the results of those tests, and be signed by the competent person who carried them out.

This is essential for insurance purposes for public liability and in case of legal action being taken for accident or negligence.

More and more people are demanding court action for negligence – do not be liable, use these regulations to keep you, your colleagues and your clients both out of danger and out of court!

Remember	
Around 1000 electric shock accidents at work are reported to the HSE each year.	

Personal Protective Equipment at Work Regulations 1992

You are required to use and wear the appropriate protective equipment or clothing during chemical treatments. Protective gloves and aprons are the normal requirements for your protection and your employer should provide these for you.

Reporting of Injuries, Diseases and Dangerous Occurrences Regulations 1995 (RIDDOR)

These regulations cover the recording and reporting of any serious accidents and conditions to the local environmental health officer, whose remit covers hairdressing salons. This officer will investigate the accident and makes sure the salon prevents it from happening again in the future. The officer can also assess the risk factors in each instance.

An accident or death at work must be reported within ten days. If the accident does not require a hospital visit, but the person is absent from work for more than three days, a report needs to be given.

If an employee reports a work-related disease, a report must be sent. Work-related diseases include occupational dermatitis, asthma caused through work, or even hepatitis. Accidents as a result of violence or an attack by another person must be reported.

A dangerous occurrence in which no one was actually injured must also be reported, for example, if the ceiling of the salon collapses overnight.

If you are a mobile hairdresser in someone's home and you have an accident yourself or injure the client, you must report it.

Employer's Liability (Compulsory Insurance) Act 1969

Employers and self-employed persons must by law hold employer's liability insurance. This will reimburse them against any legal liability to pay compensation to employees for bodily injury, illness or disease caused during the course of their employment.

Employers must insure for at least £2 million per claim, but check with your own insurance company. Also follow the recommendations of your professional association.

It is worth remembering the following points:

- A legal claim made against your salon could result in very large financial losses and possibly the sale of the owner's business or even private home.
- Public prosecution results in a heavy fine for those not having this essential insurance cover.
- Damage to the salon could be so great that the business may never recover.
- Some cases take up to ten years to come to court and with inflation the claim against you could be very much more than your original cover if you only go for the minimum requirements.

Insurance

Professional indemnity insurance

Every single professional hairdresser should have this insurance protection, regardless of how few or how many treatments they carry out.

The best deal for all insurance policies is usually found via your professional body, who will be able to offer the best rates as they negotiate on behalf of members and get a considerable discount.

As an employee you need to check with your employer whether you are covered on the business insurance, or if you need to organise your own cover. A salon owner or employer should include this liability in the public liability policy, so that *all* employees are protected against claims made by clients.

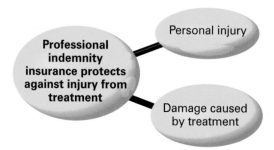

Indemnity insurance could save you a lot of money

Public liability insurance

This is not compulsory, but it is certainly advisable. It will protect the employer should a member of the public be injured on the premises. This could be something as simple as a roof tile hitting the client on his or her way into the salon. If this results in the client being unable to work for a long period of time, the client can seek legal advice and the salon owner could be sued for compensation.

Data Protection Act 1998

Businesses that use computers or paper-based filing systems to hold personal details about their staff and clients may be required to register with the Data Protection Registrar.

> **Remember**
>
> Insurance is important – protect yourself and each other.

The Data Protection Registrar will place your business on a public register of data users and issue you with a code of practice, which you must comply with, stating:

- you must keep information secure
- you must ensure information is accurate and relevant to your needs
- you must comply with individuals' requests for information that you are holding on them, failure to do so means you are contravening the Act.

Contact: Data Protection Registrar, Springfield House, Water Lane, Wilmslow, Cheshire. SK9 5AX. (Tel. 01625 545745)

The information held by an organisation on computer about any one of us can be revealed if requested within 40 days for a fee not greater than £10.00. It is possible to gain compensation through a civil court action if you feel there has been any infringement of rights in which information that was given for a specific purpose has been abused.

Health and safety rules

These will encompass all aspects of the Health and Safety at Work Act, plus COSHH and the Electricity at Work Act.

You should be in no doubt about:

- your responsibility
- salon procedures
- treatment safety
- equipment safety
- protection against cross-infection.

Salon procedures for health and safety

Client safety:
- positioning of client
- minimum risk of hazard within the salon
- correct use of equipment and products
- correct use of products
- correct evacuation procedures.

Storage procedures:
- electrical equipment
- chemicals
- valuables
- stock
- money.

Stock regulations:
- COSHH regulations are followed
- first aid procedures in place
- stock rotation
- spillage management
- correct storage and containers.

Your employer or head of the training establishment should have all these standard procedures in place. If you are not instructed within your first few weeks of beginning your new post, then ask!

Reality check!

Your own personal details are also covered by this Act. Where are you a client? Where do you think your personal details may be kept? You are probably a patient at a doctor's practice and if so, your details will be held on record by the surgery.

Remember

Regular training is the key for following salon guidelines.

Salon/workplace policies

All salons will have their own individual policies in place and it is your responsibility to follow them, so make sure you know what your salon's policies are. All salons will require employees to follow basic rules, like reading and following manufacturer's instructions. If this rule is not followed, treatments could go wrong, resulting in loss of clients and the salon's good reputation. Other salon policies will include:

- **Smoking** – some salons are completely non-smoking zones and clients would need to be informed of this by members of staff (you). You must be fully aware of the rules and enforce them if a client decides to light a cigarette.
- **Eating and drinking areas** – the preparation of food and drinks should not be in the same area as the mixing and preparation of products. This would cause an environmental health and safety issue, as many chemical products in hairdressing are caustic and if accidentally mixed with food or drinks would cause internal medical problems.
- **Drug policies** – remember, only fully qualified, medically trained personnel are allowed to administer drugs or medicines.

Cleaning, sterilising and general care of salon tools and equipment

Sterilisation means the killing of all organisms, for example, bacteria, fungus such as ringworm, and parasites such as head lice.

	Methods
Disinfectants	These are only effective if used correctly. They must be used in the correct concentrations and tools must be left in disinfectants for the correct length of time (read manufacturer's instructions). Boiling water (60° minimum) – for towels and gowns. The hot cycle of a washing machine can be used. Disinfectant solutions, e.g. barbicide NB Brushes and combs should be washed with hot soapy water before being immersed in the solution for at least 20 minutes (read manufacturer's instructions).
Sterilising wipes and sprays	Best for metal objects, e.g. scissors, clippers and razor handles (not blades) – remove loose hairs before spraying or wiping.
Ultra-violet radiation cabinet	Suitable for all tools. However, the tools must be turned over to ensure that each side has been exposed to the light for 20–30 minutes. NB Tools must be cleaned before placing in the cabinet.
Autoclaves	Very efficient method of sterilising, especially for metal tools. However, some plastics cannot withstand the heat (check manufacturer's instructions). Autoclaves take about 20 minutes to sterilise tools.

- Brushes should be washed in warm soapy water to remove grease and products, then soaked in a disinfectant solution (barbicide) for at least 20 minutes.
- Combs should be washed in warm soapy water to remove grease and products, then soaked in a disinfectant solution (barbicide) for at least 20 minutes.
- Scissors should be cleaned regularly to remove hair cuttings and sterilised using medi-wipes or sterilising spray.
- Razors and hair shapers should be brushed free of cut hair after use. The replaceable blade must be disposed of in a sharps bin to avoid piercing the skin; this is then collected by the local health authority for incineration. The handle can be sterilised by either wiping with a medi-wipe or sterilising spray.
- Fixtures and fittings, all chairs, workstations, mirrors, hood dryers, climazones and steamers must be wiped clean daily to remove any hair cuttings, chemical and styling products, and general dust and dirt.
- Floors should be swept at regular intervals throughout the day to avoid slippery surfaces. All spills must be wiped up immediately. Floors should be bleached at the end of each day.

Check it out

Write down four of your workplace's policies and keep in your portfolio of evidence.

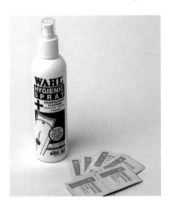
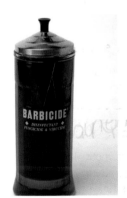
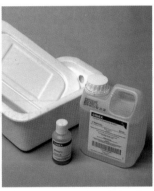

Sterilising solutions and spray

Fire policies

Fire Precautions Act 1971

By law all business premises must undertake a fire risk assessment. If five or more people work together as employees, the assessment must be in writing. Employers must also take into account *all other persons* on the premises, not just employees. This will include clients and visitors to the salon.

There must also be a fire and evacuation procedure. In every period of one year there must be at least one fire drill, which involves everyone. All staff must be fully informed, instructed and trained in what is expected of them. Some employees will have special duties to perform such as checking rooms.

All employees, trainees and temporary workers must co-operate with their employers so far as is necessary to enable the employers to fulfil the duties placed upon them by law. This means that everyone must co-operate fully in training courses and fire drills, even when everyone knows it is only a practice.

Many fire-training exercises are organised with a fire safety officer from the local fire station. Often fire engines will take part in the exercise to test the firefighters' own attendance time from the station to the premises. Everyone should be made aware of his or her own particular rules for evacuation.

When joining a salon, the new employee should be briefed on all health and safety issues, and especially in fire evacuation procedures. It is standard practice to include the information in a handbook containing all the salon's policies.

Check it out

Find out who in your college or training institution has special responsibilities during fire evacuation procedures and make a note of them for your portfolio.

Look carefully at the following example of a training institution's evacuation procedure.

Building evacuation procedures in the event of fire or bomb alert

The following procedure has been agreed and must be followed. Any staff member who does not comply is committing an infringement of the college disciplinary code. Whenever a fire occurs, the main consideration is to get everybody out of the building safely. Protection of personal or college property is incidental.

Raising the alarm

Anyone discovering a fire must immediately raise the alarm by operating the nearest fire alarm and report to the controller the fire location.

On hearing the alarm the receptionist will immediately contact the emergency services and then evacuate the building.

In the event of a fire being discovered when the reception is unmanned – the premises officer on duty will contact the emergency services and assume control.

On hearing the alarm

All those in senior positions proceed to the control point, normally at a main entrance to the building – where one person must take control of the proceedings.

All other staff: close windows; switch off machinery and lights, and close doors on leaving the room.

Assist less able colleagues, leave the building by the nearest marked route and proceed quickly to the appropriate assembly point. Staff must supervise their class.

Staff evacuating the building must check their locality is clear.

Assembly points

Everyone must remain at assembly points well away from buildings and clear of access roads.

Report to control in person or via two-way radios where allocated.

Everyone must remain at assembly points until further instructions.

DO NOT re-enter the building until you are told it is safe to do so.

An evacuation procedure

Emergency fire procedures

Fire drill dependent on the working area

- All electrical equipment to be switched off.
- Shut windows.
- Clients to be led by the stylist to a safe area. Wrap wet hair in a towel and take extra towels for warmth and water sprays in case any chemicals are nearing their full development time.
- If possible, take the client's valuable possessions with her, such as handbag, but only if it does not put the client or stylist in any danger.
- Be aware of the treatment being performed before the evacuation – if the client has chemicals on the hair, keep checking the development of the treatment and dilute the strength of the product using a water spray if necessary. This would need to be at the judgement of the person in charge of the salon – certainly a client having a perm or colour will need constant attention while waiting at the assembly point.

Sensible fire precautions

- Be informed – know what to do and where to go when the evacuation begins.
- Be sensible and do not panic – this will only make the client feel panicky too.
- Make sure that the locations of the fire alarm, fire extinguishers and fire exit are familiar.
- Never ignore smoke or the smell of burning – it is far better to have a false alarm. Better safe than sorry.
- Do not misuse or mistreat electrical appliances that are a potential hazard – always treat electrical appliances with respect.
- Do not ignore manufacturer's instructions for the storage and use of highly flammable products, which are very common within the salon.
- Do be sensible with naked flames and matches or disposal of cigarette ends – a smouldering tip can burst into flames in minutes.
- Be accountable for clients on the premises – the appointment book should be taken outside as a master check of which clients should be present.
- Do not use a lift for the evacuation – it may be that the fire affects the electrical mechanism and that then becomes another emergency.

Fire-fighting equipment

Fire extinguishers

Only a person specially trained in the use of a fire extinguisher should attempt to use one. Never put yourself or others at risk – personal safety is more important than saving material items that can be replaced.

There are different types of portable fire extinguisher for use on different types of fire – using the wrong one can make the situation worse. The latest extinguishers are coloured red with a zone or panel of colour, which indicates the contents of the extinguisher. On older models the colour of the whole fire extinguisher identifies its use.

Extinguisher	Type	Colour	Uses	NOT to be used
Electrical fires	Dry powder	Blue marking	For burning liquid, electrical fires and flammable liquids	On flammable metal fires
	Carbon dioxide	Black marking	Safe on all voltages, used on burning liquid and electrical fires and flammable liquids	On flammable metal fires
	Vaporising liquid	Green marking	Safe on all voltages, used on burning liquid and electrical fires and flammable liquids	On flammable metal fires
Non-electrical fires	Water	Red marking	For wood, paper, textiles, fabric and similar materials	On burning liquid, electrical or flammable metal fires
	Foam	Cream/yellow markings	On burning liquid fires	On electrical or flammable metal fires

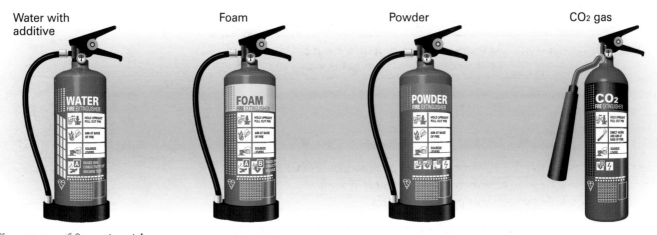

Water with additive   Foam   Powder   CO₂ gas

Different types of fire extinguishers

Fire blankets

Fire blankets are made of fire-resistant material. They are particularly useful for wrapping around a person whose clothing is on fire. A fire blanket must be used calmly and with a firm grip. If the blanket is flapped about, it may fan the fire and cause it to flare up, rather than put it out. When putting a blanket on a victim, protect your own hands with the edge of the cloth. Remember to place the blanket, never throw, into the desired position.

Sand

A bucket of sand can be used to soak up liquids, such as chemicals, which are the source of a fire. However, never risk injury. If in doubt, leave the area and phone the emergency services.

First aid

People at work can suffer injuries or fall ill. It does not matter whether the injury or illness is caused by the work they do. It is important that they receive immediate attention and that in serious cases an ambulance is called. First aid can save lives and prevent minor injuries becoming major ones.

Reality check!

Never lean over a fire. If you cannot control it, leave the room, close the door, proceed to a safe place, then phone the emergency services.

Remember

Hundreds of people die and thousands of people are injured in fires each year, many caused by lack of concentration or carelessness. It is better to prevent a fire starting in the first place, for example, use chemicals safely and maintain electrical appliances.

Even small fires spread very quickly, producing smoke and fumes, which can kill in minutes. If there is any doubt, do not tackle the fire, no matter how small.

The Health and Safety (First Aid) Regulations 1981 set out the essential aspects of first aid that employers have to be responsible for.

As a trainee or student, you must have some basic knowledge of first aid. Unless you hold an up-to-date first aid certificate, you should not treat injuries, but you should know when and how to summon a competent first aider and call for an ambulance if necessary.

Problem	First aid necessary
Chemicals entering the eye, e.g. perm lotion or neutraliser	Immediately flush the eye with cool, clean water, then summon a first aider
Scissor cut to skin	Give the client a pad to stem the flow of blood. Do not touch the wound, surrounding area or blood without gloves on. If the cut is deep or does not stop bleeding, call for first aid assistance or phone the emergency services for an ambulance
Client or colleague falls and is knocked out	Put them in the recovery position and call for medical assistance from a first aider or summon an ambulance
Client of colleague faints	Put them in the recovery position and call for medical assistance from a first aider or summon an ambulance

Common first aid problems in the salon

Reality check!

First aid in the workplace is the initial management of any injury or illness suffered at work. It does not include giving tablets or medicines to treat illness.

It is essential that sufficient first aid personnel and facilities should be available:

* to give immediate assistance to casualties with both common injuries and illnesses and those likely to arise from specific hazards at work
* to summon an ambulance or other professional help.

The number of first aiders and facilities available will depend upon the size of the workforce, the type of workplace hazards and risks, and the history of accidents in the workplace.

There are two legal aspects of first aid that you need to consider:

* **Trainees** – students undertaking work experience on certain training schemes are given the same status as employees and therefore are the responsibility of the employer.
* **The public** – when dealing with the public the Health and Safety (First Aid) Regulations do not require employers to provide first aid for anyone other than their own employees. Employers should make extra provision for the public. Educational institutions need also to include the general public in their assessment of first aid requirements.

First aid kits

The minimum level of first aid equipment is a suitably stocked and properly identified first aid container. An old biscuit tin just will not do! First aid containers should be easily accessible and placed, where possible, near to hand-washing facilities.

The container should protect the items inside from dust and damp and should only be stocked with useful items. Tablets and medication should not be kept in it. There is no compulsory list of what a first aid container should include but here are some suggestions:

- A leaflet giving general guidance on first aid (for example, Health and Safety Executive leaflet *Basic advice on first aid at work*)
- 20 individually wrapped, sterile, adhesive dressings (assorted sizes) appropriate to the type of work
- 2 sterile eye pads
- 4 individually wrapped, triangular bandages (preferably sterile)
- 6 safety pins
- 6 medium-sized, individually wrapped wound dressings
- 2 large sterile, individually wrapped, unmedicated wound dressings
- Pair of disposable gloves
- Antiseptic cream or liquid
- Eye bath
- Gauze
- Medical wipes
- Pair of tweezers
- Sterile water
- Cotton wool.

The number of first aid containers a salon or establishment has will depend upon the size of the establishment and the total number of employees in that area.

Check it out

- Who is responsible for checking the first aid box in your salon?
- How often is it checked?
- What should you do if you have used something from the box?

Make a note of this information for your portfolio of evidence.

clear plaster
fabric plaster
waterproof plaster
heel and finger plaster

elasticated roller bandage
conforming roller bandage
crêpe conforming roller bandage

crêpe roller bandage
open-weave roller bandage
self-adhesive roller bandage

eye pad
eye pad with headband
safety pins

disposable gloves

tweezers

ANTISEPTIC WIPE
Moist tissue to clean and sooth cuts and grazes

folded cloth triangular bandage
folded paper triangular bandage
cotton wool
gauze pads
wound cleansing wipes

medium dressing
large dressing
extra large dressing

Items a first aid box should contain

First aid training

First aid certificates are only valid for the length of time the Health and Safety Executive (HSE) specify, which is currently three years. Employers need to arrange refresher training with re-testing of competence before certificates expire. If a certificate expires, the individual will have to undertake a full course of training to be re-instated as a qualified first aider. Specialist training can also be undertaken if the workplace needs it.

Rectifying health and safety risks

Recording incidents

It is good practice for employers to provide first aiders with a book in which to record incidents that require their attendance. If there are several first aid persons in one establishment, then a central book will be acceptable. If you have to deal with an incident, you should record the following information:

- date, time and place of incident
- name and job of injured/sick person, and contact details
- details of the injury/illness and what first aid was given
- what action was taken immediately afterwards, for example, did the person go home, go to hospital? Was he or she taken in an ambulance?
- name and signature of the first aider or person dealing with the incident.

This record book is not the same as the statutory accident book, although the two might be combined. The information kept can help the employer identify accident trends or patterns and improve on safety risks. It can also be used to judge first aid needs assessments. It may also prove useful for insurance and investigative purposes.

Salon accident/incident report

This form should be filled in by the first aider/staff member responsible for dealing with the accident/incident. It should be completed as soon as possible after the accident/incident.

Accident procedures

Accidents happen, even to the most careful of people. In the event of an accident in the salon, stay calm and follow the salon's accident procedures.

Reality check!

If in doubt, do not treat – phone for an ambulance immediately.

ACCIDENT REPORT FORM

SECTION 1 PERSONAL DETAILS

Full name of first aider/staff member: _____

Position held in salon: _____

Date: _____

Accident (injury) ☐   Incident (illness) ☐

Time and date of accident/incident: _____

Full name of injured/ill person: _____

Staff member ☐   Client ☐   Other ☐

Address: _____

Tel. no: _____

SECTION 2 ACCIDENT/INCIDENT DETAILS

Describe what happened. In the case of an accident, state clearly what the injured person was doing. _____

_____

Name and address/tel. no. of witness(es), if any: _____

_____

Action taken

Ambulance called ☐   Taken to hospital ☐   Sent to hospital ☐   First aid given ☐

Taken home ☐   Sent home ☐   Returned to work ☐

SECTION 3 PREVENTATIVE ACTION

Preventative action implemented ☐

Describe action taken: _____

_____

Date implemented: _____

Signature of first aider/staff member: _____

Signature salon manager/owner: _____

Date: _____

An accident report form

You should be aware of all possible risks in all aspects of salon life, including:

- preparation of area
- unpacking stock
- clearing up of area
- dealing with stock/equipment/products
- putting stock away/taking stock out of storage.

Health and safety suggestions

The salon should provide lockable staff storage, filing cabinets or similar so that personal belongings can be locked away. Handbags and purses are always vulnerable to the opportunist thief, who may come in unnoticed off the street and leave with someone's valuables. If your salon does not provide somewhere secure for your belongings, you could suggest this at your staff meeting.

Staff should be discouraged from bringing large amounts of cash into work and from wearing expensive jewellery if it has to be removed during treatments and is therefore vulnerable to loss or theft.

Carry out banking of money from the till at different times of the day and do not keep too much money in the till at any one time. Removing large amounts of takings from the salon into a bank or night deposit should be done daily. Avoid taking the same route to the bank at the same time of day. Someone may be watching!

Be aware of suspicious packages left unattended – inform a supervisor and, if necessary, call the emergency services. The salon should have a list of telephone numbers by the phone in case of emergency, such as the local police station, or security guardroom – this will save time when it really counts.

Do not allow yourself to be unprotected – do not leave outside doors open when working in the salon, do not leave the till draw open, do not be naive enough to think that it could not happen to you! If unsure, seek professional advice from the local police station or crime prevention officer for personal safety hints, for staff and clients.

As a professional stylist, do not allow yourself to become a victim – follow your professional guidelines.

Personal presentation

Hairdressing is part of the fashion industry and the image you portray should reflect this. However, your personal appearance should always combine safety with professionalism. For example, high-heeled shoes are not only uncomfortable after a day's standing but also not particularly stable to walk in and open-toed sandals will not protect the toes from damage, spillage or impact injury. Shoes should be smart but essentially comfortable.

- Do not wear dangling jewellery which may be a hazard.
- Avoid stooping and slouching, which will prevent back problems occurring.

Reality check!

You should continuously review the salon for hazards that might cause an accident. For example, a lack of storage space may mean that equipment regularly gets broken – you need to review storage space to prevent this. If the only space for a trolley is next to flammable products, such as hairspray and other chemicals where there is a risk of fire, then you should review the trolley's position. If the same accident occurs more than once, then you must ask why.

All salons should have a set procedure to follow in the event of an accident. What is yours?

Reality check!

- Think ahead and be safe.
- Know what to do and be safe.
- Be responsible and be safe.

- Hairdressers often have arms and shoulders raised when cutting, perm winding, and setting. This awkward and unnatural posture often leads to hairdressers becoming round shouldered and in old age can lead to a hunched back. It is important to learn to stand with good posture while working to prevent this from occurring.
- Evenly distribute body weight by standing with both feet slightly apart – this will prevent accidents and body damage.
- Always wear the correct protective clothing to shield a uniform.
- Always wear gloves when using chemicals or if there is a possibility of coming into contact with body fluids.
- Always follow the correct disposal regulations for waste materials.
- If a salon provides a uniform as part of a corporate image, wear it with pride!
- Your hair should not interfere with any treatment you carry out to avoid the possibility of cross-infection.
- A high standard of cleanliness will ensure no cross-infection can occur:
  – Wash your hands between clients.
  – Keep your nails tidy.
  – Cover cuts or open wounds.
  – Do not attend work with an infectious disease.
  – Do not spread germs with a cold or flu.

Personal conduct

Good conduct cuts down any risks.

- Do not run or rush around the salon.
- Use equipment properly.
- Follow manufacturer's instructions at all times.
- Ensure salon and equipment are cleaned thoroughly.
- Always leave equipment ready for use by the next person.
- Do not block fire exits for any reason.
- Do not endanger anyone, even as a joke.
- Behave sensibly.
- Use proper lifting procedures.
- Take responsibility for yourself, machinery and problems such as spillage that may occur – do not expect someone else to clean up after you!
- Always treat your clients with the utmost respect.

Salon security and reducing workplace risks

There are many areas to keep secure in a business. Possible risk areas include:

- the premises
- stock and products
- equipment
- money
- display materials
- personal safety
- clients' belongings.

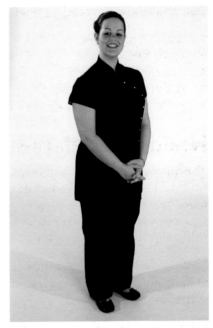

Good personal presentation gives a positive image to the salon

Reality check!

When stock is delivered to the salon it is usually left at reception for staff to check that the order is correct and then it is taken to the storage area for unpacking. Often the stock is delivered in large, heavy boxes and therefore great care must be taken by all salon employees who lift the boxes. This means bending your knees before taking the weight of the box, and keeping your back straight to avoid straining back muscles and more serious long-term back problems. See page 28 for correct lifting and handling procedures.

The premises

For insurance and mortgage applications the salon owner must have adequate security measures in place for the salon, and it is worth consulting the local police for guidance. A crime prevention officer will come and survey the premises and give advice regarding the most vulnerable areas and the most common forms of entry by a burglar.

External security

- Deadlock all doors and windows.
- Double-glazed windows are expensive but are more difficult to break into – the older the window and frame, the easier the entry.
- Fit a burglar alarm, if possible, or even fit a dummy box on the wall, which may deter a burglar.
- Closed-circuit television (CCTV) may be available if the premises are in a well-known shopping area.
- If the premises have metal shop-front shutters, use them, as they are probably the most effective deterrent to a burglar.

Internal security

- Internal doors can be locked to prevent an intruder moving from room to room.
- Fire doors and emergency exits should be locked at night and re-opened by the first person in at the start of business every morning.
- Stock and money should be locked away or deposited in the bank so that nothing is visible to entice a burglar.
- Lock expensive equipment away in the stock cupboard.
- Very large businesses employ security firms to patrol their premises at night, but, along with alarmed infra-red beams, these are not affordable for the average small salon owner. If, however, the salon is situated within a shopping centre or business park, night patrols may be included in the lease or purchase agreement or offered for a set fee per year. Costs would need to be considered, but it may save money in the long term.
- The local police station can be contacted and police patrols will regularly check the building as part of their normal evening beat.

> **Remember**
>
> A light left on in reception may deter a thief – no burglar wants to be seen

Stock and products

This includes both items on display and those in use in the salon. The smaller items may prove most irresistible to the thief as they are small enough for a pocket and are very accessible. Unfortunately, this form of theft costs many businesses a great deal of money, as stock can be expensive to replace and can be a big chunk of the capital outlay of a salon.

Another very sad fact is that the average 'thief' may be rather closer to home than is comfortable. Staff may 'borrow' an item of stock for home use and think that this behaviour is acceptable. There may be some clients who like the look of a re-sale product on display and 'forget' to pay for it!

The stealing of small items is known as pilfering. Shoplifting refers to the taking of larger items. In both cases, the salon suffers financial loss.

Tight precautions are needed to prevent the salon's stock and products from being stolen.

- Have one person (usually a senior stylist or senior receptionist) in control of the stock and limit keys and access to stock.
- Do a regular stock check – daily for loss of stock and weekly for stock ordering and rotation.

- Use empty containers for displays, or ask the suppliers if they provide dummy stock (this will also save the product deteriorating while on display).
- Keep displays in locked glass cabinets that can be seen but not touched.
- Try to keep handbags (both staff's and clients') away from the stock area, usually reception, to stop products 'dropping' into open bags.
- Have one member of staff responsible for topping up the treatment products from wholesale-sized containers.
- Hold regular staff training on security and let the staff know what the losses are and how it may affect them – some companies offer bonus schemes both for reaching targets of sales and minimising pilfering. Heavy losses may affect potential salary increases.

In the salon

Sally has recently been given the responsibility of stock control at The Crowning Glory salon. Since taking over the role, she has become suspicious that some members of staff are pilfering retail products as the stock control sheets do not match the stock in the salon. As the role is new to her and she has to work with the rest of the staff who she may be accusing of theft, she is unsure what to do.

- Hold a group discussion on what you think Sally should do to deal with this situation.

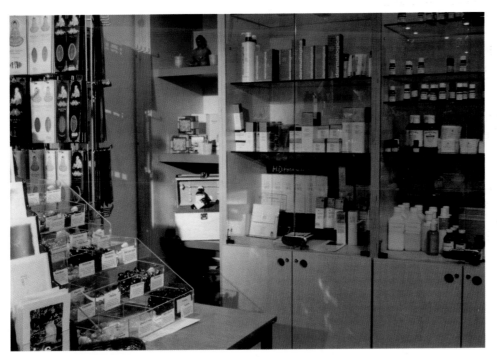

Keep displays in locked glass cabinets

Fulfil salon reception duties

Unit G4

This unit covers all aspects of a receptionist's duties. Every salon needs a welcoming reception area, overseen by a confident and effective receptionist. This is because the reception area is the first impression the client will have of the salon – and first impressions are usually lasting ones. You will need to find out your salon's guidelines for dealing with both general enquiries and specific problems that may occur. You will also have to learn how long each stylist needs for each of the services offered and how to use the appointment system correctly so that the salon is run cost effectively while maintaining client satisfaction.

What you will learn

- Maintain the reception area G4.1
- Attend to clients and enquiries G4.2
- Make appointments for salon services G4.3
- Handle payments from clients G4.4

Before starting this unit, you need to look at two essential parts of the salon's working environment:

- the receptionist's role
- the atmosphere of the salon.

The receptionist's role

To be a successful receptionist, you will need to know everything that the job role demands. You should be aware of the limitations of your authority and know when to ask the manager or salon owner for help.

Some receptionists are employed for their managerial and office skills and they may not be professional stylists. However, to be able to book in a client and talk about treatments, all receptionists should have some knowledge about the treatments shown on the salon price list and products used in the salon.

Knowledge of the treatments will not only allow you to talk with confidence about each treatment, but will also enable you to book appointments correctly, schedule the working day into a logical sequence and advise clients. All this can only be achieved through good training, which should be seen as an investment for the future and the healthy growth of the business. If the receptionist is *not* a hairdresser, he or she should have all the treatments (where possible) as a client to enable him or her to understand fully what is involved and to be able to talk about the treatments.

A further role of the receptionist is to carry out skin tests on clients wishing to book for colouring processes (see unit H13 page 239).

The importance of the receptionist

- As the receptionist, you will be the first person the client sees or hears on the telephone. You are therefore the ambassador for the salon.
- The receptionist represents the entire business and first impressions do count!
- The atmosphere of the salon – good or bad – is set by the receptionist.

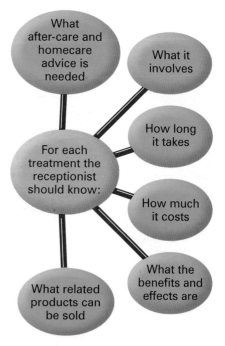

The receptionist should be able to talk knowledgeably about treatments and retail products available in the salon

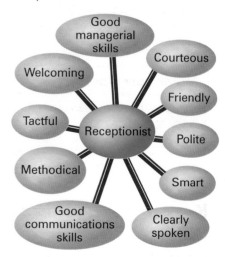

The qualities of a good receptionist

- The receptionist can make or break the success of the business. How well you do your job will determine how smoothly the salon will run.
- The receptionist is the lynchpin of the salon, holding everyone (both clients and staff) together.
- The reception area is the central pivot that the business revolves around, and its success will largely depend upon the skills of the person in charge of it.

The atmosphere of the salon

The reception area should be as welcoming and friendly as possible. The decor should be light and gentle on the eye and be a positive reflection upon the rest of the salon. The area should be very clean, warm, and tidy, and clients should be able to wait in comfort. It should be inviting and encourage the customer to want to stay.

Check it out

Think about the qualities and skills of the receptionist in the salon where you work, or you may prefer to consider another salon where you have had some experience as a client. Note down his or her qualities. You will need to refer to them as evidence collection for this unit.

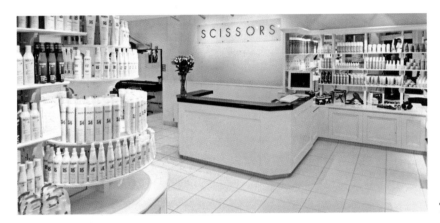

The reception area should be welcoming

Maintain the reception area   G4.1

Part of a receptionist's job is to ensure that the reception area is clean and tidy at all times, as this is the clients' first impression as they walk through the door. Promotional display stands need to be well stocked to allow clients to see what products are available for them to buy in order to maintain treatments carried out in the salon. Making sure that you have all the correct stationery to carry out your job efficiently and knowing the salon's policies on client care are the key to offering a professional service.

What you will learn

- Keeping the reception area clean and tidy
- Keeping stationery stock up to date
- Product displays
- Legislation affecting retail products
- Client hospitality and client care

Keeping the reception area clean and tidy

From your own experiences you may have come across salons that do not appear to be professionally run. This may be for a number of reasons, but may have been as a result of a bad impression when entering a salon.

Look at the reception area in your salon and see how many positive points you can identify about how your reception is kept clean and tidy.

Hopefully you should have found the following positive points:

- Magazines are up to date and stacked neatly.
- All finished coffee cups are removed and washed up.
- Client's coats are taken from them upon arrival and hung up.
- If there are cushions in the seating area, these are 'plumped' and neatly arranged.
- Tables are kept dust free.
- The floor area is hoovered or swept regularly.
- Reception area is kept free of obstructions.

What you may have found are the following negative points:

- Dirty cups left from previous clients.
- Magazines scattered over dusty tables.
- Client's coats left on seating areas.
- Hair on the floor all around the salon.

Out of the two lists, which one portrays a more professional caring image?

When maintaining the reception area think how and when you can carry out the jobs required of you in order to keep the reception area clean and tidy. Should you be hoovering around clients' feet? Should you wait until you have enough cups to make it worthwhile washing up? The answer is NO. Common sense is required on your part so that the jobs you carry out maintain a professional reception without making clients feel uncomfortable or in the way.

Cleaning the floor and dusting can be carried out last thing at night or first thing in the morning before clients arrive. Cups and saucers can be picked up in a regular hourly roundup to ensure you do not run out. Magazines can be tidied when cups are collected from reception. Coats can be taken from clients when you know that they are having a treatment.

Keeping stationery stock up to date

You will need certain stationery items when you are working on reception.

These will probably include:
- a memo pad for taking messages
- treatment sales dockets
- retail sales dockets
- appointment cards
- price lists
- a price list for retail products
- a cashing-up summary sheet.

When you are taking a message for a stylist, either over the phone or from a client in person, you will need to take all of the relevant details. Which item of stationery will you need from the list above?

If you ran out of the correct forms on reception and the message was written down on a scrap piece of paper, the chances are that the message would be lost. It is important to make sure that you have all of the relevant forms and stationery so that reception can function professionally.

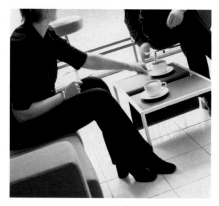

Make sure all finished coffee cups are removed and washed up

Remember

The reception area is the first impression a client gets of a salon and it needs to be the right one.

Reality check!

It is important that you use the correct stationery so that the salon's records are kept accurate and up to date.

Your job may be to ensure that there are enough price lists for clients to be able to take them away with them if required. They may be regular clients and know the prices of their own treatments, but what about if they want to introduce family or friends to the salon?

Each stylist may have his or her own treatment docket pad or retail docket pad: this is to help the salon work out different stylists' commission on retail sales. If you have not notified the person in charge who orders in the stationery that one particular stylist was running low on his or her own coloured dockets, the salon's commission scheme could be completely worthless.

These are just some examples of how important it is to make sure that you know what stationery your salon uses.

Product displays

Another important job of the receptionist is to make sure that all product display stands are kept well stocked with the right levels of stock at all times.

If you are selling products to clients you will need to make sure you are knowledgeable about what the products do and the suitability of products for different treatments so that you can make the correct recommendations.

Using a copy of the grid below, make a list of all the products your salon has for sale; the benefits of each product and what treatment the product is suitable as a follow up for. You will also need to research the cost of the product to the client.

Check it out

Find out who you report stationery shortages to within your salon and what is the minimum amount of stationery that the salon may keep at any one time.

Check it out

Find out what retail products you have available in your salon.

Product type	Benefits of the product	Follow-up product to treatment received	Cost

Product knowledge is essential when selling to clients

You will also need to be aware of the following laws and regulations when selling products.

Legistlation affecting retail products

Sale of Goods Act 1979 and Sale and Supply of Goods Act 1994

Three main points:

1   Goods must be merchantable: reasonably fit for normal purpose and not faulty, that is, a hairbrush should not fall apart the first time you use it.
2   Goods must be fit for any purpose made known, either expressly or by implication, for example, a neck cream should not be used on hair.
3   Goods must be as described, for example, a natural bristle hairbrush must not be made of plastic bristles.

Trades Descriptions Act 1987

It is a criminal offence for a trader to make false claims about goods or services offered for sale. You must not say, for example, that an anti-ageing cream will make you look ten years younger. Suggest that services, treatments and products *may* help the client to look younger.

The Consumer Protection Act 1987

The three parts of this Act fall under both criminal and civil law.

1   Product liability: a faulty product is one that does not reach the standard of safety you are generally entitled to expect. A customer can claim compensation if the faulty product causes death or personal injury.
2   It is a criminal offence to sell unsafe goods; products must meet a general safety requirement. Traders are strictly liable if they break the general requirements and can be fined or imprisoned. Retailers supplying consumer goods can argue that they took reasonable steps to avoid committing the offence, that is, instructions or warnings were given, specific circumstances were taken into account.
3   It is a criminal offence for a trader to give consumers a misleading indication about the price of goods, services or facilities. Always have an up-to-date price list on display and products with the correct price (including VAT) attached to them. Any special offers must be clearly displayed and worded.

If you are selling products you will need to make sure that you keep a check of the amount of stock you have. This will ensure that you do not run low on products and miss the chance of selling opportunities to clients.

> ### Check it out
>
> Who do you report stock shortages to in your salon and what is the minimum amount of stock you can run to?

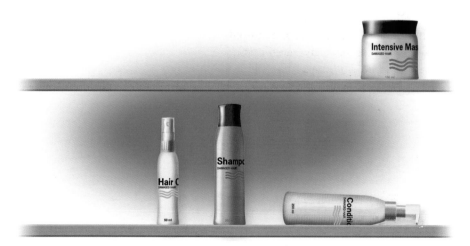

Clients may be disappointed and selling opportunities missed if the stock cupboard is bare

Client hospitality and client care

We have all been into a shop at one time or another where the staff have been more interested in discussing the previous night's events than serving us. How has this made you feel?

Good hospitality and client care are essential to ensure clients will return time and time again and the salon will prosper.

Most salons will offer drinks to their clients. At some salons they may be free of charge while at others there may be a small charge. You may find that salons that do not charge for drinks may only offer them to clients who are having chemical processes or a treatment over a certain period of time.

Would it make sense to offer a hot drink to a client who is only having a dry trim? By the time you boil the kettle and make the drink he or she may be leaving the salon. However, a client may only be having a dry trim, but if the stylist is running a little late and the client has to wait, you may decide that it is appropriate to offer him or her a drink whilst waiting. You need to use your common sense when deciding.

Hospitality extends beyond offering a client a cup of tea! Make a list of how else you can make a client feel welcome when he or she enters your salon. Some of the things you have on your list may include:

- greet every client with a smile, even when you answer the telephone, because this reflects in your voice
- make sure you have positive body language by looking the client in the eye and sitting up straight at reception
- always ask the client how you can help
- offer to take the client's coat and ask him or her to take a seat
- offer the client a drink or magazine whilst he or she is waiting
- find out how long the stylist is going to be and inform the client of this
- if the client has to wait a little longer than usual check that he or she is fine.

> **Check it out**
>
> What is your salon's code of practice for hospitality and client care? Should you rush over to a client and greet him like a long-lost friend or relative, or should you politely greet the client as he approaches the reception area by asking if you can help him?

> **Check it out**
>
> Find out what beverages your salon has to offer and what they charge, if anything.

Attend to clients and enquiries

G4.2

Receiving clients into the salon is rather like welcoming a guest into your home. The hospitality and friendliness should be the same. Whether it is the client's first visit, or fifteenth, the polite and welcoming atmosphere should be the same. This is achieved through verbal and non-verbal communication skills, listening skills and questioning techniques. In this element you will look at good practice in handling a range of clients and enquiries.

> **What you will learn**
>
> - Handling enquiries
> - Confirming appointments
> - Recording messages

Handling enquiries

The approach to clients and all visitors to the salon can be summed up in the word PLEASE, which stands for:

- Posture
- Listen
- Expression
- Appearance and attitude
- Speech
- Eagerness to help others.

Posture should be good and body language open. Nothing is more off-putting to a visitor than someone slouching over a desk. It says, 'Can't be bothered with you,' and sends out entirely the wrong message.

Listen with your ears, 'listen' with your eyes by looking at the client to show you are paying attention, and 'listen' with your body language so that you are saying, 'You are important to the salon and I am taking notice of you.'

Expression should be welcoming, smiling and open, not hostile with a frown or scowl.

Appearance and attitude should reflect total professionalism and reflect the high standing of the salon.

Speech should be clear, without a patronising tone and jargon free! (Do not use technical terms that the client will not understand.)

Eagerness to help others is an excellent quality – use it whenever you can!

When greeting clients you need to quickly identify the enquiry.

- Is the client in your salon because he or she has come to make an appointment, or has an appointment?
- Is the client there to pick up a price list?
- Is the client a regular client who has called in to purchase some retail products?
- Is the client actually a representative from a company wishing to see your boss to show a new range of products?
- Has the client come in to complain about a previous service?

Balancing the needs of individuals

Customers may have special needs that have to be considered. For example:

- Clients with physical disabilities may require some help negotiating doorways and getting into the salon. Always offer to help, but do not assume the client cannot manage – and never patronise or 'talk down' to the client.
- Clients who are hard of hearing are usually good lip readers, so the receptionist should face the client and speak clearly; this allows the client to see the words forming. Depending upon the severity of the disability, a notepad could be provided to jot down a message. A price list can be a good visual aid to help clarify the client's needs.
- Visitors from overseas may have slight problems being understood, although some cultures have a better command of English if they have been taught it in school. Again, speak clearly, use visual materials to help clarify what is required and seek help if available.
- Older clients may have problems with mobility or hearing, but do not assume this to be the case – do not pre-judge!

Check it out

How many other reasons can you think of as to why a client would be in your reception area? How many of these reasons can you deal with and which ones need to be referred to a senior member of staff?

Reality check!

Making a client angry is one way to lose business.

Dealing with telephone enquiries

Good telephone communication skills are very useful for business, and it is worthwhile learning how to use the telephone well.

Good telephone manner

There are some key steps to acquiring a good telephone manner, ensuring that the person on the end of the phone is treated courteously, efficiently and accurately. These include the following.

- Always have a pen and paper handy so that you are prepared to take messages.
- Answer the phone promptly, even if you are busy. If you do feel harassed, pause, take a deep breath before lifting the receiver and put a smile in your voice – it is very easy to sound abrupt on the telephone.
- Identify the salon quickly, after making sure you are connected properly and the caller can hear you.
- Be cheery – no matter how pressurised you may feel, it should not be obvious from the tone of your voice. No one wants to be greeted with a miserable sounding receptionist! Redirect the call quickly, if going through to another extension. If the call cannot be put through, ask if the caller wishes to leave a message.
- You may answer the telephone to an unhappy or disgruntled client. Below is a list of points to remember.
- Stay polite at all times.
- Take down as much information as you can about the problem.
- Take the client's details and contact number.
- Reassure the client that someone who can deal with the complaint will phone him or her very shortly.
- Inform a member of staff **immediately** after the phone call.
- Know the limits of your own authority.

Dos and don'ts when using the telephone

- **Do** answer with a smile on your face – just as if you can see the caller's face.
- **Do** write a message clearly so that it can be read easily and make sure that it includes all information such as the name of the caller.
- **Do** remember that all calls are from existing or prospective clients.
- **Do** ask to use the phone if you need to make a quick personal call.
- **Do** remember that there might be telephone calls outside of office hours or when everyone is genuinely busy. An answer machine is a simple solution. Revenue may be lost if there is no one to answer that important phone call.
- **Don't** sigh into the phone – it gives the impression that the caller is a nuisance and that you are doing a huge favour by answering.
- **Don't** be curt, rude or irritated when you first pick up the phone – you never know who is on the other end and no one deserves rudeness.
- **Don't** lie to the caller – if you do not know something or where someone is, then be honest. If you make something up, you will only get caught out and lose credibility.
- **Don't** ever slam down the phone in temper, cut someone off, or talk about the caller in a rude manner – the caller will most certainly hear and be offended.
- **Don't** use the telephone for long-distance or private calls. Itemised phone bills now show who made a call, for how long and to whom. No employer would mind the odd local call or emergency message, but do not abuse an employer's goodwill.

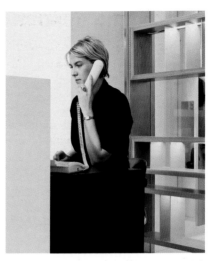

Good telephone skills are essential

Reality check!

It can be just as easy to give a bad impression over the phone as it is in person – perhaps more so, because the caller only judges what is heard and may not know the background leading to an irritable telephone manner.

Check it out

Make a list of all the enquiries you answer throughout a working day. How many were telephone enquiries? How many were face-to-face enquiries? Keep a note of these by writing down a brief account of the nature of the enquiry, the client's name and the date and time, and include this as evidence for your portfolio.

Confirming appointments

You should always confirm the details of an appointment with a client to make sure that you have understood each other. By doing this, you are double-checking that all of the information received is accurate and that the client is happy with the date and time of the appointment. You should remember to do the following:

- Repeat back to the client the details of the appointment by stating clearly the date, time and service he or she will be receiving. Most salons have an appointment card system.
- If there is a potential problem with the stylist's column in the appointments book, discuss this with the stylist *before* confirming the appointment.
- Make sure that any confidential information is recorded in the appropriate place and not broadcast to the whole salon!

What is confidential information?

This includes the client's address, telephone number, health status, medication and any other private information you might have access to. You are allowed to give these details to authorised people only, such as the salon owner, manager or employees. No person outside of the salon must have access to your clients' personal details.

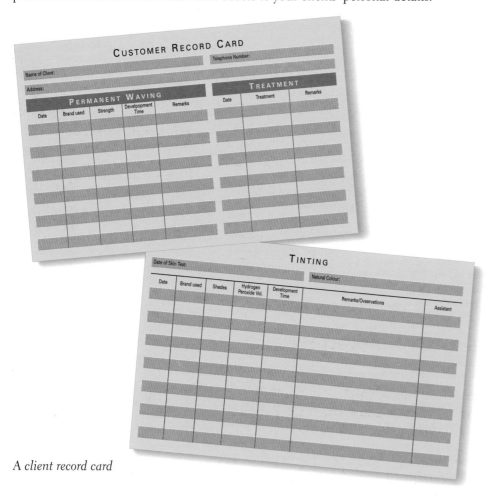

A client record card

Remember

Appointments are essential to your salon. They enable the salon to run efficiently. Without them, the salon would not be able to function.

Make sure you know how your salon appointment system works.

Reality check!

If you do not keep your clients' personal details private, you are breaking important laws of confidentiality. If your clients' details are kept on paper or computer, you must follow the requirements of the Data Protection Act.

Recording messages

As a receptionist, you will be required to take messages for other members of staff. You will also need to produce evidence of this for your portfolio, so make sure you keep a copy of any messages you have passed on.

It is very important to write down the whole of the message at the time it is given to you. It is unlikely you will remember it word for word, so make a habit of writing down all the information immediately. You will need to include:

- who the message is for – there is no point taking a message if you do not know who to pass it on to!
- the caller's name, address (if necessary) and telephone number (there may be more than one Mrs Allen, for example)
- the date and time of the call
- how important the message is – for example, it may be urgent
- a brief description of the nature of the message
- whether the caller required a reply – in this case it is essential to have the caller's telephone number.

It is important to listen carefully and ask the caller to repeat any part of the message you did not understand or hear properly. Always repeat the message back to the caller to make sure you have all the correct details – especially the phone number.

MESSAGE	
FOR	*Deepak*
FROM	*Mrs Alessi*
TEL. NO.	*0208 321 145*
TELEPHONED ✓	PLEASE RING ✓
CALLED TO SEE YOU ☐	WILL CALL AGAIN ☐
WANTS TO SEE YOU ☐	URGENT ☐

MESSAGE: *Needs to speak to you asap – you can call her on the tel. no. above up to 5.30pm*

DATE: *10.05.02*   TIME: *9.03am*

RECEIVED BY: *Amber*

Recording a message

Make appointments for salon services

G4.3

You have looked at the approach you need to take when dealing with clients, both face to face and on the telephone, when they enquire about their appointments or make new ones. You are now going to explore how to make appointments for clients and ensure the smooth running of the appointment system.

What you will learn
• Good practice in dealing with appointment requests
• The right way to schedule appointments

Good practice in dealing with appointment requests

It is usual for the appointments for each stylist to be kept in a large book, usually with a column for each stylist. This allows the stylists to see at a glance what services are booked in for the day and enables them to make the appropriate preparation.

The golden rule in all salons is: have an appointments system and use it correctly. Pages in the appointments book should be set out for several weeks in advance so that clients booking ahead or for special occasions (such as weddings) can make appointments with confidence. This also allows the stylist to book out time for holidays and personal appointments.

When booking an appointment, you should include the following details:

- name of client
- telephone contact number
- type of treatment.

If the salon has a system of coding, then use it – it will make life easier. For example:

H/L = highlights
P/W = permanent wave (perm)
C/B/D = cut and blow-dry
W/C = wet cut

D/T = dry trim
S/S = shampoo and set
B/D = blow-dry.

The right way to schedule appointments

You will also need to know how long to book each appointment for. You should allow for:

- greeting the client and consultation
- client preparation during the treatment
- client receiving homecare and aftercare.

Below is a typical page taken from an appointments book.

Remember

Always deal with requests from clients promptly and politely.

Reality check!

If you do not allow enough time for the stylist's first treatment of the day, he or she will overrun, making the next appointment late. This could continue all day and the knock-on effect may be that the last client is kept waiting far too long. The stylist becomes stressed under pressure, the client may feel rushed, and the benefits of the treatment will be lost!

DATE **18th June – Monday**
STYLISTS

	1	2	3	4	5	6

Time	1 – Leah	2 – Andrew	3	4	5 – Shelly	6
8		Leah	Andrew		Shelly	
9	Mrs Taylor P/W		Mrs Dodds S/S		Mr Davies TR / Mrs Singh	
10	Neut C/B/D P/W		Miss Potts Semi colour C/O S/S		Mr Rees flat top	
11	Mrs Rahim W/CUT		Rinse C/B/O colour		Danni Graham x 2 TRIMS	
12	LUNCH	LUNCH			Mr O'Hara C/B/D	
1	Mrs Westerby Hi-lights (top) Mr Westerby D/TR		Mrs Moorman full head		LUNCH	
2	Rinse C/B/D //// Hi-lights		foils x 2 colours		Tedore long hair S/S	
3	Mrs Champion Re-growth colour		Rinse Restyle colour		C/O + Hair up	
4	Mrs Pattell C/B/D		Rinse C/B/D colour		Mrs Adam B/dry	
5			Mrs Palmer cancellation required with Nicola after 3pm for wet cut			
6						
7						
8						

Page from an appointments book

Some salons do not have appointment booking facilities; they rely on staff being available to receive clients who walk in off the street. The advantage of this system is that the workload can be easily distributed between staff and the manager allocates the jobs as fairly as possible. The disadvantage is that regular customers do not always get the same stylist. This type of system therefore does not suit all clients.

Booking appointments

When booking an appointment:

- fill out the details in pencil – this allows changes, such as a cancellation, to be made without making the page messy and illegible
- use a simple code to identify any potential problems – for example, C = cancellation, L = late arrival, A = client has arrived, and so on
- make sure that everyone can easily understand start and finish times
- make sure that all names and numbers are clear and legible
- allow the hard-working stylist a break for lunch – do not be pressured by a persistent client into giving a lunchtime appointment to a stylist who has no other break throughout the day
- try to stagger the stylists' lunch breaks so that there is always a stylist to cover a busy lunchtime session
- give an appointment card to the client with all the details recorded on it – they then have a record of when to come in, it confirms the appointment for the client, and cuts down the possibility of a missed appointment.

Always remember to double-check the appointment with the client. If a client's husband phones up to book his wife in but is not sure whether she wants a cut and blow-dry or a dry trim, how will you know how much time to book out for the appointment? What would you do in this instance?

One possible solution would be to tell the husband that you will make an appointment for the shorter service for the time being until he can confirm with his wife. This will ensure that the stylist is not sitting around having an unwanted tea break!

When booking appointments for clients, it is important to make sure that you take all of the clients' details accurately. You need to make sure you are booking them in for the right amount of appointment time and for the service that they want.

Confirming appointments

Whenever you book an appointment for a client, always read back the appointment details to confirm that you have the right information.

Missed appointments and clients without appointments

Every salon should have a policy on missed appointments. Some salons have a small cancellation charge if the appointment is missed, rather like the dentist. There is usually no cancellation fee if the appointment is cancelled with 24 hours' notice. Both staff and clients need to be clear on this policy and it should be displayed in the reception area.

Be prepared to fit in a client who arrives without an appointment. You should always check the appointments book before fitting the client into a suitable slot – and then inform the stylist who may not be aware that a client is waiting.

Check it out

- What system does your college/salon/training institution have in place for dealing with clients who may turn up without an appointment?
- How much time does your salon allocate for each of the different services offered?

Please retain this card for future appointments		
Date	*Time*	*Stylist*

If appointments are missed or not cancelled within 24 hours of the appointment, a charge will be applicable

Appointment card

Remember

Calls may come in out of working hours or when everyone is genuinely busy. An answer machine is a simple solution.

Remember

When you fit in a client without a booking, use a code to alert the stylist that the client is waiting. If the client is new to the salon, he or she may require hair and skin tests before certain treatments can be carried out. You would, therefore, need to allow more time for tests and for the initial consultation.

Handle payments from clients

G4.4

It is important that a salon has a safe and secure system for the processing of payment transactions. Most salons have an electronic till and some salons have a computerised till to:

- help calculate the client's bill
- help the receptionist double-check the correct amount of change
- provide a receipt for the client
- provide a till reading of the salon's daily takings
- securely hold the clients' payments and till float.

The reception area is also an excellent place to display a range of retail products, as the client may decide while he or she is paying for the treatment to try the product that has been recommended by the stylist.

What you will learn

- Calculating the cost of treatments
- Methods of payment
- Handling discrepancies
- Managing transactions securely

Calculating the cost of treatments

No matter how much a treatment costs, from a small child's trim to a full head of woven colours, it is always important to treat clients in a courteous manner. The client should be treated as courteously at the end of the treatment as at the beginning and should feel that the treatment received was excellent value for money!

In the salon

Vanessa was coming to the end of a long day; she was tired and ready to go home. So that she could get away on time, she had started to cash up. This was a little premature as not all of the clients in the salon had finished their treatments and they still had to pay.

When one client came to reception to pay for a dry trim, which was £7.50, Vanessa was really annoyed that the client did not have the correct amount, as it would affect her float money.

'It is only £7.50, haven't you got the right money?' asked Vanessa.

The client looked surprised and rummaged around in her handbag to find some more change. When she left the salon she looked embarrassed.

- Should Vanessa have cashed up this early?
- How should Vanessa have dealt with this situation?

It is important to remember that all clients should be treated courteously no matter how much or little they have spent. You should always make clients feel important and thank them for their business.

As the receptionist, you should know which treatments the client has received in order to total the bill accurately. If your salon charges for extras such as tea, coffee and biscuits you should make sure these are added to the final bill. You need to ensure clients know of any extra charges that may be added to their bill for refreshments. The stylist and receptionist should liaise to ensure the client is charged correctly.

Methods of payment

The way the client pays is very much his or her choice and you must be prepared and able to cope with any payment method. The main methods your client will use to pay are:

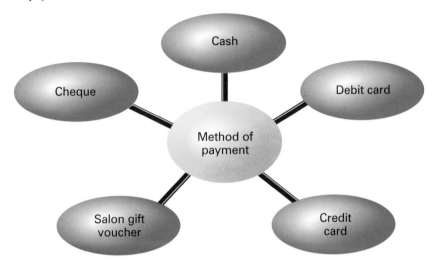

All are equally acceptable and should be handled with care.

Cash

There are several things to be aware of when a customer pays with cash. Large banknotes e.g. twenty or fifty pounds should be checked to make sure they are genuine and not counterfeit. You need to check for the following:

- Look for the watermark – every note has a watermark, which can be seen when the note is held up to the light.
- Look for the metallic strip which is woven into the paper – it should be unbroken.
- Compare the feel of banknote paper – often a forged note is not printed on the same quality of paper and may have a thin papery feel.

The police often circulate a list of forged notes to be on the look out for. The banknote numbers are on a stop list and this list should be kept near the till so that numbers can be compared.

If you are given a forged note, quietly ask the client to step into the office, away from reception, to avoid embarrassment. The client may have been given the money from another source. Ask a supervisor or the salon manager or owner to deal with the situation. You should then return to your duties at the front desk. In most cases, the client will not be aware that the note is forged, so it is not up to you to accuse him or her. It is important, however, that the note is removed from circulation and the police are informed.

Even when accepting money from very regular customers, it should still be checked thoroughly.

Remember

A client may visit your salon frequently and £7.50 adds up over the months, whereas a client spending £50.00 may only come to you once in a blue moon! Both are of equal importance.

Remember

Never feel embarrassed when checking money. It will save the salon from financial loss and protect the customer.

Reality check!

Payments for all treatments should be acknowledged, either by a handwritten receipt or a printed one from the till, regardless of which type of payment is used.

Dealing with cash involves a lot of responsibility and care must be taken to avoid errors.

Procedure for handling cash payments

- Place the client's money on the till ledge to ensure you remember what amount you have been given. Do not place the money straight into the till draw as this may lead to confusion – was it a £10 note or a £20?
- Count the change required from the note and then re-count it into the client's hand.
- Place the client's money in the till drawer and close it.
- Give the client the receipt to confirm the cost of the treatment, how much was given to you, and the change to be given.

Cheques

A cheque is equivalent to a letter to the bank telling it to pay a certain sum to a specified person. Most banks and building societies offer a cheque service, although a debit card service is also available (see page 62).

A cheque payment is very acceptable, providing certain checks and precautions are carried out. Always check that:

- the date is correct – day, month and year (this is especially important just after New Year!)
- the name of the salon is spelt correctly – the client could be offered a stamp with the full name pre-printed on it
- the amount is correct and that the amount in words and figures are the same
- the signature is included and that it matches the one shown on the client's cheque guarantee card.

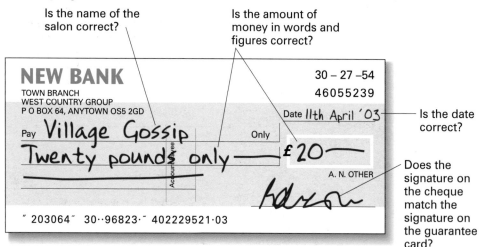

Always check cheques very carefully

What is a cheque guarantee card?

A cheque guarantee card should always support a cheque to the bank. It has two functions:

1. It acts as proof of identity.
2. It guarantees that the bank will honour the cheque up to the limit of the card. The limit on most bankcards is now £100.

There is always the exception to the rule and you may find you have a client whose limit is only £50. What happens if the total cost of the treatment exceeds this amount? If you have a situation where you have asked a senior member of staff for authorisation and he or she declines, how would you inform the client?

You should always check the expiry date on the cheque guarantee card – written as 03/04 for example, which is the month and year the card needs to be re-issued. You also need to check that the signatures match and that the card type is the same as the cheque, for example, an HSBC cheque is supported by an HSBC cheque guarantee card.

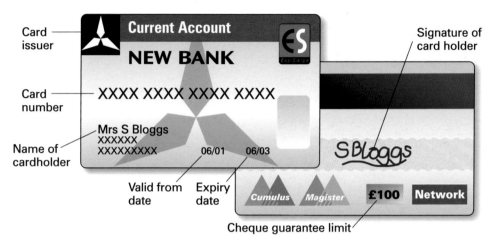

Card issuer — Current Account NEW BANK
Card number — XXXX XXXX XXXX XXXX
Name of cardholder — Mrs S Bloggs
Valid from date — 06/01 Expiry date — 06/03
Signature of card holder — S Bloggs
Cumulus Magister £100 Network
Cheque guarantee limit

A cheque guarantee card is usually the same as a debit card

The cheque is then treated exactly like cash, put into the till, a receipt given, and the till closed.

Credit cards

Credit cards are becoming as common as any other payment facility. All leading banks and a variety of other financial institutions offer credit cards to those customers

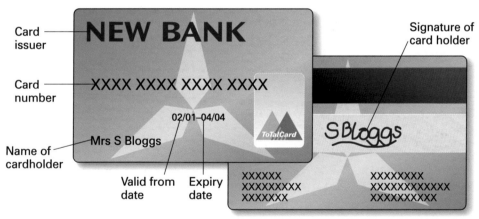

Card issuer — NEW BANK
Card number — XXXX XXXX XXXX XXXX
Name of cardholder — Mrs S Bloggs
ToTalCard
Valid from date — 02/01–04/04 Expiry date
Signature of card holder — S Bloggs
XXXXXX XXXXXXX
XXXXXXXXX XXXXXXXXXXXX
XXXXXXX XXXXXXXXX

A credit card

whom they consider creditworthy. Larger salons will usually accept credit cards, although small salons might not do so.

So how do credit card payments work? If your salon has a contract with a credit card company, it will usually display a sign stating that credit cards are accepted. The customer's card is 'swiped' through a computerised till connected to the credit card company. Once the credit card company authorises payment, usually within a minute or two, the client signs the credit card receipt agreeing to make the payment. The salon gives a copy of the credit card receipt to the client and keeps one for its own records. The credit card company will then pay for the goods or services the client

Reality check!

If depositing money at the bank, avoid using a big bank bag, which advertises exactly what it is you are carrying! Never take the same route to the bank at exactly the same time every day. Someone may be watching and being a victim of a snatch robbery would be a dreadful experience. Do not be a willing victim – be safe!

Remember

Remember to check credit cards just as you would cash or a cheque:

- Is the card in date?
- Is the name or title clear and as you know the client?
- Does the signature match the name on the front of the card?
- Is the card on a stop list issued by the local police?
- Is the hologram on the front clear and definite?
- If the card passes all these security checks, then carry on and process.

has bought by transferring the money electronically to the salon's bank account and the client will be billed by the credit card company at a later date. This is an efficient way for the salon to receive payment; in return, the credit card company charges the salon a handling fee of 1.5 or 2 per cent.

Debit cards

This is when payment is made electronically, transferring money straight from the client's bank account to the salon's account. This saves the client having to write a cheque. Debit cards are usually the same card as the cheque guarantee card.

To take a payment using a debit card, swipe the card through the computerised till unit, using a sliding action, so that the information stored on the magnetic strip on the back of the card can be read. The details are then printed onto a duplicated slip, which you should ask the client to sign. Tear the slip off the till and hand back both the card and the top copy of the slip, which acts as a receipt, to the client.

Salon gift vouchers

Some salons offer vouchers for clients to buy as gifts. The vouchers may be used to pay for a treatment or part of a treatment. They should be treated as cash and must be stored securely, either in the till, a locked drawer, or a safe that has restricted access. It is a good idea to number gift vouchers for security purposes. When used as payment, the voucher should be placed in the till after being marked to show it has been used.

Handling discrepancies

Unfortunately, there may be times when payment discrepancies and disputes arise. They should be dealt with calmly, without causing too much embarrassment to the client. Possible problems may include:

- if the currency is invalid – perhaps a foreign note or even a forged note
- if an invalid credit/debit card is presented – it may be out of date or not match the cheque details
- if a cheque is filled out incorrectly or does not have a current cheque guarantee card
- suspected fraudulent use of a payment card – perhaps it has been put onto the stop list.

Managing transactions securely

It is important to ensure the safety and security of the reception area, as this is usually a requirement of the salon's insurance policy. If money is left on show, rather than safely locked in the till, it could be targeted by thieves. As the receptionist, you are responsible for the security of the salon's takings and this should not be taken lightly. It is advisable to be alert to all those who use the till to make sure transactions are correctly processed.

At the beginning of the day it is the receptionist's job to go to the bank to collect the change (daily float) for the till. It is also important to ensure that there is always sufficient change in the till. If you run out, you may need to ask a nearby shop for change. If you think you are going to run out, you should report this to a senior

Reality check!

Be careful with debit and credit cards. All the information they contain – usually the holder's account number and expiry date of card – is stored on a magnetic strip at the back of the card. If this strip comes into contact with a magnet, the information is destroyed. Even the magnetic clasp on a purse or handbag is enough to disable all information. Some retail stores use a magnet to remove security tags, this can also interfere with your debit card!

Check it out

If your salon sells gift vouchers, who has the authority to issue them? How are they processed through the till?

Reality check!

In the event of a payment discrepancy that you are unable to resolve, you should refer to the salon manager or owner. As long as you stay calm and professional and report the incident promptly to the correct person, you will have acted within the limits of your authority.

member of staff. It is helpful to keep some additional change in the salon to avoid this problem. However you need to remember to replace the change when it is used.

To give you an idea of the amount of change that may be required for the day, refer to the following list.

- 1 x £10 note
- 2 x £5 notes
- £30 in £1 coins
- £5 in 50ps
- £3 in 20ps
- £2 in 10ps
- £1 in 5ps
- £1 in 2ps and 1ps.

It will depend on the structure of the salon's price list as to how much change your float will require. For example, if your salon's prices all end in 95p, you will need to have extra five pence pieces in the till.

At the end of the day's business, the till must be totalled and the takings should match the recorded amount taken, either through the till roll or a docket system. If a float has been used to provide a base of change at the beginning of the day, then it needs to be deducted. This can then be used for the next day's trading and the balance of the takings should be paid into the salon's bank account.

Most large banks offer a night-safe facility, in which the takings can be deposited. It is not ideal to keep large amounts of money on the premises over night, as there is always the risk of a burglary.

Check it out

Carry out the following checks in the salon where you work:

- What is the value of your salon's daily float?
- If you noticed the till getting short of change, how would you deal with the situation?
- Who would you refer a payment discrepancy to if you could not resolve the situation yourself?

Give clients a positive impression of yourself and your organisation

Unit G5

This unit is all about communicating with clients and giving a positive impression of you and your salon whenever you deal with a client. Most successful salons earn their reputation through providing an excellent personal service. You are, therefore, responsible for playing your part in earning a good reputation for your salon through every client you come into contact with.

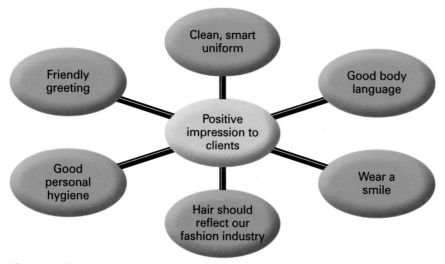

Elements of a positive impression

What you will learn	

- Establish effective relationships with clients G5.1
- Respond appropriately to clients G5.2
- Communicate information to clients G5.3

Establish effective relationships with clients

G5.1

When you work in hairdressing, it is very important that you are able to get on with anyone who walks through your salon's door. As a stylist, you should be pleasant, patient and helpful to everyone coming into the salon. It is only through trust and effective communication that you can start to build a relationship with your client and it is vital that you start to build this from your client's first visit to your salon. It is also important to continue to build upon relationships with well-established clients. They should be made to feel special when visiting your salon or they will try the salon around the corner; do not become complacent with well-established clients.

What you will learn

- Appearance and behaviour
- Greeting clients
- Valuing and respecting your client
- Identifying your clients' needs
- Working under pressure
- Keeping clients informed and reassured
- Responding effectively to client behaviour

Appearance and behaviour

We have already discussed appearance in Unit G1 as your appearance also affects health and safety.

A new client's first impression of you will be visual, i.e. how you look. Therefore it is really important for you to make the right impression by making every effort to look your best while you are at work.

However, it is not just how you look that will make an impression on your client. How you behave will have a massive influence on how your client views you as a person and will reflect on your salon. As a mature adult you will be expected to act sensibly and professionally at all times so that you don't endanger anyone in the salon. This will also create the correct and positive image that your salon owner/manager will want you to help achieve.

Check it out

What are your salon's rules for stylist appearance and behaviour? Write them down and keep in your portfolio of evidence. Why is it important to follow these salon rules?

Greeting clients

Most salons have a procedure for greeting clients, but if the salon is busy it is usually whoever is free who greets the client first. Make every effort to stop what you are doing, excuse yourself from the client you are working with, if necessary, and greet the client as soon as he or she walks into the reception area. The client may have entered the salon to book an appointment, to cancel an appointment, to have a treatment or for a general enquiry; whatever the client's needs, he or she is entitled to a prompt and welcoming greeting.

Valuing and respecting your client

Clients can choose from a number of different salons, all offering the same services. They choose your salon for many different reasons and can just as easily go to another salon if they do not feel valued or respected.

It may be helpful to define valuing and respecting.

Valuing = to hold a client in high esteem, to attach importance to a client.

Respecting = to hold a client in high esteem, to avoid harming, degrading, insulting, injuring or interrupting a client.

The way you communicate with your client must always be respectful. It is not appropriate to argue with a client in the salon, even if you do not agree with his or her beliefs or opinions. Your client is paying for a service, not to listen to your views or opinions (unless they are asked for, of course). This is a good reason why subjects such as religion and politics should be avoided during general conversation.

Check it out

- List two ways of making your client feel respected.
- List two ways of making your client feel valued.

Identifying your clients' needs

In Unit G7 you will cover in detail client consultation and analysis of the hair and scalp. You must make sure you identify your clients' needs and also confirm their expectations so that you are positive you know their requirements. This can only happen by effective communication.

Working under pressure

At many times throughout a normal salon day you will be under pressure from time, from other members of staff and from clients. You need to learn how to cope with pressure without becoming stressed. Talk to other members of the salon staff to find out how they cope with the salon's daily pressures.

It is also important to be helpful and courteous to clients at all times even when you are under pressure at work.

Check it out

Sit back to back with a colleague. One of you needs a pencil and paper (the stylist). The person without pencil and paper (the client) must try to explain a hairstyle to their colleague without the use of style names, facial expressions or hand gestures. The partner must try to draw the hairstyle.

This can be quite a hard task depending on how good the communication from the client is. This is very true in real salon life.

In the salon

Danielle had been running late all day due to getting up late, missing her bus and arriving 40 minutes late for work. None of her colleagues were prepared to help her out with her clients as they were fed up with covering for her constant lateness. Just before lunch she was hurriedly blow-drying Mrs Dudley's hair and not really listening to the conversation Mrs Dudley was trying to have with her. She just kept smiling and saying 'Oh, lovely' every so often as she was too busy worrying about the two clients she was keeping waiting and the lunch date she had with her boyfriend Robbie. Eventually she realised Mrs Dudley was crying and turned off the hairdryer to ask what was wrong. Mrs Dudley explained, through sobs, that she was trying to tell Danielle that her husband had just died and all Danielle could say was 'Oh, lovely'! Do not let time pressure be your downfall!

- What should Danielle do to ensure she is not late for work?
- What should you do if you cannot hear your client's conversation?
- What will happen if Danielle is consistently late for work?

Keeping clients informed and reassured

It is important to communicate effectively with your client throughout the treatment. Think of the whole treatment as being split into three, therefore your treatment has:

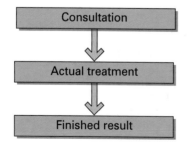

It is important to inform and reassure your client throughout the treatment, not just at the beginning. Explain what you are doing and why you are doing it, as most clients are interested in what hairdressers do. Some clients may need more reassurance than others as they may already have some previous knowledge of hairdressing treatments and will understand why you have used a particular product for example. Other clients may be totally confused by the whole process, so some explanation of what is happening during the treatment will be helpful.

<table>
<tr><td>

Remember

Hairdressers train for a long time to learn what they are doing and why they need to do it, so do not assume the client also knows!
</td></tr>
</table>

Responding effectively to client behaviour

Many different clients will enter your salon. You will need to learn how to deal with all kinds of behaviour. You will find that people have varying degrees of tolerance and understanding – it stands to reason that you will encounter some angry and confused clients.

Here are some definitions to help you:

Confused = muddled, perplexed, bewildered, mixed up or mistaken.
Angry = feeling angry or showing anger. Extremely displeased.

Confused clients will need a lot of reassurance and you may need to explain more than once why you are doing something e.g. why you need the head in that position. Try to have patience and be understanding. Remember not to use technical terms as although professional terms are useful to 'us', they can cause confusion to clients with no technical background or understanding.

Angry clients will need to be handled very carefully. Try to establish why they are so angry and put yourself in their position – would you be angry too? A client could be angry because the result of the treatment is not what he or she had hoped or asked for. Carrying out a thorough consultation and not dismissing your clients' wishes can usually avoid this. Sometimes a client may become angry because he or she has been kept waiting for an appointment. Even if the delay is no fault of your own, always apologise and make your client as comfortable as possible by offering refreshments and magazines. If a client becomes angry at any point during the treatment, always remain calm, even if you are being shouted at. Getting angry yourself will not help the situation. If you feel you cannot deal with the situation yourself, you should ask the client to take a seat and find someone who can help you.

Respond appropriately to clients   G5.2

This means you should always be polite, assist when your clients need attention, and respond promptly and positively to your clients' questions. You should always check with your clients that you have fully understood their needs and treatment expectations and allow them time to consider your explanations. If your clients do not fully understand, you should give further explanation to help clarify the situation, or this could result in unhappy and dissatisfied clients.

<table>
<tr><td>

What you will learn

• Responding to clients' needs
• Selecting communication techniques
• Responding positively and promptly to clients
• Checking clients' needs and expectations
</td></tr>
</table>

Responding to clients' needs

When a client indicates that he or she needs attention, it is vital that you respond to the request immediately. Do not assume that the request is insignificant or unworthy of your time, as it may be a matter of urgency to avoid a potential accident. A client may feel perm lotion burning her neck and if not treated immediately it could result in a serious hairline burn.

Selecting communication techniques

Whatever your position in a salon, you will need to communicate with others. You will come across a wide range of clientele and it is essential to identify your clients' needs and pitch your communication at the right level. For example, an elderly client may not be very interested in which nightclub you recently went to but a teenage client might be. You may be the only person an elderly client has seen all week and he or she would probably welcome conversation, whereas a client booked for a relaxing scalp massage may prefer a quieter, less stimulating chat. If your business is to be successful, you will need to communicate effectively and appropriately with all clients.

Responding positively and promptly to clients

Very often clients will ask questions about the treatment they are having and you need to be confident in your knowledge and understanding of the treatment to be able to answer the questions. If you do not know the answer, be honest and try to find someone who does know the answer.

It is also a good idea not to talk too technically about treatments to clients in case they misunderstand the information. It is much better to give a simplified version and know that your client fully understands the implications of the treatment. Also allow your client enough time to consider the information given instead of getting him or her to make a rushed decision. Experience shows that clients usually regret a hasty decision.

All clients like to have the 'feel good factor', as we all like to be made to feel special. What makes you feel special?

Negative reactions to questions will disappoint your client. Even if you do not think your client's suggestions for a re-style are suitable, respond in a positive way by suggesting a more appropriate style tactfully. Do not just dismiss your client's views.

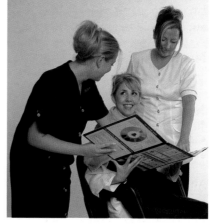

Always talk simply to your client so that he or she understands the implications of the treatment

Checking clients' needs and expectations

Some clients that come into your salon will be very nervous and will say as little as possible. Make sure you know exactly how they want to look when they leave your salon before you start the treatment.

As a quality check after a treatment you should ask yourself:

- Would I like to be treated in the same way I have just cared for the client?
- Would I pay for the treatment I have just given to the client?
- Did I communicate effectively with the client?
- Could I have improved upon the quality of my service?
- Was it as good as it could have been or was it rushed?
- Has the client re-booked?

Communicate information to clients

Have you ever had your hair done and felt that the stylist did not take enough time and effort to listen properly to how you wanted your hair to look? This was probably due to lack of communication and shows how important it is to communicate effectively with your clients.

What you will learn	

- Communication techniques
- How to give clients information
- Checking client understanding when information may be complicated
- Explaining to clients when their needs cannot be met

Communication techniques

Communication may be verbal, non-verbal or written.

Verbal communication

Verbal communication is what you say. It needs to be:

- clear
- to the point
- easily understood – using everyday language and avoiding technical terms where possible
- friendly in tone.

Eye contact with your client is important. For clients who may be hard of hearing, eye contact often reinforces the message.

Non-verbal communication

This is another term for body language. Your body conveys messages by:

- posture
- facial expressions
- tone of voice
- gestures.

Although a client may say that he or she is not nervous about having a particular treatment but facial expressions, twitching or fiddling, may tell you otherwise! These unconscious gestures tell you a lot more about your client than verbal communication and the stylist should be aware of body language and develop an intuition to act upon it.

Watch for signs that understanding is not clear or the client is not satisfied or following what you are saying.

Positive body language involves expressions and gestures such as smiling, nodding in agreement, lots of eye contact and open gestures, for example, arms uncrossed.

Negative body language includes frowning, tension, no eye contact and closed gestures such as the arms crossed.

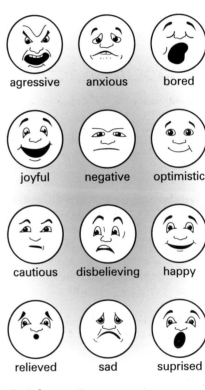

Facial expressions

Remember	

Your body language conveys how you feel. You may put your client off by aggressive stances, frowning and not making direct eye contact.

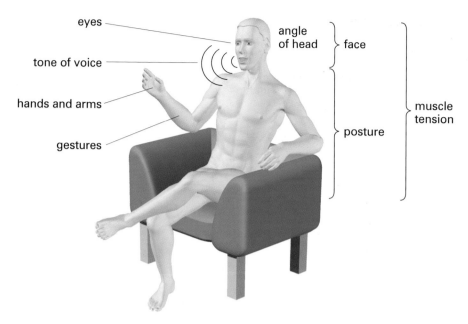

Areas of the human body that send out non-verbal messages

The ability to listen

Effective communication is a two-way process. You need to have good listening skills. This means:

- knowing when to stop talking and listen to what is being communicated
- listening with interest and understanding
- providing encouragement and confirming you have taken in the conversation, for example, by nodding or agreeing with the point raised.

Listening is a good skill to develop and differs from hearing. It is so easy to talk and not really listen. Always maintain eye contact with the person who is speaking and let the person finish the sentence – never interrupt. Really understanding what the client is trying to say may mean you pick up on what the client is not telling you too!

Do not plan your reply while you are being spoken to as you will not have all the facts until the client has finished.

In the early stages it is quite a compliment if the client wants to talk freely to you, but it may be some time before you fully gain the client's trust and confidence.

Observation skills

It is important to assess your client's body language in order to interpret if he or she is comfortable with any suggestions you make regarding his or her hair.

How to give clients information

There are many different ways to give clients the information they need about products or services offered in your salon. The most commonly used method is by talking to your client and explaining different offers you may have on products or treatments. Other methods could include printing information on the back of appointment cards, sending out information fliers stating promotional offers, or posters in salon windows. All these methods would offer information to your client and he or she could then ask for further clarification from you if necessary.

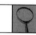

Check it out

With a partner, listen to each other for a full five minutes, without interrupting, cutting across his or her conversation, or putting together an answer before your partner has finished speaking. This is actually very hard to do. Make notes about how you performed. What did you find difficult?

Checking client understanding when information may be complicated

Clarification means checking the details given by the client to ensure the information you receive is correct. You need to do this whenever information is being passed on to you. This needs to happen at all stages of client contact. Here are some examples.

- When the client makes a telephone booking, the date, time, nature of treatment and client name and phone number should be repeated back to the client as confirmation.
- When the client arrives at reception for the appointment, the time of the booking and the name of the stylist may be repeated to the client.
- When the client is having a consultation, repeating back the information you have been given allows you to clarify information such as, 'So, Mrs Jones, your hair has been dry for some time, is that correct?' This also gives the client opportunities to respond to your open questioning techniques and encourages a good relationship to build up.

Explaining to clients when their needs cannot be met

Sometimes it is not possible to carry out your client's wishes. This could be because the client's hair is too damaged for the perm he or she has requested; it could be due to a contraindication (see Unit G7) such as head lice, or simply because the hairstyle the client has chosen would not be achievable because his or her hair is too fine.

Whatever the reason, it is important for you to explain clearly and fully the reasons why you cannot carry out the treatment. You should be able to offer some advice to help the client's situation. For example:

- Hair too damaged for perm – advise a course of restructurant conditioning treatments
- Head lice present – seek medical advice from GP or pharmacist
- Hair too fine for chosen style – help, advise, and choose suitable style for fine hair
- Face shape not suitable for the client's chosen re-style – advise more suitable style to compliment and enhance the face shape
- Client wants to go blonde but natural hair colour is too dark – advise a more suitable and achievable hair colour
- Client wants to keep the length but her hair is very split and damaged – explain that the hair will break off if the damage is not removed
- Client wants an appointment but you are fully booked – try to accommodate your client with another member of staff.

Remember

Always try to explain fully the reasons why you cannot meet your clients' needs. Always be polite and tactful in your explanation and remember to treat your client with the utmost courtesy, otherwise you might just seem plain rude.

Promote additional products or services to clients

This unit deals with the different ways you can promote the products and services offered by your salon. The promotion of additional services and products will generate additional revenue for the salon. It will also help to encourage clients to use the recommended home haircare products to maintain the hard work carried out in the salon and prolong the lifespan of perms, relaxers and colours. Hairdressing is a very competitive market and salons must continually update their marketing of products and services if they are to grow, thrive and become market leaders in the ever-changing world of fashion.

What you will learn

- Identify additional products or services that are available G6.1
- Inform clients about additional products or services G6.2
- Gain client commitment to using additional products or services G6.3

Identify additional products or services that are available

G6.1

Not all treatments are suitable for all clients. For example, some treatments require a skin test prior to the appointment to assess the sensitivity of the skin to hair colours. If a client has a treatment that is not suitable, he or she will not be pleased. It is also important to suggest the correct products to clients, as incorrect product advice will result in bad-hair days and unhappy clients.

Before you start to identify additional products or services for your client, check:

- that the treatment you are thinking of offering is suitable to your client's needs, for example, you are trying to help maintain the client's hairstyle so there is as little maintenance as possible. If you suggest a perm, will this make the hairstyle last longer or will it make the hair harder for the client to blow-dry?
- that the product you are recommending is the most suitable one for your client's hair. Do not get into the habit of recommending mousse to every client, as mousse does not suit all types of hair texture. Think about the strength and the consistency of the individual products in your salon and how they maintain different hairstyles to achieve different looks and effects.

Reality check!

It is very important that you are fully aware of the services and products your salon offers – or business might be lost. This should include treatment processes and the advantages and disadvantages of each.

What you will learn

- Updating salon information
- Checking new product or service details
- Identifying individual clients' needs
- Spotting client opportunities
- Complaints procedure
- Legislation

Updating salon information

As a member of the salon team, you are responsible for making sure all the appropriate information regarding the products and services offered by your salon is up to date. Do not leave this job to one person as all staff benefit from this information and everyone should take an active role. This could involve checking manufacturers' and wholesalers' price lists, contacting company representatives for posters or promotional leaflets, visiting wholesalers for special offers, or simply updating the salon's price list.

Checking new product or service details

If you are unsure of a new product or service offered by your salon, you must be confident enough to ask another member of your team. It could be that new stock arrived on your day off and you are not sure whether it is suitable for your client or not.

Everyone is entitled to time off for holiday leave and often during this time new products or services can be introduced. If you have missed vital training on how to offer a new service, you should be able to arrange an in-house training session with a more experienced member of the salon team who has already carried out the service and attended the initial training.

Other ways of keeping up to date with new products and new techniques are to read industrial magazines such as the *Hairdressers Journal* and to make regular visits to trade events such as Salon International, which is held yearly. Regular salon training sessions will allow company trainers/technicians to keep all members of the salon team up to date with new launches of products and equipment.

Reality check!

Never be afraid to ask if you are unsure. This helps prevent mistakes from occurring in the salon.

Identifying individual clients' needs

Even when you are training there are opportunities to identify products or services suitable for your client. It may be when:

- gowning – if you noticed your client was suffering from dandruff, you could recommend an appropriate shampoo to use at home.
- during shampooing – if you noticed a build-up of styling product, you could recommend a clarifying shampoo to use at home and more appropriate styling products to help reduce the build-up. The shampooing stage may be the longest amount of time you spend with some clients, so there may also be the opportunity to discuss future services. General questions such as:
  - 'How has your hair been behaving this week?' may lead to you being able to suggest a service the client is not booked in for.
  - 'Are you having a holiday soon?' may be an opening for your client to buy some ultra-violet protective products to help protect against sun and sea damage.
- seating your client for the next service – you could talk about the products displayed on the work station and ask if the client has tried any of the new range.

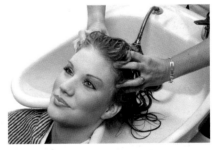

Shampooing gives you an opportunity to discuss future services

General conversation about a product may spark the client's interest and he or she may be encouraged to buy. Try to judge your client's body language and if you feel some helpful advice would be appreciated, try to use your verbal communication skills to their best advantage by describing all the benefits your client would get from purchasing something new, different and exciting!

Be confident in your knowledge of the product or service and with your approach to your client, as this will instill confidence and the client will be more likely to follow your advice.

Spotting client opportunities

Spotting an opportunity to offer a client an additional service or product can be quite simple. If a client is waiting in the reception area and is looking at the product stand, this is an ideal opportunity for you to go over and offer your professional advice. Do not jump in with a massive sales spiel, but talk to your client on an individual basis, asking about his or her needs and requirements. You should then have enough information to be able to identify which products or services are suitable for your client's needs.

Remember

Do not become too bossy and offhand in your manner or you may irritate your client.

Retail products

Product	Hair type	How to use	Benefits to client
e.g. Wella-Flubber			Really firm hold which lasts all day

Retail product knowledge is essential when recommending products to clients

Check it out

Using a copy of the chart opposite, make a list of all the retail products in your salon. Write down which hair type they are suitable for, how to use them correctly and the benefits to the client.

In the salon

Miss Burton has arrived for her appointment to have a beauty treatment. While waiting for her therapist, she asks for some advice on her hair, which has been dry since her foreign holiday two weeks ago.

Write down the advice you would give Miss Burton for:

- retail products sold in your salon
- additional services to help repair the dryness.

Keep this piece of work in your portfolio of evidence.

Complaints procedure

If a complaint arises, however minor, it is important to follow the correct salon procedure:

- Deal with any complaints pleasantly and in a professional manner.
- Calm the client and remove him or her from the reception desk to a more private area.
- Listen to your client. Be objective and not defensive – the complaint may be valid.
- Be prepared to apologise if you are in the wrong and offer some form of compensation – a free treatment, perhaps.
- Try to reach a mutually satisfactory outcome. This will minimise the damage that a complaint may have on other clients and prevent legal action being taken.
- Should the complaint be about another member of staff, ask the staff member about it later in a calm manner. Do not blame a colleague in front of the client.
- Record the complaint in the customer comments book.
- Know the legal implications of further action.

Legislation

The Consumer Protection Act 1987

This Act follows European Laws to safeguard the consumer in three main areas:

1 Product liability
2 General safety requirements
3 Misleading prices.

Before 1987 an injured person had to prove a manufacturer's negligence before suing for damages. This Act removes the need to prove negligence.

A useful definition is:

Injure = do physical harm or damage to.

This could be a client getting injured as a result of incorrectly using a product that was bought from your salon. He or she should have had clear information and advice on how to use the product correctly so that an injury didn't occur.

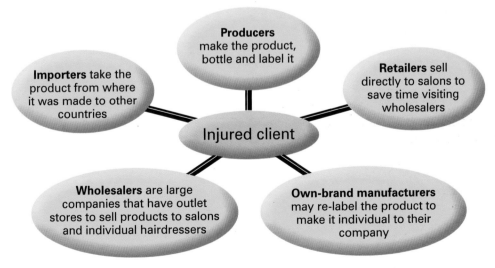

An injured person can take action against any one of these groups of people

In the salon this means that only reputable products should be used and sold and care should be taken in handling, maintaining and storing products so that they remain in top condition. It is important that all staff are aware of handling, maintaining and storing when selling products and when using products in a treatment.

Cosmetic Products (Safety) Regulations 1996

These regulations are all part of consumer protection. The EU has laid down strict regulations about the composition of products, labelling of ingredients, how the product is described and how it is marketed. American cosmetic companies have had to list all ingredients on their labels for years and Europe is now following suit. This is ideal for the easy identification of products that clients/customers may be allergic to such as lanolin.

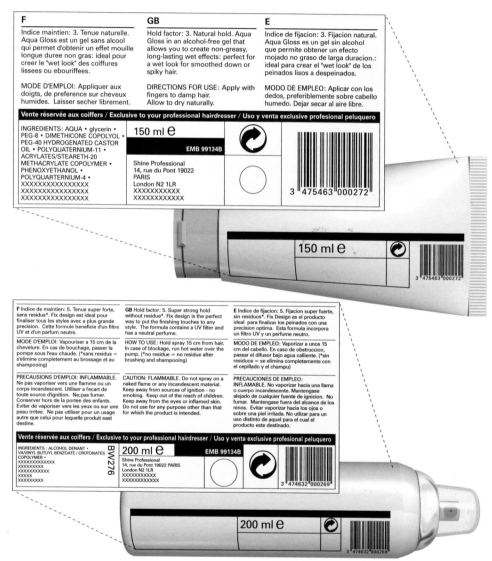

Remember – always read the manufacturer's instruction leaflets and labels

Trades Descriptions Act 1968 (and 1987)

This Act is concerned with the false description of goods and it is important to realise the relevance of this Act.

It is illegal to mislead the general public. This also applies to verbal descriptions given by a third party and repeated. So, if a manufacturer's false description is repeated, you are still liable to prosecution.

The law states that the retailer must not supply information that is in anyway misleading or falsely describe or make false statements about either a product or a service on offer.

The retailer must not:

- make false contrast between present and previous prices
- offer products at half price unless they have already been offered at the actual price for at least 28 days prior to the sale.

Be careful when using statements saying something is 'our price'. Comparison of prices can be misleading and can be illegal – be sure that the product is identical in every way. You should also check that products are labelled with their country of origin.

Sale of Goods Act 1979, Sale and Supply of Goods Act 1994

This Act has several others under its umbrella of protection:

- The Supply of Goods and Services Act 1982
- The Unfair Contract Terms Act 1977
- The Supply of Goods (Implied Terms) Act 1973.

The Sale of Goods Act recognises the contract of a sale between the retailer and the consumer when purchasing a product. This applies when the salon sells a product to a client, but it can apply to us all as consumers when we purchase any goods. (This Act is a good one to quote when returning something to a shop!)

The Act states that the retailer:

- has a responsibility to sell goods of the very best quality that are not defective in any way
- must refund the money for the purchase if it is found to be defective (some retailers will only offer an exchange of goods if there is no receipt)
- must then make a complaint to the supplier.

The Supply of Goods and Services Act 1982

This Act also deals with rights for the consumer and also the trader's obligations towards the consumer. It has two branches: goods and services.

Goods

This allows the consumer to claim back some or all of the money paid for goods. When we buy something in good faith we expect it to be of merchantable quality, fit for the purpose for which it was sold and as described in the advertising. This applies to all goods, regardless of whether they are on hire, in part exchange, or as part of a service.

Services

This means that the person or trader providing a service (such as a hairdresser) must charge a reasonable price, provide the service within a reasonable time and give the service with reasonable care and skill. This means no two-hour haircuts, no charging over-the-top prices, and no slap-dash treatments!

Your customer can complain and contact the Trading Standards Office if they feel they have a case against you. Be careful!

The Unfair Contract Terms Act 1977

This Act was prior to the Sale of Goods Act 1979 and defined the term 'of merchantable quality' for the first time.

The Supply of Goods (Implied Terms) Act 1973

This Act attempts to exclude or restrict statutory terms related to title, description and fitness of the goods.

Both of these Acts covered consumer rights before the Sale of Goods Act 1979, when definitions became tighter and the law was better defined regarding consumer rights.

Inform clients about additional products or services

G6.2

This element deals with how to inform and advise your clients of suitable products or services that they would not normally have. It is important to use the correct approach when advising clients so that they can fully understand and appreciate the information you are giving them. It is not appropriate, for example, to interrupt another conversation or to pounce on a client as soon as he or she enters the salon to try to sell products.

What you will learn
• Appropriate timing and methods of communicating with clients
• Giving accurate and sufficient information to clients

Appropriate timing and methods of communicating with clients

When you decide to give your client information or advice on additional products or services, timing is crucial. If a client feels hassled, he or she will certainly not buy anything you suggest. Choose a time when your client is relaxed and there is sufficient time to evaluate your advice. During shampooing is an ideal time as your client should begin to relax whilst being massaged.

Good times to give the client advice on additional products and services include:

- while the client is waiting for a treatment
- during the initial consultation
- during the shampoo process
- during the treatment, especially during waiting periods such as processing a chemical treatment
- while the client is paying for a treatment.

Remember, this is only a guide and you should be determined by your client's mood, body language and general signals.

Opposite is a flow chart to help guide you through the stages of positive promotion of products or services to your client.

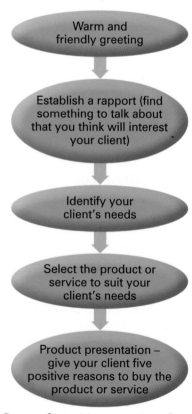

Stages of a positive promotion of products or services

Sometimes it is not possible to speak to every client individually due to the pressures of time in your salon, but you can still promote products by use of good visual aids and posters. Other ways in which you can communicate service or product information to clients is by giving them newsletters or promotional fliers before they leave the salon, or by mailing out information to existing clients. This can be done by using the clients' details stored on a computer database to mail out salon promotions at different times throughout the year. Some salons find this a very effective method of giving clients promotional deals. Some salons put promotional posters in the salon window to entice clients to ask about the latest treatment being offered. Whichever method you choose, make sure you make it work by being enthusiastic and motivated when a client shows interest.

Giving accurate and sufficient information to clients

Now that you know when to give advice on products and services, you need to understand why it is important to give accurate and sufficient information to your clients. You are governed by law when giving your clients advice and the law says you must give correct advice and not mislead your clients into buying something that is not suitable for them. This could lead to prosecution. If your advice is accurate and sufficient, it will enable your client to make an informed decision on whether they wish to buy an additional service or product. Always be clear in your mind what you want to say about a product or service and make sure your client understands by simple questioning techniques.

Treatment timings

The timings of treatments should be given accurately. Do not mislead clients or underestimate how long a treatment may take as you will not be believed next time. In addition, the smooth running of the salon will be disturbed if timings are not given correctly. Time is money and to be cost effective, timing must be accurate. Standard timings help maintain the quality in the salon, so that all stylists offer the same time for each treatment. All clients are then treated equally and get the same value for money.

Frequency of treatments given should also be negotiated with the client and is dependent upon:

- time available
- financial considerations of the client
- the condition of the hair.

See pages 55–7 for a guide to filling out the appointments book. You should take into account the length of a treatment when booking in clients.

Prices

Prices vary from salon to salon and area to area. The salon should always display a price list where it can be seen clearly by clients and potential clients. This allows clients to view for themselves the costs and may also be additional advertising!

The cost of a treatment given should be accurate, with no hidden extras.

Check it out

Design a promotional leaflet or poster for your salon. Decide if you are going to promote a service or a product and make it as attractive and interesting as possible to grab the attention of your clients. Keep this as evidence in your portfolio.

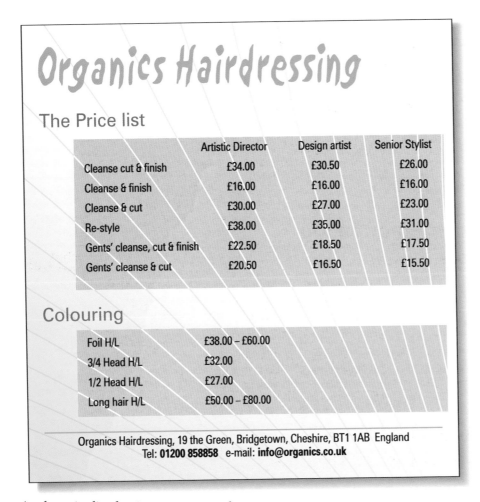

Organics Hairdressing

The Price list

	Artistic Director	Design artist	Senior Stylist
Cleanse cut & finish	£34.00	£30.50	£26.00
Cleanse & finish	£16.00	£16.00	£16.00
Cleanse & cut	£30.00	£27.00	£23.00
Re-style	£38.00	£35.00	£31.00
Gents' cleanse, cut & finish	£22.50	£18.50	£17.50
Gents' cleanse & cut	£20.50	£16.50	£15.50

Colouring

Foil H/L	£38.00 – £60.00
3/4 Head H/L	£32.00
1/2 Head H/L	£27.00
Long hair H/L	£50.00 – £80.00

Organics Hairdressing, 19 the Green, Bridgetown, Cheshire, BT1 1AB England
Tel: **01200 858858** e-mail: **info@organics.co.uk**

A salon price list showing treatments and prices

Special offers

If the salon has any offers to pass on to the client then the stylist needs to be aware of these. This helps promote the offer and provides a chance to sell additional treatments that the client may not be aware of.

There is legislation concerning sales prices, so be careful when advertising a sale in your window (see page 75)!

Retail sales

Many salons offer a full retail sales service to complement the products used in a treatment. Be aware of what your salon sells, if it is in stock and what its benefits and selling points are. If your client asks for your advice before buying a product and you are unable to give it, you may lose a sale.

Product knowledge

Be sure the information, benefits and effects you are claiming are true. It is also professional to ensure that the product you wish to sell to your client is in stock. Selling an unsuitable product just to close the sale is very bad practice and the client will lose faith in you.

Regular training and visits from manufacturers will ensure that your information is up to date and accurate. Many companies are happy to visit colleges to introduce product training.

Check it out

If you are employed in a salon, put the salon price list and all the advertising material the salon may have in your portfolio. Regardless of whether you can actually perform the treatments or not, you need to be aware of all the salon services offered. If you do not understand some of the treatments on the price list, ask your manager for a demonstration during staff training, or ask a more experienced stylist for a full explanation.

If you are not employed in a salon, collect two price lists from salons in your area and compare their services, presentation of price list and range of treatments. Discuss in class the differing services and the reasons why you think the differences occur.

Remember

It is very important that the stylist understands the treatments he or she is talking about. Do not make anything up – this is very unprofessional and can be dangerous. Always refer to the manufacturer's instructions and product information if you are unsure.

Always try to be as professional as possible. Always treat your client with the utmost respect, as without clients you would not be employed. As the old saying goes: 'Treat others how you wish to be treated yourself.'

Advice

Remember that clients are paying for your skills and expertise (your knowledge) and your ability to address their particular problems. All clients should be treated with the same respect and courtesy, regardless of how trivial their questions may be.

When giving advice never patronise the client. You may not know if the client has professional knowledge greater than yours!

Be both honest and realistic with aims and objectives of the treatment. Remind the client that results may take some time and may not be instant, for example, during a course of conditioning treatments to help restore moisture and strength to the hair.

Gain client commitment to using additional products or services

G6.3

What you will learn
• What to do if the client shows no interest • Delivery of the product or service • When referral is necessary

What to do if the client shows no interest

If your client is not interested in what you have to say regarding additional services and products, you need to ask yourself some questions:

- Is the information I have given relevant to my client's needs?
- Am I explaining myself clearly enough?
- Am I talking to my client at the right level, or am I being too technical?
- Is this the right time to give my client advice?

If the honest answer to these questions is no, you may wish to:

- make the advice more relevant to your client's needs
- make your explanations clearer to your client
- avoid technical terms when dealing with clients who have no previous background in hairdressing
- stop the conversation until the client is fully relaxed and ready to listen to your advice.

If, after trying another tactic, your client still has no interest in your advice, you should not pursue it any further as it could lead to embarrassment for both you and your client. Tactfully change the subject to something you know your client will be entertained by or interested in.

Delivery of the product or service

If, following your advice, your client has agreed to purchase something in addition to the original treatment, you need to check his or her understanding regarding delivery of the additional service or product. Is the client going to have to wait for the service, and if so, for how long? Always explain fully to avoid any misunderstandings.

In the salon

Mrs Truman is a regular client at Bentley's Beauty and Hair Salon, where she has a weekly blow-dry. Recently her stylist, Bob, has been using the salon's new ceramic straighteners on Mrs Truman's hair and she has taken Bob's advice and ordered a pair for use at home. Unfortunately, the salon has been experiencing problems obtaining the ceramic straighteners from the supplier, as the demand for them has been huge. As the straighteners are very expensive, Bob had to ask Mrs Truman for payment to secure the delivery and ensure the salon was not out of pocket.

Instead of explaining that there was a problem with delivery of the straighteners, Bob tried to avoid the conversation as he found it embarrassing to think that his client had paid £100 to the salon four weeks ago and had still not received her goods. This caused confusion, as no one had given Mrs Truman a plausible explanation as to why she was still waiting for the straighteners that she was desperate to have. Therefore, Mrs Truman cancelled her order of the straighteners and decided to go to another local salon to see if they could organise an order for her.

- How could this situation have been avoided?
- If your client is not a regular visitor to the salon, what would you need in order to contact them?

You should, obviously, take responsibility for any client's order of additional products that you have dealt with. If there is a problem with delivery of the item, you should inform the client immediately to avoid misunderstandings. Ensure you do as much as possible to help the situation by knowing how to contact wholesalers, suppliers and salon representatives.

If your client has booked an additional treatment, it is your responsibility to do your best to ensure you arrange an appointment to suit your client's needs. This may sometimes take a little effort on your part to juggle the appointment system to ensure you accommodate your client's needs. A little extra effort goes a long way and will ensure a 'feel good factor' for your client.

When referral is necessary

The needs of each client will vary and you need to be able to give correct information on all additional services and products offered in your salon, even if you are not competent yet to perform them.

If you do not know, you must be professional enough to admit this and ask a salon manager or more experienced member of staff to help. As a trainee stylist, you should be pleasant, patient and helpful to everyone coming into the salon, even if you are unable to fulfil the client's needs. Never dismiss a client and always be as helpful as possible.

Remember

Never make something up about any service or treatment you are unsure of. This will lead to problems occurring and is considered unprofessional behaviour!

Advise and consult with clients

Unit G7

This unit is all about getting you started as a hair stylist. Before you begin to assess any client's hair or prepare for a treatment, you need to have a clear understanding of the underlying principles of what you are doing. Before any successful treatment comes a thorough and in-depth consultation with your client. During this consultation you will need to assess the hair and scalp thoroughly by looking for indications of infections or infestations and assess the condition of the hair and scalp for the intended treatment, whilst listening intently to your client's ideas and wishes and taking into account his or her body language. This is no mean feat and takes some practice to get everything co-ordinated to achieve a successful consultation. You need to be able to consult with clients over non-technical (shampooing, conditioning, blow-drying and setting) and technical units (cutting, perming, relaxing and colouring) before you can be deemed competent by your assessor in this unit for your NVQ qualification.

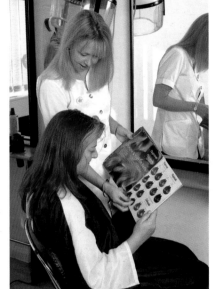

What you will learn
• Identify what clients want G7.1
• Analyse the hair, skin and scalp G7.2
• Advise your client and agree services and products G7.3

Identify what clients want

G7.1

This element will guide you through listening and questioning techniques that will help you to identify your clients' needs. At first, some students find it difficult to talk to clients, which makes it almost impossible to carry out a thorough consultation. It may help if you practise a consultation on a colleague or friend before you are faced with a 'real' client!

What you will learn
• Assessment techniques and questioning the client
• Questioning techniques
• Clarification techniques
• Observation techniques
• Effective communication and listening skills
• Treatment and client expectations

Assessment techniques and questioning the client

Have you ever had your hair done and felt that the stylist did not take enough time and effort to listen properly to how you wanted your hair to look? In this unit you will be given information and tips to help you to ask the right questions so that you meet the needs and wishes of the clients.

It is vital you understand the importance of consultation and analysis before you start the practical skills units. By learning to carry out a thorough and in-depth consultation you will have built an excellent foundation for your future career as a professional stylist.

Most successful salons earn their reputation through providing an excellent personal service. The consultation should be carried out thoroughly and the service should be free. A consultation should be carried out prior to the initial treatments and enables the client and stylist to meet to obtain the correct information to determine a successful treatment.

A good stylist will use all the skills shown in the spider diagram opposite and follow the client's body language to help obtain the information required for an effective treatment plan. Both the client and stylist should agree in advance on the treatment to be carried out, how much it will cost and how long it will take.

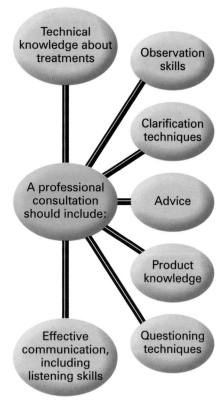

The skills required in a professional consultation

Questioning techniques

Asking questions is a skilled task. If you really want to find out what your client thinks and needs from you, you need to ask him or her questions. The types of questions and how you ask them will dictate the reply you get, so it is important that you give some thought to your questioning technique.

The information you obtain should be included on the client's record card, which you will be filling out as you discuss details in your consultation. Use the record card as your guide. If your client is new to the salon, you will need to make a new record card; if your client is a regular visitor to the salon, you will need to update the record card at every visit – making sure you have the correct card for your client!

You will need to ask the client for his or her personal details such as address and telephone number. Then you have to decide which type of questioning you should use to obtain further information about the client and his or her needs. There are two types of questions: closed and open.

- **Closed questions** usually only need one word answers. For example, 'Have you used a permanent colour on your hair?' This type of question confirms or eliminates information: 'Yes, I have' or 'No, I haven't'. Sometimes you will need to ask a closed question if you just require facts, but try to keep this type of questioning to a minimum.
- **Open questions** help to make the conversation flow as they require a fuller response. For example, 'How are you today?' Since open questions encourage more detailed answers, they are good to break the ice with, as the client cannot respond with a simple yes or no.

In the salon

A professional stylist will use open, or leading questions to help put a new client at ease. For example:

'What's the weather doing out there now?'
'Where did you manage to park the car?'
'How far have you come?'
'How did you hear about us?'

Rather than:
'Did you get the bus?'
'Is it still raining?'
'Have you been here before?'
'Is this your lunch hour?'

- Can you spot the differences?
- Try making up some of your own open and closed questions and try them out within your group.

Clarification techniques

Clarification means checking the details given by the client to ensure the information you receive is correct. You need to do this whenever information is being passed on to you. This needs to happen at all stages of client contact. Here are some examples.

- When the client makes a telephone booking: the date, time, nature of treatment, client name and phone number should be repeated back to the client as confirmation.
- When the client arrives at reception for the appointment: the time of the booking and the name of the stylist may be repeated to the client.
- When the client is having a consultation: repeating back the information you have been given allows you to clarify information, for example, 'So, Mrs Jones, your hair has been dry for some time, is that correct?' This also gives the client opportunities to respond to your open questioning techniques and encourages the build-up of a good relationship.

It is also important to encourage your client to ask about any areas he or she is not sure about. You can usually tell by a client's facial expression or body language if he or she is confused.

Observation techniques

It is important to assess your client's body language in order to interpret if he or she is comfortable with any suggestions you are making.

It is also vital to fully observe the hair's condition, growth pattern, porosity, elasticity and texture. Refer to pages 88–91 for information on how to carry out these tests.

Effective communication and listening skills

Communication is a two-way process and the ability to be an effective listener means:

- knowing when to stop talking and listen to what is being communicated
- listening with interest and understanding
- providing encouragement and confirming you have taken in the conversation, for example, by nodding or agreeing with a point raised.

Listening is a good skill to develop and differs from hearing. When you hear something your brain does not necessarily process the information. Whereas if you listen, you have to concerntrate in order for your brain to process, make sense of and store the information in your memory. It is so easy to talk and not really listen. Always maintain eye contact with the person who is speaking and let the person finish his or her sentence – never interrupt. Really understanding what the client is trying to say may mean you pick up on what the client is not telling you too!

Do not plan your reply while you are being spoken to as you will not have all the facts until the client has finished.

It is vital to your salon's business interests that all members of the team communicate effectively with clients and with each other. Clients will not return to your salon if they do not feel valued; effective communication is a way of letting your client know he or she is valued. Poor communication between clients and salon staff may lead to misunderstandings and potentially unhappy clients.

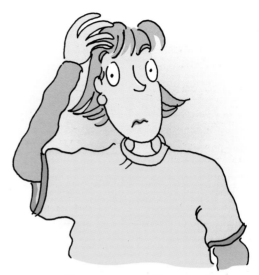

Encourage your client to ask questions if they seem confused

Remember

It may be helpful to use visual aids to help clients with decision-making, for example, colour charts or hairstyling magazines. Clarification of information also gives you the chance to help clients examine their lifestyle, health and homecare routine.

Say what you mean to your client clearly and use your facial expressions and body language to give meaning to the conversation. This will also show your client you are interested in the conversation. Always try to gauge your client's mood and adapt your conversation if he or she is in a quiet frame of mind. Some clients may not wish to discuss their feelings and you must respect this and not be embarrassed by silent pauses in the conversation. As you gain experience with clients, you will learn to listen to your clients' tone of voice and be able to steer the conversation away from the topic that is causing an emotional reaction. This can be done by carefully and subtly changing the focus of the conversation to something else.

If a client is new it is quite a compliment if he or she wants to talk freely to you, but it may be some time before you fully gain the client's trust and confidence. When your client does confide in you, it is important to observe the rules of client confidentiality. Clients must be able to rely on you not telling anybody anything they may tell you. This includes:

1   their address and telephone number
2   information about illness or disorders
3   personal confidences.

Treatment and client expectations

It is very important that the stylist understands the treatments he or she is talking about. Do not make anything up – this is very unprofessional. Always refer to the manufacturer's instructions and product information if you are unsure.

Be careful not to use technical terms that your client may not understand. You will confuse and possibly concern your client by saying 'I'm just going to apply the ammonnium thioglycollate to your hair', instead of, 'I'm just going to apply the perm lotion to your hair'.

Reality check!

In reality, it is easy to run out of time for a thorough consultation as 'time is money' in the salon. However, it is vital to the success of the treatment that you allow your client sufficient time. A client will have a 'feel good factor' if you spend sufficient time analysing his or her treatment needs. Remember, a happy client becomes a regular client.

Analyse the hair, skin and scalp   G7.2

Now that you have learnt how to talk to your client during the consultation, you need to know what to look for during the hair, skin and scalp analysis. In this element you will learn what to look for and how to avoid cross-infection of infestations and infections, in order to achieve a successful treatment result.

What you will learn

- Visual checks and tests necessary for hair, skin and scalp
- How to identify factors that will affect future services and product choice
- Protecting yourself and your client – when to refer to a GP

Visual checks and tests necessary for hair, skin and scalp

Now that we have discussed how to communicate with your client, it is time to carry out the very important client consultation. At this point it is essential to look at your client's record card to view any previous information written that may affect the service you are about to carry out. Always remember to record all relevant information about the treatment and tests you have completed for future reference.

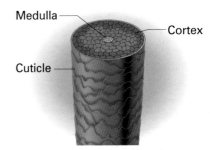

The hair shaft differs in texture

Visual checks are of great value to hairdressers as we are such visual people, working in a very visual industry. It is very important to look closely at the hair and scalp during the consultation and to take into account the following factors.

- **Porosity** – the condition of the cuticle scales; how smooth or rough the hair feels.
- **Texture** – how thick or fine each individual hair is (see the illustration). This will depend on the number of cuticle layers and whether there is a medulla present. Texture may affect the porosity and elasticity of the hair.

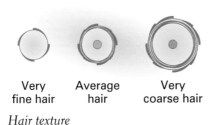

Hair texture

- **Density** – the amount of hair. How much hair there is per 2.5 cm^2 is important to consider when re-styling. Often a client has a picture of a hairstyle on a model who has lots of thick, lustrous hair. If the client has very fine, sparse hair, you will not achieve the same look!
- **Length of hair** – Is it the same length all over the head? Long hair will have been shampooed and dried hundreds of times. It may have had many chemical processes on the older ends, which will affect the condition of the cuticle and the cortex.
- **Growth patterns** – the direction in which hair grows from the scalp is important to consider before many treatments, for example, cutting a crown area too short may produce a spiky area that is not manageable for the client (see page 177).
- **Curl** – how much natural wave or curl the hair has, or is it permed?
- **Elasticity** – this is important to determine the strength of the cortex. Hair in good condition is springy and bouncy – this is because the hair has good elasticity. It can stretch up to one third of its length when dry (half its length when wet) and then return to its original length. Hair with poor elasticity will overstretch and then snap, for example, over-bleached hair.
- **Face shape** – the shape of the face is important when looking at suitable hairstyles to maximise your client's best features (and minimise any prominent ones, for example, a large nose would be accentuated by hair swept off the face). Look at the illustrations of face shapes on page 88 – these should help you to analyse your client's face shape. An oval-shaped face suits most hairstyles and this is the face shape stylists try to create using hairstyles to minimise square jaw lines and long and round faces.
- **Previous and existing chemical treatments** – is there any perm, colour, relaxer on the hair? This is vital to assess correctly or there may be disastrous consequences.
- **Natural hair colour** – this is important when colouring or lightening the hair. This is discussed more thoroughly in Unit H13.
- **Lifestyle** – your client needs a hairstyle that he or she can manage. If you create a style that is high maintenance, the client may not have the time, energy or skills to recreate the style every day. Try to suit the needs and personality of your client by creating a style that is versatile and workable.
- **Head shape** – if a client has a flat crown area, you may need to compensate for this by leaving the hair longer on the crown when cutting or using smaller perm rods on the crown when perming.

Oval

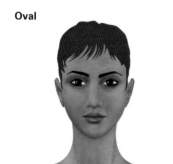

This face shape and bone structure is considered to be the ideal face shape. The chin tapers gently from a slightly wider forehead. Ideal for any hairstyle

Round

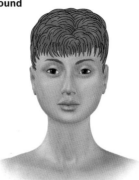

The face is usually short and broad with full cheeks and round contours. Width at the top of the head should be provided with height from the hair, which should be worn close at the sides.

Square

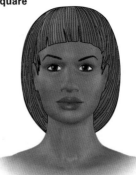

The forehead is broad, corresponding with an angular jawline. This face shape should have a little height without width and the hair should taper well towards the jawline.

Oblong

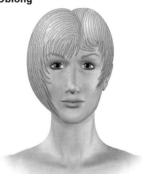

This face shape is narrow. Width is needed to shorten the face length. A fringe would be suitable with short hair. Asymmetric (unbalanced) styles also suit this face shape.

Heart shaped

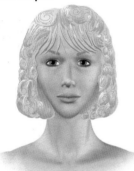

This shape usually has a wide forehead with the face tapering to a long jawline, rather like an inverted triangle. The aim of the hairstyle is to reduce the width across the forehead, emphasising the jawline.

Diamond shaped

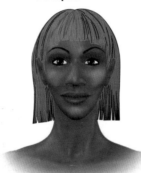

The forehead in this bone structure is narrow with the cheekbones extremely wide tapering to a narrow chin. The hairstyle should aim to minimise the width across the cheekbones. A central fringe should be worn with hair full below the cheeks but flat at the cheekbone line.

Pear shaped

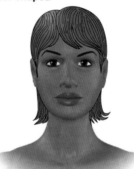

The forehead is narrow and the face gradually widens to the angle of the jaw which is broad and prominent. The hairstyle should create the impression of width across the forehead and make the jawline seem narrower. The hair should be swept off the forehead to create an illusion of width with a reverse flicking fringe.

Triangular shaped

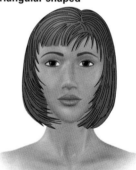

This is similar to the heart-shaped face, but not as soft. The aim of the hairstyle is to reduce the width of the jawline, by emphasising the forehead. The hair should be worn close at the cheek bones with fullness in the jawline area.

Face shapes

Elasticity test

This tests the internal strength of the hair. Hair that has been damaged due to chemical treatments may have lost much of its natural strength. This will be due to the internal chemical links and bonds in the cortex of the hair becoming broken and damaged. Consequently, this type of hair may stretch up to two-thirds of its original length and may even break off. Therefore, it is important to carry out this test before using chemical processes. Hair that is in good condition will stretch and then return to its original length.

Method

Take one strand of hair and hold each end firmly between the thumb and forefinger of each hand and gently pull. If the hair stretches more than half of its original length then it is over elastic and may snap or break during chemical processing.

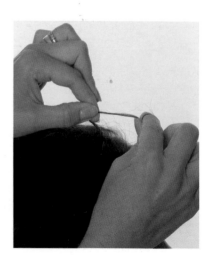

An elasticity test being carried out

Porosity test

This tests the condition of the outer layer of the hair shaft – the cuticle (see page 11 for more information on the cuticle). Porous hair will absorb water and chemical products more quickly than non-porous hair. If the cuticle is closed, flat and undamaged, the hair will feel smooth and look shiny. However, once the hair is chemically or physically damaged, the cuticle scales will become raised and may even be missing. Any chemical products that are then added to porous hair will be absorbed unevenly and may produce uneven curl or uneven colour results. This is why special perm lotions for tinted and highlighted hair are used. They are weaker in strength and are less likely to over process and give a poor result.

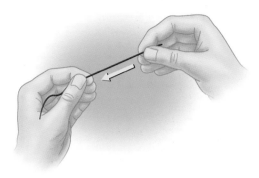

The porosity test

Method

Take a strand of hair and hold it by the root (where the hair grows from) between the thumb and forefinger of one hand. Run the forefinger and thumb of your other hand from the root down to the point (where the hair has been cut). If the hair feels rough and bumpy, the cuticle scales are raised and open and this is an indication of porous hair. If the hair feels smooth, the cuticle is flat and closed and the hair's cuticle region is in good condition.

Skin test

This test is a necessary safety precaution. It is carried out to check if the client is allergic to colouring products and should be carried out 24–48 hours before the colouring process.

Any colouring product, which requires hydrogen peroxide to be mixed with it, produces a chemical reaction that may cause some clients to have an adverse reaction such as irritation or swelling. In very severe cases, clients may have difficulty breathing due to swelling in the neck area – this is avoidable if you carry out a skin test before treatment.

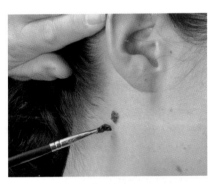

Carrying out a skin test

The manufacturer's instructions will always advise if a skin test is required, so always read these carefully.

Sensitivity to colour can sometimes cause an allergic reaction such as dermatitis. It is recommended that a skin test be carried out every six months, even on regular clients.

If a skin test is not carried out, you might make your insurance policy null and void, which would make you personally liable for any claim made against you.

Method

Use water and cotton wool or an alcohol wipe to thoroughly cleanse a small area of skin behind the ear or in the crook of the elbow. Mix together a small quantity of colour (a dark shade should be used) with a few drops of 20-volume hydrogen peroxide. Apply a small amount of tint (the size of a five pence piece) to the chosen area and allow to dry. Advise the client to leave the test on the skin for 24–48 hours unless there is any irritation.

Positive reaction – redness, soreness, itching, inflammation. If any of these occur, the client should immediately wash the area clean of the tint. If the area is very sore, the client may need medical advice. **If the client has a positive reaction, DO NOT proceed with the colouring process and advise him or her to use calamine lotion to soothe the area.**

Negative reaction – the skin appears normal when the test is removed and, therefore, the colouring process may proceed.

When the client returns to the salon, note the reaction on the record card and analysis sheet. The recorded information must include the date of the test and the result.

Test cutting

This is to test for the suitability of colouring products on hair and to check if the colour will have the desired result. It involves taking a small amount of hair and treating it with any of the following products:

- temporary colour – coloured setting lotion or coloured mousse
- semi-permanent colours – colour that lasts between four to twelve shampoos
- permanent colours – tints that are mixed with hydrogen peroxide
- bleaches – used for lightening the hair's natural colour.

Method

Take a hair cutting from an unnoticeable part of the head and place masking tape over one end of the hair to secure. Mix a small amount of the intended product in a tint bowl and make sure the test cutting is completely covered with product. Check manufacturer's processing time instructions, but remember that there will be no heat from the scalp to help with the development of the colour. Once processing time is complete, rinse semi-permanent, permanent and bleach products (temporary colours are left on) and dry the test cutting. Examine and record the result.

Incompatibility test

Some chemicals do not work well together (incompatible) and may have a bad reaction if one is used over the top of another. Some colours, for example, contain metallic salts, which are incompatible with other chemicals.

You should carry out an incompatibility test before perming, colouring or bleaching if you are unsure of the products already on the hair or if the hair has a doubtful history.

Method

Mix together (preferably in a glass bowl) 10 ml of hydrogen peroxide and 10 ml of alkaline perm lotion. Place a small cutting of hair in the solution and wait. If heat is given off, the lotion fizzes and the hair breaks, dissolves or changes colour, then this is a **positive reaction** and the hair should **NOT** be permed or coloured with a product containing hydrogen peroxide.

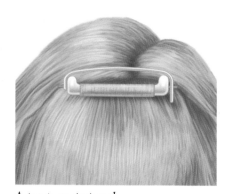

Incompatibility test being carried out

Pre-perm test curl

When handling fragile, porous hair or hair with a doubtful history, it is advisable to wind, process and neutralise one or more small sections of hair. The results will be a guide to the best rod size, processing time and lotion strength to use. This test will also give a good indication of the condition resulting after the perming process and will determine whether the hair is suitable for this treatment.

Method

It is not always suitable or possible to carry out a test curl on the head, so a cutting of hair may be taken and tested separately, but remember there will be no scalp heat to help the processing.

- Wind the hair around two or three rods of your chosen size.
- Apply perm lotion and leave to process for the manufacturer's specified time.

A pre-perm test curl

- Carry out a development test curl to see whether processing is sufficient. If so, rinse, neutralise for the time specified by the manufacturer, remove rods and evaluate curl result.

Strand test

A strand test is taken to check the development of colouring products while the colouring process is being carried out.

Method

Remove some of the semi-permanent colour, permanent colour, bleach, colour stripper (colour reducer) or relaxer from a strand of hair with a damp piece of cotton wool.

Check to see whether the product has developed properly and if you are happy with the result.

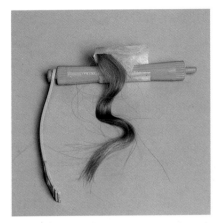

Pre-perm test result

Development test curl

This test is carried out during the processing of the perm to check whether the desired development has been reached.

Method

- Always wear gloves to carry out this test.
- Hold perm rod and undo rubber fastener.
- Unwind the curler one and a half turns, holding firmly.
- Push the hair towards the scalp allowing it to relax into an 'S' shape movement. Be careful not to pull the hair as it is in a very fragile state.
- When the size of the 'S' shape corresponds to the size of the curler, the processing is complete and should be stopped to avoid over processing.

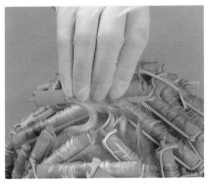

A *development test curl*

Always take test curls on different areas of the head as one area may be ready before another and this would cause an uneven curl result.

The temperature of the salon will make a difference. Perms will process quicker on warm days than on cold days.

Pre-relaxer test

This is done to test for the suitability of products, development time and resulting condition of hair.

Method

Take a small section of hair from where the most resistant area is and pull through a slit in a piece of aluminium foil (placed as close to the scalp as possible). Apply relaxer to the strand and leave for two to three minutes.

If the test gives a satisfactory result, proceed with the treatment. If not, repeat the strand test, leaving the relaxer on a little longer.

Note: When carrying out subsequent processes do not re-treat this section of hair, as it will become over processed and may break.

How to identify factors that will affect future services and product choice

Contraindications

A contraindication is the presence of a condition that makes the client unsuitable for treatment. A contraindication means that treatment should not take place at all or that the treatment needs adapting.

A treatment is normally unsuitable because the client has a medical condition, which may be external and visible or it may be 'hidden' and discovered during the consultation.

Why conditions prevent treatment

- The disease could be contagious and, therefore, there is a risk of cross-infection to both stylist and other clients, e.g. head lice.
- The condition may be made worse by a treatment, e.g. open cuts or abrasions on the scalp.
- There may be a reaction later, which puts the client's health at risk, e.g. allergic reactions to colours.

A thorough consultation prior to any treatment being given should reveal any contraindications.

A stylist should not name specific contraindications when referring a client to a GP. You do not have medical qualifications with which to make a diagnosis and it is unacceptable to cause the client concern, which may be unfounded.

If the contraindication is small and localised in one area, treatment may take place with some adaptation. For example, eczema in its dry state may be treated, but when in its wet and open state it is a contraindication to treatment.

Protecting yourself and your client – when to refer to a GP

It is vital that you are able to identify the infections and infestations shown in the following chart and know what action should be taken. Cross-infection of some of these conditions can be prevented by good hygiene. Many diseases are also significantly reduced by vaccination. Precautions can be taken against both hepatitis B and tetanus.

Reality check!

To prevent cross-infection, follow good hygiene practices in the salon at all times:

- Maintain own personal hygiene.
- Always carry out a thorough consultation with clients.
- Ensure good, effective salon hygiene.
- Maintain and clean equipment regularly.
- Maintain client hygiene – make sure anything that comes into contact with the client, such as towels, is clean and used only for that particular client.
- Protect the salon against possible risks through thorough training of all staff to include how to recognise disorders and diseases and the steps to take if any are found.

Remember

A thorough consultation before the treatment will stop the risk of cross-infection within the salon.

Reality check!

If you treat a client and ignore the contraindication present, you are responsible and could be sued for negligence. Seriously ill clients are unlikely to come in for their treatment, but even if the client appears to have no health worries, you must check – it is your responsibility! The client may not be aware of the problem.

Condition	Description	Cause	Treatment
Pityriasis capitis (dandruff)	Small, itchy, dry scales (white or grey)	Overactive production and shedding of epidermal cells – stress related	Dandruff shampoo, e.g. selenium sulphide or zinc pyrithone; oil conditioners or conditioning creams applied to the scalp
Seborrhoea (greasiness)	Excessive oil on the scalp or skin	Overactive sebaceous gland – stress related	Shampoos for greasy hair; spirit lotions

Condition	Description	Cause	Treatment
Psoriasis	Thick, raised, dry, silvery scales; often found behind the ears	Overactive production and shedding of the epidermal cells – possibly passed on in families, recurring in times of stress	Medical treatment; coal tar shampoo
Male pattern baldness	Receding hairline, thinning hair, baldness	Hereditary, i.e. passed on in families	Medical treatment is being developed
Sebaceous cyst	A lump either on top or just underneath the scalp	Blockage of the sebaceous glands	Medical treatment may be advised; treat gently during salon services
Fragilitis crinium (split ends)	Split, dry, roughened hair ends	Harsh physical or chemical treatments	Cutting and reconditioning treatments
Damaged cuticle	Cuticle scales toughened and damaged, dull hair	Harsh physical treatments	Reconditioning treatments; restructurant
Alopecia areata	Bald patches	Shock or stress	Medical treatment; high frequency treatment
Trichorrhexis nodosa	Hair roughened and swollen along the hair shaft, sometimes broken off	Harsh use of chemicals; physical damage,	Restructurant; reconditioning the cut hair whenever possible
Monilethrix	Beaded hair – a very rare condition	Uneven production of keratin in the follicle – hereditary	Treat very gently within the salon
Tinea capitis (ringworm)	Pink patches on scalp, develops onto a round, grey, scaly area with broken hairs – most common in children	Fungus (not a worm) – spread by direct contact (touching) or indirectly through brushes, combs or towels	Highly contagious; medical treatment required
Impetigo	Blisters on the skin, which weep and dry to form a yellow crust	Bacteria entering through broken skin	Highly contagious; medical treatment required
Pediculosis capitis (head lice)	White or light brown specks attached to the hair shaft close to the scalp; often at nape of neck and behind ears; itchiness – very common in children	Small parasites (with 6 legs, 2 mm long), which bite the scalp and suck blood from the host. The females lay eggs (nits), which stick to the hair close to the scalp (they need warmth to survive). Cannot jump but are spread by direct contact (head to head) or indirect contact (from brushes, combs, etc.). Can live for 2 days off the scalp. Once infected, lice multiply rapidly	Highly contagious; refer to pharmacist
Folliculitis	Small yellow pustules with hair in centre	Bacterial infection from scratching or contact with infected person	Medical treatment required
Warts	Small, flesh-coloured raised lumps of skin	Virus spread by direct contact or touch	Only contagious when damaged; treat with care in salon

Condition	Description	Cause	Treatment
Scabies treatment	Red irritating spots and lines on the skin	Animal parasites (itch mites) burrowing in the skin	Highly contagious; medical required
Barber's itch (sycosis)	Small yellow spots around the follicle; general irritation and inflammation; possible burning sensation	Bacterial infection of the hair follicle; generally found in beard area	Medical treatment required

Conditions, infections and infestations of the hair and scalp

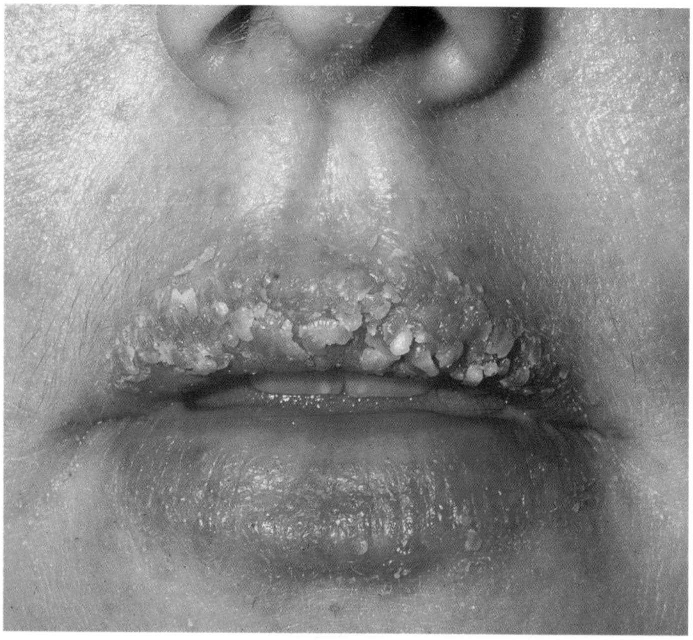

Impetigo

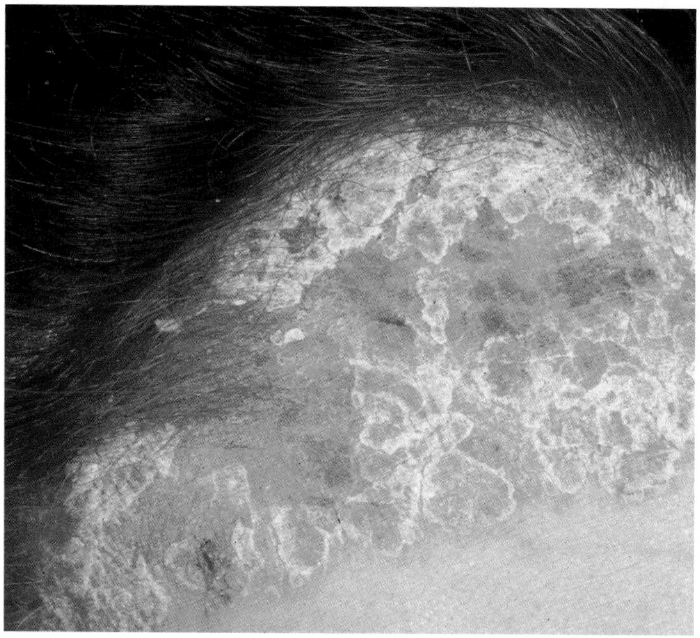

Psoriasis

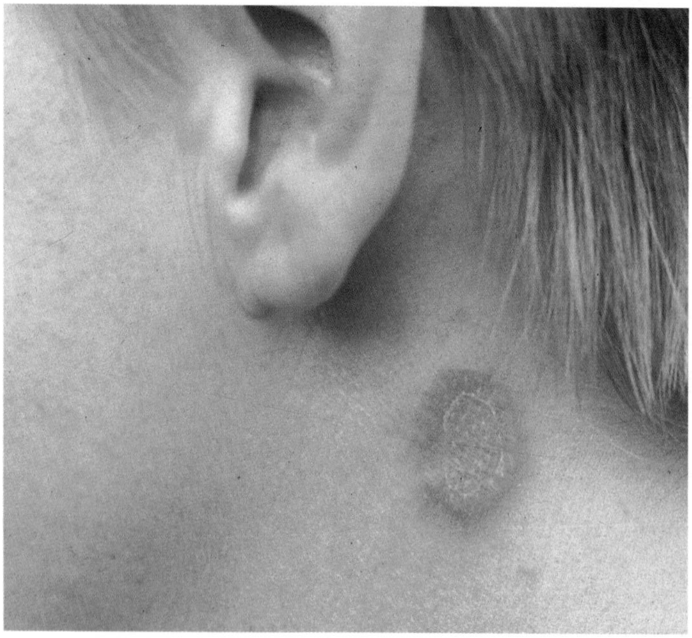

Ringworm

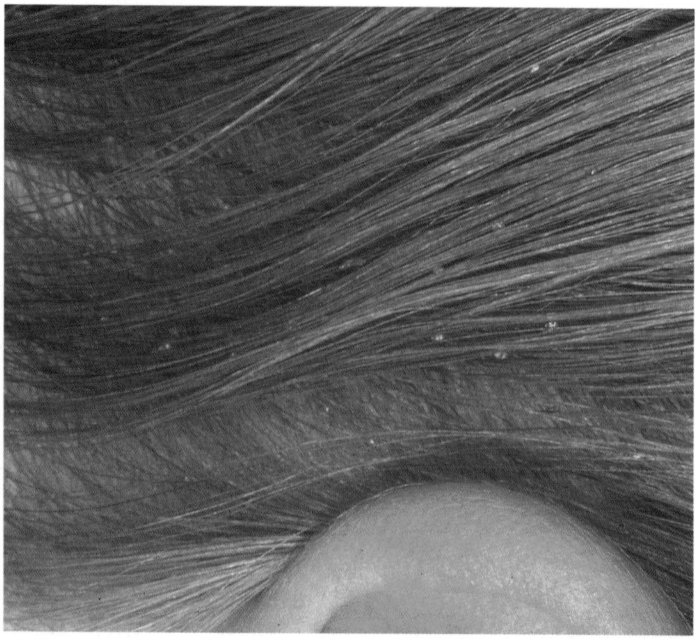

Head Lice

Advise your client and agree services and products

G7.3

In this element you will learn how to give correct recommendations to your client. It is very important to advise the correct products and services for your client to enable successful home maintenance of the treatment. This will promote a longer lasting, more effective treatment and will encourage the client to return for further treatments and products, which in turn will increase the revenue of the salon.

What you will learn
• How to make successful recommendations for your client
• How to meet the needs of your client
• Discussing cost and duration of treatments
• Ensuring client records are completed correctly
• How to maintain client goodwill, trust and confidentiality

How to make successful recommendations for your client

Be sure the information, benefits and effects you are claiming are true. It is also professional to ensure that the product you wish to sell to your client is in stock. Selling an unsuitable product just to close the sale is very bad practice and the client will lose faith in you.

Regular training and visits from manufacturers will ensure that your information is up to date and accurate. Many companies are happy to visit colleges to introduce product training.

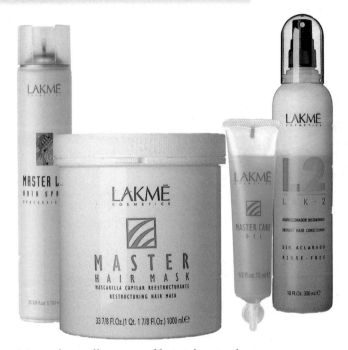

Most salons sell a range of hairstyling products

How to meet the needs of your client

Remember that clients are paying for your skils and expertise (your knowledge) and your ability to address their particular problems. All clients should be treated with the same respect and courtesy, regardless of how trivial their questions may be.

When giving advice never patronise the client. You may not know if the client has professional knowledge greater than yours!

Be both honest and realistic with the aims and objectives of the treatment. Remind the client that results may take some time and may not be instant, for example, during a course of conditioning treatments to help restore moisture and strength to the hair.

Salon services

As a stylist, you should be pleasant, patient and helpful to everyone coming into the salon.

The needs of each person will vary and you need to be able to give correct information. If you do not know, you must be professional enough to admit this and ask a salon manager to help. Never make something up!

Suitability of treatment

Not all treatments are suitable for all clients. Some treatments require a skin test prior to the appointment to assess the sensitivity of the skin to hair colours. If a client has a treatment that is not suitable, he or she will not be pleased.

Agreeing outcomes

It is important to ensure your client is fully satisfied with the outcomes of the service and products used. You must make sure you have met your client's needs fully to ensure a successful salon visit. If your client is not satisfied for any reason, this can be addressed and a note made on the record card for future reference.

Discussing cost and duration of treatments

Standard timings help maintain the quality in the salon, so that all stylists offer the same time for each treatment. All clients are then treated equally and get the same value for money.

Frequency of treatments given should also be negotiated with the client and is dependent upon:

- time available
- financial considerations of the client
- the condition of the hair.

See page 56 for an example of a page from an appointments book. You should take into account the length of a treatment when booking in clients.

Prices

Prices vary from salon to salon and area to area. The salon should always display a price list where it can be clearly seen by clients and potential clients. This allows clients to view for themselves the costs and may also be additional advertising!

The cost given for a treatment should be accurate, with no hidden extras. See page 80 for an example of a salon price list showing treatments and prices.

Special offers

If the salon has any offers to pass on to the client then the stylist needs to be aware of these. This helps promote the offer and provides a chance to sell additional treatments that the client may not be aware of.

There is legislation concerning sales prices so be careful when advertising a sale in your window (see page 77)!

Retail sales

Many salons offer a full retail sales service to complement the products used in a treatment. Be aware of what your salon sells, if it is in stock and what its benefits and

Reality check!

It is very important that you are fully aware of the services your salon offers – or business might be lost. This should include treatment processes and the advantages and disadvantages of each.

selling points are. If your client asks for your advice before buying a product and you are unable to give it, you may lose a sale.

Ensuring client records are completed correctly

Good record keeping is essential to any hairdressing salon. The function of a client record card is to:

- record relevant client details (for example phone number) so that you can contact the client if necessary
- provide full and accurate information, which will ensure client safety
- ensure consistency of treatment regardless of who performs the treatment
- record the date of each treatment
- record changes to the treatment
- safeguard the salon and the stylists – to prevent clients taking legal action for damages or negligence.

The client record card should be filled out in full for every treatment the client has. It should be written accurately, neatly and legibly. For an example of a client record card see page 54.

Most salons use a number system (see below) to store client information or keep records on computer for safekeeping and for easy retrieval. You need to be aware of the Data Protection Act 1998, which is designed to protect individuals from misuse of the information held about them (see pages 98–9 for more details).

A salon needs to store record cards in such a way that they are accessible to the receptionist and stylist, but not so open that others can view them. A locked filing cabinet or drawer with limited access is ideal.

Salons generally use one of two methods to file records:

1 a number system – client 1, client 2, and so on
2 in alphabetic order, using the first letter of the surname – if two names begin with the same letter, then the second letter is used and so on. Where several clients have the same surname, they are filed alphabetically by their initials.

Be very careful which client is which! Always take the client's initial and full name, along with address details. Repeat the details back to the client to double-check that there is no confusion with clients of the same name.

The information stored on a record card

The more detailed the record card is, the better picture the stylist will have of the client. It also enables different stylists to treat one client knowing all possible details that may affect the treatment outcome.

A typical record card should include:

- the client's name, address and contact number
- the client's occupation
- a client record number

Remember

Information on record cards should be kept private and confidential. If confidentiality is broken, it is an offence to the client and might lead to loss of clientele and earnings. If confidentiality is broken, it is an offence under the Data Protection Act (see Unit G1) and the salon or stylist may be liable to prosecution.

- contraindications, for example, head lice, cuts or abrasions, and so on, if present
- previous treatments and products, and their success or problems
- treatments carried out and date they were carried out
- cost and estimated time or length of a course of treatments
- outcomes/result and effectiveness of treatment
- aftercare recommended
- homecare, which is relevant and achievable to the client
- recommendations for further treatments
- purchases of products or additional treatments.

All these details should be checked regularly, even with a very regular client.

Many manufacturers of hairdressing products supply record cards to salons and they can be purchased in bulk, for ease of use.

> **Remember**
>
> A record card is a vital ingredient for successful salon management.

How to maintain client goodwill, trust and confidentiality

In the salon

Simone is taking Janice's column of clients while she is on holiday.
Mrs Jordan has booked for a perm and Simone has read the record card prior to Mrs Jordan's arrival at the salon. She has organised everything necessary for the perm including the perm rods and perm lotion that were used the last time Janice permed Mrs Jordan's hair six months ago. Mrs Jordan arrives at the salon and Janice carries out the perm. However, the result of the perm is very unsatisfactory and Mrs Jordan's hair feels like cotton wool. After discussion with Mrs Jordan and the salon manager it is discovered that Janice had carried out bleach highlights on Mrs Jordan two months ago and had then coloured over this with a permanent tint as the client felt it was too light. Neither of these treatments were recorded on the record card.

- Mrs Jordan has been a regular client at the salon for the past ten years. How can the salon go about regaining her trust so that she will come back again?
- What gestures of goodwill could they show her?

Develop and maintain your effectiveness at work

Unit G8

This unit is all about you – how to take responsibility for improving your performance at work and how to work well with your colleagues. Any personal improvement will help 'you' make a positive contribution to the overall effectiveness of the salon. You may be asking, 'How will this help me to become a good stylist?' The answer is that being able to be objective about your own performance i.e. standing back and viewing your behaviour from the outside, will help you to develop your personal and emotional attitudes, improve your relationships with your colleagues, and encourage a positive working atmosphere within the salon.

What you will learn

- Improve your personal effectiveness at work G8.1
- Work effectively as part of a team G8.2

Improve your personal effectiveness at work

G8.1

Developing yourself as a person and your skills as a stylist are essential if you are going to play an active part within your salon. This element looks at ways in which you can improve your work, both through making the most of your salon's appraisal system, working towards targets, and also by taking advantage of training opportunities while you are at work. It also considers the importance of keeping up to date with developments in the hairdressing industry.

What you will learn

- Carrying out your job role to salon and National Occupational Standards
- Identifying your own strengths and weaknesses – the appraisal system
- Seeking guidance when instructions are unclear
- Seeking feedback on your performance
- Asking colleagues for help
- Making and taking opportunities to learn
- Reviewing developments in hairdressing regularly and keeping your skills up to date
- Agreeing and reviewing targets regularly to develop your future personal development plan

---

Carrying out your job role to salon and National Occupational Standards

It is very important to understand your job role within the salon. If you do not understand what is expected of you while you are at work, how can you possibly fulfil all that is expected of you by managers and colleagues?

Once you have a defined job role, it is much easier to be an effective member of the salon team. As a trainee within the salon, you will be expected to assist all other members of the salon team. Once you have assisted with the treatments carried out in the salon, you will have an understanding of what the treatments involve. This will then allow you to anticipate the needs of the treatments and of your colleagues carrying out the treatments and to therefore give prompt assistance.

If you are unclear about your job role, it is vital that you approach your salon owner or manager to get clear guidelines of what you are expected to do during your working day/week. If you do not have a clear understanding of your responsibilities, your colleagues may view you as lazy when you do not carry out a task that is expected of you. It is also important to carry out the tasks expected of you to salon and National Occupational Standards. For example, there are correct methods, techniques and sequences of carrying out hairdressing tasks and these have been written into the National Occupational Standards that make up your qualification and are there for a specific reason. If you decide to neutralise 'your way' instead of following your salon's guidelines and those laid down in the National Occupational Standards, you will create problems for your client, your salon and yourself. If you always work to the highest possible standard, you will become a professional, skilled hairdresser who is known for high standards of work and is highly sought after by clients.

Identifying your own strengths and weaknesses – the appraisal system

If you keep making the same mistakes and clients complain or stop coming into the salon, something is obviously wrong! Spotting your own mistakes and then changing how you do a particular job to make sure you get it right in the future is one way of tackling this. However, it is not always easy to be inward looking and this is where a good manager will help by giving you regular work-related reviews or appraisals of your performance at work.

Many large companies provide self-appraisal forms for the employee to fill in and a joint performance appraisal form, which the manager discusses with the employee. An appraisal involves a discussion of your performance from which you as an employee will benefit as well as your employer. It is important to react in a positive way to any feedback or review. Nobody likes criticism, but it is important to listen carefully to what is said.

Appraisal is not just about achievement within your job role or how many sales you may have completed – that is really only half the purpose of being a stylist (although an important one for the business!). It is also about your development as an individual. It opens up many areas of discussion between a manager and an employee, including future plans. It should highlight how well you as an individual are coping within your job role, whether the salon is asking too much of you, and provides you with an opportunity to offer your opinions on improvement. Appraisal should be viewed as a two-way discussion, not simply a reprimand for poor performance at work!

An appraisal or team review should happen regularly, perhaps once a month, or every three months.

- It should be held at a mutually agreed time.
- It should be constructive and open, not conducted in fear of job loss.
- It should be objective and as non-personal as possible.
- It should be a review for both parties, not simply a judgement of the employee's performance.
- It should be constructive and positive.
- It should leave the employee feeling enthusiastic, not depressed.

> **Reality check!**
>
> You should view performance appraisals as a positive way of learning and progressing in personal growth and maintaining good working relationships.

Self-appraisal – taking opportunities to review and target set

Self-assessment form for appraisal Strands

Salon:

Date:

Position held:

Hair stylist:

Please add comments on how you feel you are progressing in each area listed

Appearance:

Absences:

Time keeping:

Job performance:

Sales:

Strengths:

Weaknesses:

Any areas of change:

Staff development request:

Action plan for next review:

A self-appraisal form

Check it out

- Look at Masako Miyazaki's self-appraisal form.
- What do you think she is hoping to achieve from the appraisal?
- What strengths and weaknesses has she identified?
- Analyse your own performance by copying and completing the blank self-assessment form.

Self-assessment form for appraisal Strands

Salon: Strands

Date: July 2003

Name: Masako Miyazaki

Position held: Senior stylist

Please add comments on how you feel you are progressing in each area listed

Appearance:
Good, I try to look professional every day.

Absences:
Could be better, as unfortunately I had a week off with flu last month. I haven't had any time off this month.

Time keeping:
Could be better, as I have been late five times this month.

Job performance:
Good, I feel my regular clients always ask for me, and I have worked hard this month.

Sales:
Good, as above, my sales are from my regulars.

Strengths:
I am confident with my treatments and I especially enjoy trying new styles.

Weaknesses:
Time keeping, I have missed my bus quite a lot in the mornings.

Any areas of change:
I have been helping to cover for Jane who has been off ill this month.

Staff development request:
I would like to go on a fashion colouring course if possible, as many clients are booking in for partial colours.

Action plan for next review:
To improve on time keeping and to do my course.

A self-appraisal form used to review and target set

A self-appraisal form includes whatever the employer/manager feels is relevant to the job role.

When identifying strengths and weaknesses try to be honest with yourself. Do not focus only on your bad points – be constructive. Look at Masako Miyazaki's self-appraisal form – she balances negative with positive comments. You should have an equal balance of strengths and weaknesses

Seeking guidance when instructions are unclear

If you have been asked to perform a specific task but are unsure what you have to do, it is important to find out more information from the relevant person to make the instructions clearer. You should, in the first instance, ask the person who gave you the task to do to clarify the instructions so that you fully understand what is expected of you. Only when you have a clear understanding of the task can you carry this out to the highest standard. Do not be afraid to ask – your colleagues would rather you ask than make a mistake!

Seeking feedback on your performance

To help develop your skills, you need to identify your strengths and weaknesses. Nobody expects you to become an instant expert – you will gain more knowledge and experience over time in the salon. However, you should make sure that all the skills and knowledge you have are up to date. Regular training, reading trade journals and attending trade shows and exhibitions will help you to do this. Be enthusiastic to learn new skills and regard it as a challenge rather then a chore.

A self-appraisal form enables you to identify your strengths and weaknesses and from this you may set short-term and long-term personal targets. A joint review of your performance with your manager, assessor or tutor, should then identify whether your personal targets are realistic and achievable using the SMART formula (see below).

Short-term goals are easier to measure and judge than long-term goals. Achieving these will encourage you to improve further. A short-term goal for the stylist Masako, for example, is to complete a fashion colouring course and gain her certificate. This is rewarding and achievable. A series of short-term goals can also help you achieve a long-term goal.

Long-term goals are not so easy to measure and may be harder to keep in view. They require much more dedication to achieve. A long-term goal for Masako may be to gain two more years salon experience then apply for a job as a stylist on an ocean liner.

Case study: Masako's performance appraisal

Using the SMART theory for Masako's performance appraisal will help her and her manager/assessor decide how best to help Masako achieve her targets. The main problem seems to be her late arrival in the salon on some mornings and it is good that Masako has identified this as a weakness – especially if she is relying on the good-will of her colleagues to prepare her clients for her when she is late.

Specific – Is her target specific? Yes, but she needs to identify how she intends to tackle her poor time keeping.

Measurable – She must aim to improve her time keeping by 100 per cent, that is, she must not be late at all (only in exceptional circumstances)!

Achievable – Do not aim for something that cannot be realised. Masako should be able to improve her time keeping. She could also have a short-term target to double her retail sales for the next month.

Remember
Short-term goals are like the carrot dangling on the stick! They provide incentive and reward.

SELF APPRAISAL

The purpose of this Self-Appraisal Form is to help you reflect on your job performance and prepare for a performance appraisal interview. Use this form as a basis for key points you may wish to raise with your manager during the interview.

Remember, the three main objectives of an appraisal interview are to:
> *1. Assess past achievements/failures*
> *2. Consider the need for further training/development*
> *3. Specify way in which future performance can be improved*

1.   What parts of your job do you consider you have performed well?

   I am confident with most treatments, however,
   I still find colouring hard and sometimes need
   help with layered cuts

2.   What parts of your job do you feel you could have performed better?

   I don't feel I'm very good at reception duties
   as I'm not very confident when making
   appointments.

3.   Comment on your overall level of job satisfaction.

   I really enjoy my job and like assisting the other
   members of the team. Thursday is the best day as this
   is my 'training evening'.

4.   Indicate aspects of your work you particularly like/dislike.

   I really like putting long hair up. I dislike setting
   as I find it difficult to fit the rollers in.

5.   What factors, if any, have made your work difficult to perform?

   My confidence level. I need more practice with
   cutting and colouring. Perhaps a cutting/colouring
   course would help. More guidance needed on
   reception duties.

A performance appraisal form

Realistic – Is Masako's aim to improve her time keeping realistic? Masako lives some distance from the salon in a rural area where there is only limited public transport. She does not own a car. The bus service runs every hour on the hour, so if Masako misses the 8am bus she cannot get to the salon in time. Masako needs to make more of an effort to catch the 8am bus. If she is prepared to do this then her aim is realistic.

Timed – Masako should aim to improve her time keeping over the next month when her self-assessment and review will be ready to be done again. This will help her to gauge how well she is doing.

Now Masako has analysed the problem, she needs to find ways to help her achieve her aim. These could involve any of the following:

- set her alarm clock to go off half an hour earlier on working days
- ask if another member of staff (or friend or neighbour working nearby) could offer her a car share, perhaps splitting the petrol costs
- learn to drive so she is no longer reliant on public transport
- change the appointment booking-in system at the salon, so that she starts at 9.30am when she can realistically get to work and then either finish half an hour later or have only a short break for lunch
- cycle to work and get fit at the same time!

> **Check it out**
>
> - Look at the self-assessment appraisal form that you completed earlier.
> - How would you tackle your weaknesses?
> - What short-term and long-term targets could you set to develop your strengths?

Asking colleagues for help

Some people find it hard to ask others for help, however, in hairdressing you must be able to ask your colleagues for help for many different reasons. When you are training it is really important to be able to ask your colleagues to help you learn if you are finding certain tasks difficult. Remember – even the most famous hairdressers were trainees once and had to learn what you are learning. Some of you will find some parts of your hairdressing qualification harder than others, but practice makes perfect, and if at first you do not succeed, try and try again (and if you still find it hard – ask for help!).

Making and taking opportunities to learn

You may need to seek help from the relevant person in your salon if you are unable to obtain learning opportunities relating to your work. This will probably be your salon owner or manager as only he or she will be able to help give you the opportunity to learn if there is any cost involved. You may, however, be able to shadow another more experienced member of the team, which should provide you with a learning opportunity. Observing a talented stylist can help you to learn techniques and different methods of working. You must take every opportunity to learn, as it is very easy to sit back and think you know enough, but in our ever-changing industry there is always something new to learn!

> **Remember**
>
> Do not become a 'stuck in a rut' hairdresser – be the best you can be. It only takes a little effort to be creative and your career will be much more enjoyable.

Reviewing developments in hairdressing regularly and keeping your skills up to date

Hairdressing is a rapidly changing industry. If you wish to be a part of a busy salon that offers the latest trends and services, you will need to regularly update your skills by attending workshops and courses in cutting, colouring, and so on. Various companies and suppliers, such as Wella or L'Oreal, run such courses.

You should also purchase and read trade journals. These will give you the latest information and often include step-by-step photos of new techniques. At work, you should set aside time to discuss new products that may be coming on to the market with manufacturers' representatives who may call at your salon.

You need to be aware of what is happening in the industry to enable you to offer the best and most current services to your clients. For example, if a client came into your salon with the latest copy of a fashion magazine and asked you to reproduce one of the hairstyles shown inside but you did not have the expertise to carry out this service, how would you feel? What image would you be portraying of the salon? Would the client have confidence in you and come back? Self-development and training are important to make sure you do not become stale or lose interest or clients by poor product knowledge or skills.

Agreeing and reviewing targets regularly to develop your future personal development plan

Linked into the appraisal system of monitoring performance is the setting of targets for an action plan to improve performance at work. Here are some **SMART** guidelines to help you:

Specific – have particular aims in mind rather than too grand an idea. Set a goal specific to you, for example, 'I want to complete two assessments each week.'

Measurable – make sure you are able to measure your aims with a start and a finish. Assessments can be measured against the NVQ performance criteria and ranges. You must know where you are now and where you want to be. For example, product sales might be on average £50 per day and a ten per cent increase would take that to £55 per day.

Achievable – aim for something that can be realised. You could have a short-term target, for example, to complete an NVQ unit by a certain date.

Realistic – be sensible in your aims, for example, doing ten cuts per hour is not realistic. How long would it take you to cover all the performance criteria and ranges in one unit?

Timed – you should set a timescale in which to achieve your target, for example, 'By next month I will improve my timekeeping by 50 per cent,' or, 'By Christmas I am going to have my portfolio for Unit G1 ready to be signed off by my assessor.'

How often you decide to review your set targets is up to you and your salon, but short-term targets are usually easier to manage.

You are in control of your own destiny. If you regularly review how you are doing at work you will be more focused on achieving set targets. Do not let opportunities pass you by because you are too lazy to have a development plan for your future.

Work effectively as part of a team

G8.2

Creating and maintaining good working relationships with your colleagues involves developing a variety of personal skills, including those of a good communicator, so that you can play your part in creating a happy and harmonious working environment.

What you will learn
• Agreeing, working together and achieving objectives
• How to be an effective team member
• Politely asking for help and information
• Responding to requests willingly and politely
• Anticipating the needs of others and offering prompt assistance
• Making effective use of your working day
• Reporting problems to the relevant person
• Resolving problems with colleagues effectively
• Being friendly, helpful and respectful to your colleagues

Agreeing, working together and achieving objectives

Every salon will have its own working philosophy. Generally this will be to anticipate and fulfil clients' needs within a healthy and happy salon environment thereby promoting a thriving business. In order to achieve your salon's objectives, you and your colleagues need to agree ways of working together in the salon towards a common goal. A salon team will always be made up of people with different strengths and weaknesses and it is important to make full use of everyone's strengths and try to improve the weaknesses. A team will also be made up of different personalities and it is important for everyone to get on when working together as part of a team. The team will only be effective if everyone feels they are working equally and resentment will build up if some team members are not working as hard as others. Make sure you are an effective team member by working as hard as you can. Regular team meetings (ideally weekly) will help to maintain a good working relationship, as any problems can be sorted out in a business-like forum.

How to be an effective team member

On joining a salon you will become part of a team and will be expected to work with other team members – your colleagues – to ensure the smooth running of the salon.

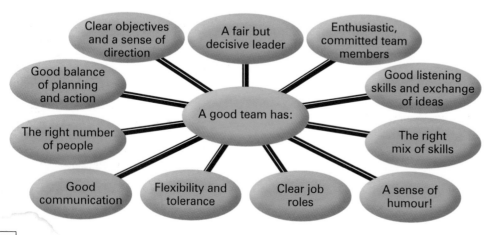

Qualities a good team should have

The pie chart opposite shows how we see one another, in other words, what we are judged upon. If we act irresponsibly, it may affect the whole team.

Team spirit can be lost:
- if one member of the group works on his or her own, that is, not as part of the team
- if there is a breakdown in communications
- if team member(s) are unwilling to be flexible and tolerant of others' mistakes
- when there is too much work for too few people
- when job roles become blurred and people encroach upon areas they should not.

As a team member, it is your responsibility to know:
- who all the staff are in the salon
- who is responsible for what
- who to go to for information and support.

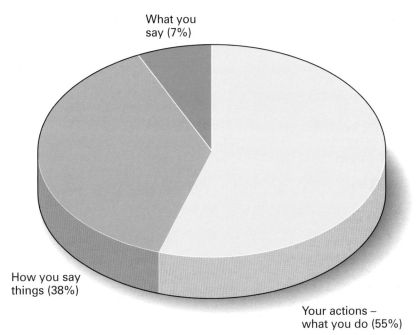

How we judge other people and how they judge us

What you say (7%)

How you say things (38%)

Your actions – what you do (55%)

Politely asking for help and information

Good communication between colleagues builds good relationships that will be reflected in the smooth running of the salon.

In the salon

You have been working for four hours without a break and are looking forward to finishing your next client because then you will have the time to stop for a drink. When the client arrives you discover that she is expecting a cut and blow-dry – she was wrongly booked in for a trim – so you will not get that break after all. You see that another member of staff is free. If she would shampoo for you then you would have a chance to make a drink.

- Do you sit the client at the washbasin, hope your colleague sees her and offers to shampoo her hair?
- Do you say to your colleague, 'Michelle, would you mind shampooing my next client for me so I can make myself a quick drink'?
- Give reasons for your answer.

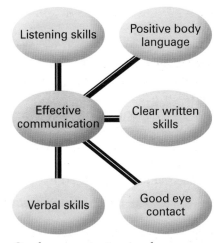

Good communication involves many skills

Listening skills

Positive body language

Effective communication

Clear written skills

Verbal skills

Good eye contact

Unless your colleague is telepathic or highly perceptive he or she will not necessarily know that you need a drink. You should be able to ask for assistance when necessary and perhaps next time Michelle needs assistance you can return the favour.

If you need help or information, you should ask for it – politely. Stating why you require assistance will explain to other members of staff how they are helping you. Being polite and professional at all times will promote team spirit.

Remember
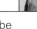

Treat others as you wish to be treated.

Remember

Never attempt to do a job that you have not been trained to do.

Responding to requests willingly and politely

When a colleague asks for your help you should respond willingly and politely to the request. If you do not, you will not be working as an effective team member and will not pass this unit of your qualification. How your colleagues perceive you at work is very important to your working professional life. You should always want to be known as a polite and willing trainee, and if you are not, you will not last very long in this industry. Salon owners, managers and other members of staff do not have to put up with grumpy, rude trainees.

Anticipating the needs of others and offering prompt assistance

When you can see that your colleagues need your assistance it is up to you to offer help and to know whether you are capable of doing that particular job. In order to anticipate the needs of other members of your team, you need to understand your job role and responsibilities within the salon. Once you have worked in the salon for a while you will get to know when certain colleagues' need your help. At first they may need to ask you for help, but you will soon learn when you are needed and this will allow you to anticipate your colleagues' needs and offer your assistance. When you know a colleague needs help it is important to stop the job you are doing (if possible) and give immediate assistance. Try to prioritise the jobs you are responsible for so that you can be as effective as possible in the salon and to all members of your team.

Being capable and competent means doing a job as well as you have been trained to do. Do not attempt to bluff your way through a job – this could put a client or colleague at risk.

Being responsible for your actions involves taking responsibility for any mistakes you may make and taking the appropriate action to minimise any further damage.

Making effective use of your working day

In a busy salon you will be asked or instructed to carry out many different services. Your job list may contain a number of items and instructions may be fired at you in quick succession. Don't panic! Here are some guidelines to help you.

- Make a list of the jobs you have been asked to do.
- Check with the relevant person that you have written them all down.
- Ask which ones are priorities, i.e. which ones need to be done first.
- Tick off the jobs/services as you carry them out.
- If you are unsure of any of the tasks that you are expected to carry out, confirm with another member of the team before you begin.
- If a list has been left for you and you cannot understand the writing, ask a colleague to have a look.

Reality check!	

Always make sure you understand what is being asked of you – the ability to listen carefully is an important skill. Show that you understand by nodding your head, for example, or if you do not know or understand something, do not guess – ask!

Remember	

Never try to cover up mistakes – this will only make things worse.

Remember	

Never carry out a task if you are unsure. Always check with a colleague who has more experience or is in authority so that you get it right.

In the salon	

1 Your manager leaves you a list of jobs to do while she is away on holiday. You are not sure whether any of the jobs require immediate attention or if they are of equal importance. Who would you refer to?
2 The manager is out of the salon and you need to clarify an issue straightaway. Who would you refer to?

In the salon

Scenario A

A colleague asks you to start an application of a full head bleach and you agree to do so. You have mixed the product and are halfway through the application when the stylist tells you that you have used too weak a strength of hydrogen peroxide and, as a result, the hair will not lift quickly enough. She is going to have to re-mix the product and start the application again. As she will have to use two lots of product but can only charge the client for one, you will have to foot the bill for the first wrong application.

- In your group, discuss how this situation might have been avoided.

Scenario B

A colleague asks you to phone a supplier and order some stock. When the stock arrives you find that you have ordered too much. The company will not take back the extra stock and the salon owner is not very happy because she will have to pay for stock that she does not want.

- In your group, discuss how this situation might have been avoided. Think about the limits of your responsibility.

Scenario C

You cut a teenager's hair. At the end of the service she tells you that her mum is going to come in later to pay. You allow the client to go and the mother never comes into the salon with the money. Your manager is upset because you have cost the salon money and tells you it will be deducted from your wages!

- In your group, discuss the limits of your authority in this situation.

Check it out

Write a list of your responsibilities in your current working role. Do you have the authority to carry out these tasks? If in doubt about your responsibilities, who would you ask for confirmation? (Helpful hint: if you have a job contract, this should contain a job description.)

Remember

The more skills you have to offer as a stylist, the more employable you are.

Reporting problems to the relevant person

There is always a hierarchy within a salon and it is important for you to know the correct channels to go through when you experience a problem. This means you need to know **who** you should approach with a particular sort of problem. For example, if it is a problem concerning work schedules, you may need to contact the salon manager to help you resolve the situation. However, if you have a wages problem, you may need to speak to your salon owner who holds the purse strings. You should find out who does what in your salon so that you know who to approach with different problems. If you approach the wrong person with a problem, it could make the problem even worse.

Imagine the following scenario: an angry client comes into the salon complaining that the perm you carried out over a month ago has dropped and she has an uneven curl result. She demands her money back. It is not within the limits of your authority to do this, so here are some guidelines to help you handle this difficult situation.

- Be sympathetic and listen carefully to the client.
- Ask her politely to take a seat while you find someone in authority to speak to her.
- Inform your employer or the most senior member of staff that you have a client at reception who would like to discuss her last perm as there seems to be a problem. You should then explain the situation in as much detail as possible so your superior is able to talk knowledgeably to the client.

- You should be present at the following discussion so that you can see what the exact problem is and how the problem is dealt with. Only offer input to the conversation if asked.

Here are some of things you should not do.

- Do not get angry with the client.
- Do not be rude and tell her that nothing is wrong with her hair.
- Do not lie and say there is nobody who can deal with her and ask her to come back on your day off!

In another situation, a regular client comes into the salon for a treatment without an appointment. You should never make a client feel unwelcome and should try to be as accommodating as possible. If it really is not possible to fit the person in at that time, make an appointment. This also applies to a client who is late for an appointment or where a stylist has been over-booked. Re-scheduling appointments can work both ways. It might be as a result of staff sickness – clients may have to be juggled into other time slots. If you always deal with clients in an open, genuinely apologetic manner, most will be flexible!

When a client changes a booking, again be flexible. If time permits and the client's needs can be accommodated, then do so. The receptionist will need to be made aware, so that the time slot isn't double-booked. Flexibility is the way to encourage new and repeat business.

Resolving problems with colleagues effectively

If you have a problem with another member of the team, it is important to approach that person first. You should think carefully about what you are going to say and make sure your timing and the situation are appropriate. For example, wait until you are alone with your colleague and go somewhere where you are out of earshot of the rest of the salon. Be mature in your approach and never start shouting. Say what you need to say calmly and this should help you to resolve the situation. Listen to your colleague's point of view as well and try to get a 'win, win' situation by resolving the problem so that you can continue to work with each other without bad feeling. If you feel you cannot deal with the situation, you may need to involve your salon manager.

Being friendly, helpful and respectful to your colleagues

Working in a commercial salon is different from working in a college or training institution. You will, however be expected to work sensibly, responsibly and as part of a team at work and at college. There will be many instances where a colleague may require your help. This does not mean that your colleague is failing to do his or her job properly. It might be because:

- a treatment/service took longer then anticipated
- a client may have been a few minutes late and, as a result, affected the stylist's timing
- a chemical process may have processed more quickly or slowly than anticipated
- a stylist has been inadvertently double-booked and has two clients at the same time.

Any one of these factors could contribute to a colleague needing your assistance. Here are some ways you could offer to help:

- shampoo a waiting client
- make the client a drink so that the stylist does not have to stop to do this and will then be able to begin the service straightaway
- rinse a colour or perm if it had processed more quickly than first thought
- take one of your colleague's clients if the client is agreeable.

Being part of a team means that if you are asked for assistance, you give your help willingly and courteously (politely). By being fully aware of what is happening in your working environment you will be able to anticipate your colleagues' needs. You should aim to offer assistance before being asked for it. This is called using your initiative i.e. taking the first step or action without being prompted to do so.

If a job needs doing, carry it out without being asked. This will prove to your employer that you can be relied upon to work effectively and practically at all times.

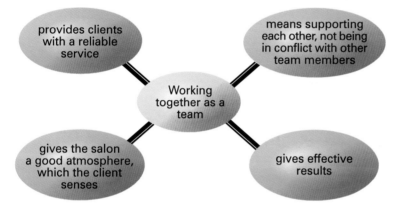

The importance of working as a team

When you leave college or a training institution, you will be the newest, least experienced member of staff. It may take time to build up a regular column of clients and, as a result, you may be the person who has the most free time to be called upon. When you build up a client base and you are busy, the team will recognise this and somebody else will do the job.

When working under the guidance of a colleague, you should:

- accept that your colleague is in charge
- take instructions and act upon them
- communicate effectively
- take responsibility for your job role and do it to the very best of your ability.

In the salon

You have been already been asked several times today to wash up the tea and coffee cups used by both staff and clients. Your supervisor has just asked you to wash up yet again! You think that it is time someone else did this chore.

- Do you moan to your supervisor and say someone else should take a turn?
- Do you willingly get on with the washing up without grumbling?
- State your reasons for your answer.

practical SKILLS

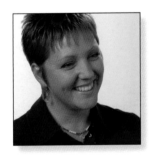 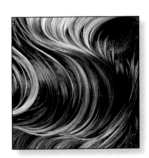 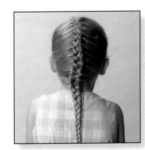

Shampoo and condition hair and scalp

Unit H9

Shampooing and conditioning are an essential part of most hairdressing treatments. In order to make hair more manageable for blow-drying, setting, cutting, perming, relaxing and some colouring processes, the hair must be thoroughly cleansed of all dirt, natural grease and products such as hairspray, mousse and wax. (If you need to refresh your memory, revisit 'Facts about hair and skin'). If any of these are left on the hair before further treatments, such as perming, they will cause a barrier between the hair and the chemical and the perm will be unsuccessful. It is very important to be able to analyse your client's hair and scalp type correctly in order to choose the appropriate products to suit the client's needs – every head is individual and will be slightly different. If you use the wrong shampoo, conditioner or scalp treatment, you can create problems for your client. For example, if you used a shampoo containing oil (coconut oil shampoo) for a greasy hair and scalp, you will just add to your client's grease problem.

A good shampooing technique has the added bonus of relaxing the client – as you massage the shampoo throughout the hair and scalp, you sooth the nerve endings and muscles within the scalp. If clients require a more intensive massage, a deep penetrating conditioning treatment will also help to improve the internal structure of the hair.

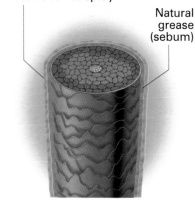

Styling products such as mousse and hairspray

Natural grease (sebum)

A hair shaft before shampooing

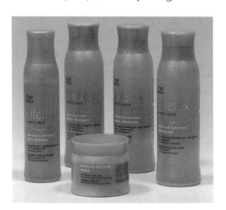

A range of shampoo and conditioning products

What you will learn 
• Maintain effective and safe methods of working when shampooing and conditioning hair H9.1
• Shampoo hair and scalp H9.2
• Condition hair and scalp H9.3

Maintain effective and safe methods of working when shampooing and conditioning hair

H9.1

As shampooing and conditioning are the first hairdressing services you will carry out, it is important that you understand your salon's rules and regulations on health and safety. You need to follow these rules to ensure the wellbeing of yourself and your client. This is the first step towards becoming a professional stylist, as the standards set by qualified staff should ensure that the quality of all services are maintained at a high level.

What you will learn
• Carrying out a consultation and choosing suitable products
• Preparing and positioning the client for a shampoo and conditioning treatment
• Health and safety issues
• Replenishing low levels of resources
• Re-ordering products
• Completing client record cards after shampooing and conditioning

Carrying out a consultation and choosing suitable products

Once you have gowned the client, you should carry out a thorough consultation to assess your client's needs, choose and organise appropriate products and equipment, and think through and plan the treatment.

During the consultation for a shampoo and/or conditioning treatment, you should assess:

- hair condition – is it normal, dry, damaged or frizzy? Does it need moisture adding? Does it snap when you test its elasticity? How does the cuticle region feel?
- scalp condition – is it dry, normal, greasy or dandruff affected? Also ask your client if he or she is experiencing any scalp-related problems at the moment.
- hair type – is it Asian hair, African Caribbean hair or European/Caucasian?
- hair texture – is the hair fine, medium or coarse?
- previous chemical treatments – you must ask your client if you are unsure what is already on the hair and check:
  - for any contraindications. Refer to 'Facts about hair and skin' to refresh your memory
  - purpose of treatment (prior to a perm, for example)
  - subsequent treatments.

You will then have the information to enable you to:

- choose products to suit the client
- organise your working area with all necessary products and equipment for the treatment (for example, steamer to aid penetration of intensive conditioning treatments)
- discuss the treatment plan with the client
- start a record card
- begin the treatment.

Preparing and positioning the client for a shampoo and conditioning treatment

The client should be protected with a gown, towel around the shoulders, and a disposable plastic shoulder cape, secured by a sectioning clip. It is important not to place the sectioning clip too high under the client's chin or it will become uncomfortable if the client bends his or her head forward. The plastic shoulder cape will protect the client's clothing. It is very important to position your client correctly at the basin to ensure a watertight seal around the neck. Your client should be seated comfortably in the backwash basin chair. You should guide your client back by supporting his or her shoulders. Position the client's neck correctly by making sure there are no gaps between the neck and the edge of the basin. If there are, your client will most certainly get wet! It is an important point to make sure your client is positioned correctly before turning the water on.

Health and safety issues

Manufacturer's instructions

Before using any shampooing or conditioning product, you must read the manufacturer's instructions. These give you the information to use the product properly (as intended) and will result in the treatment being as successful as possible.

Remember

G5.2 covers generic consultation very thoroughly. If you need to refresh your memory on consultation techniques, refer to page 83.

Reality check!

It is frustrating to choose a product that suits the client's needs, only to find the last of the product has been used and not replaced or re-ordered. You must always follow your salon's rules for stock control so that this does not happen.

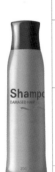

Shampoo
Damaged Hair

Effect
Damaged hair is thoroughly nourished, gently cleansed and repaired. Hair is easier to comb too.

Application
Apply a small amount to damp hair and distribute evenly. Massage gently into a lather. Rinse thoroughly and repeat if necessary.

250 ml

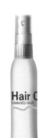

Conditioner
Damaged Hair

Effect
Penetrating deeply into the damaged hair, the nutrient complex rebuilds hair from within, leaving it easier to comb.

Application
Distribute sufficient product evenly through towel-dried hair and gently massage. Leave for 1–3 minutes. Rinse thoroughly.

250 ml

Hair Oil
Damaged Hair

Effect
This highly effective formula penetrates deep into the hair structure. Regenerates and seals damaged hair shafts and ends, helping to prevent further damage.

Application
Depending on length and amount of hair, distribute and work in at least 5 pump depressions to dry hair. Do no rinse out.

50 ml

Reality check!

If you do not follow the manufacturer's instructions when using a product and a problem results, the manufacturer will take no responsibility. The responsibility falls on you, as the stylist, to use a product exactly as instructed. Failure to do so might be considered as negligent.

Shine Polisher
Damaged Hair

Effect
The ideal preparation before styling. This highly effective complex strengthens damaged hair from within, restoring stability and shine.

Application
Apply a small amount to the palms of the hands and work into dry hair.

150 ml

Intensive Mask
Damaged Hair

Effect
Intensive, long-lasting nourishment. Repairs and cares for damaged hair, sealing the hair's structure to help protect against further damage.

Application
Apply sufficient product and distribute evenly through towel-dried hair and gently massage. Comb through and leave for approximately 5–10 minutes. Rinse thoroughly.

150 ml

Always follow manufacturer's instructions

Water safety

It is essential that clients' safety is a priority during their time in the salon. When shampooing and conditioning, you are using water and possibly electrical equipment (such as a steamer), both of which can cause serious accidents if health and safety rules are not followed.

Workplace environment

Standard health and safety rules to follow

- The salon must always be kept clean and tidy.
- Any spillage of water or product on the floor is a potential hazard and should be wiped up immediately.
- Your work area should be kept clean and tidy throughout the service and any waste should be removed immediately after shampooing and conditioning.
- Always make client comfort an important issue and position your client carefully at the basin before you begin shampooing.
- You should position yourself to ensure good posture whilst working to avoid discomfort and the risk of injury.
- Any shampooing or conditioning product entering the eye should be flushed immediately with clean water and first-aid attention sought.
- A client suffering from an infection or infestation must not be treated in the salon, as the problem is likely to cause a cross-infection to other clients, colleagues and yourself.

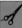

In the salon

Sobia is the new apprentice at Eclipse Hair Salon. Pepe, a junior stylist, has asked her to shampoo a client. Although Sobia has been shampooing for a couple of weeks, she is still training. She begins to apply water to the hair when she notices tiny things crawling on the top of the client's head. She is unsure what to do, so she excuses herself from the client to seek advice from Pepe. He immediately realises that the client has head lice so no further treatment can take place that day. He tactfully and discretely informs the client (who now has wet hair) of the situation and recommends that she visit a pharmacist to obtain a suitable treatment to kill the parasites.

In your group, discuss the following:

- How could this situation have been avoided?
- Some equipment has already come into contact with the client. What action should be taken to prevent cross-infection of the infestation to other clients and staff?

Control of Substances Hazardous to Health Regulations 2003

The Control of Substances Hazardous to Health Regulations – commonly known as COSHH – require employers to control exposure to hazardous substances in the workplace. Most of the products used in the salon are perfectly safe, but some products could become hazardous under certain conditions or if used inappropriately. For example, hairspray is a potentially explosive gas and will explode with force if placed in heat (such as a fire or even on top of a hot radiator). All salon employees should be aware of how to use, store and dispose of products through staff training sessions (see Unit G1 for more information on health and safety in the salon).

Electricity at Work Regulations 1992

The Electricity at Work Regulations are concerned with general safety when using electricity. In a hairdressing salon, they are particularly concerned with the use and maintenance of electrical equipment. All electrical equipment must be checked regularly for electrical safety by a competent person (not necessarily a qualified electrician but someone who must be capable of attending to basic safety checks). In a busy salon this may be every six months. If electrical equipment is found to be faulty, it must be withdrawn from service and repaired.

Your own safety

As mentioned in the Workplace Environment section, it is important to work throughout the day maintaining correct posture. You should try to keep your back as straight as possible when working and if you need to bend, always bend your knees and not your back. Another occupational hazard is dermatitis. This is a skin condition usually found on the hands, which is irritated by the constant use of water and hairdressing products. Always dry your hands thoroughly after shampooing and regularly protect your skin by using a barrier cream to help prevent any dryness from occurring.

Replenishing low levels of resources

In order to minimise any disruption to your client's treatment and your treatment plan, always replenish resources, such as cleanly laundered towels and gowns, regularly throughout the day.

Reality check!

When conditioning hair you may need to use electrical equipment to aid the treatment. Always dry your hands before plugging in electrical equipment and make sure you have made any necessary safety checks for frayed wires. Never use equipment you have not been trained to use.

Around a thousand electric shock accidents at work are reported to the Health and Safety Executive each year.

Re-ordering products

If you use the last of a shampoo, conditioner or scalp treatment (product or equipment) during a treatment, you should make sure that the item is replaced. If you run out of the only product suitable for your client's needs, you will be unable to provide the client with an effective treatment.

You may not be responsible for the re-ordering of products and equipment, so make sure you know the system to follow and use it to ensure you are not the one causing an 'out-of-stock problem'.

Completing client record cards after shampooing and conditioning

It is important to record all treatment details, even for shampooing and conditioning, for future reference. This is because you are unlikely to remember which products you used on the client's previous visit to the salon. Unless you have a record of the conditioning treatment used last time, you cannot evaluate if it was successful or whether you need to change to another product.

Before shampooing and conditioning

Gown client appropriately.
Carry out a thorough consultation.
Follow your salon's health and safety rules and regulations.
Know the salon's shampooing and conditioning products and what they are able to do to the hair.
Choose appropriate products to achieve client's requirements and optimum condition.

Client Record Card

Name: Jasmine

Address:

Post Code: .... Telephone: ....

Date	Treatment/Product/Perm Colour/Condition etc	Application/Rod size/Timing/Result	Student
25 April	Deep conditioning treatment	Good result	Alice

Client Record Card

Name: Jasmine Hubert

Address: 123, Russell Street
Fareham

Post Code: PO12 6JS Telephone: 936221

Date	Treatment/Product/Perm Colour/Condition etc	Application/Rod size/Timing/Result	Student
25/4/03	Deep conditioning treatment: Clynol Corregin 1·4 shampoo → Corregin 2·4 condition → Corregin 3·4 scalp tonic	shampooed twice massaged for 10 mins + under steamer for 10 mins applied to towel dried hair + left in Successful result - hair felt smooth + shiny Recommended a course of 6 treatments over next 6 weeks.	Alice Anderson

Compare these record cards for the same client. The client says she found the conditioning treatment she had last time to be very beneficial. Which card would you prefer to use?

Shampoo hair and scalp

H9.2

Shampooing is a very important and beneficial part of a hairdressing treatment. It is an essential start to many other treatments as it removes general dirt, natural grease, and any styling and finishing products that your client may have used such as mousse, wax and hairspray. It is probably one of the first treatments you will learn. It can take some time to perfect as there are many things to consider all at the same time, such as trying to keep the client's face and clothing dry, using the correct products, performing a good massage, and also learning how to handle the hair!

It is important to use the correct shampoo for the client's hair and scalp condition. You will need to learn which shampoos are suitable for specific hair and scalp conditions. Knowing the products will also enable you to give good homecare advice so that clients benefit from using the most suitable products at home. It is also important to use the correct shampoo immediately before a chemical treatment such as perming. The wrong type of shampoo may affect the perm and result in an unsuccessful curl.

The massage techniques you need to learn for this element are very important, as clients will judge the quality of their shampoo by the massage (as well as by how dry they stay!).

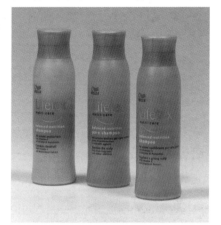

Shampoo products

What you will learn

- Preparing for shampooing
- Knowing shampoo products
- Massage techniques for shampooing
- Shampooing procedure – ensuring client comfort

Preparing for shampooing

It is important to know and follow your salon's rules for preparing the client and yourself for shampooing. You should always gown the client correctly.

Shampooing fixtures and fittings

Before beginning the shampoo, decide whether to use a frontwash basin or a backwash basin.

A frontwash basin is more suitable for:

- people who have back or neck trouble
- people too small to lean into a backwash basin, for example, children.

A backwash basin is more commonly used because:

- it prevents water and chemicals entering the client's eyes
- it is more comfortable for most clients
- the client's clothing is less likely to get wet.

Check it out

Write down all the areas you need to assess during your consultation with the client.

Remember

When using a frontwash basin always give your client a towel to protect the eyes and face from chemicals or water.

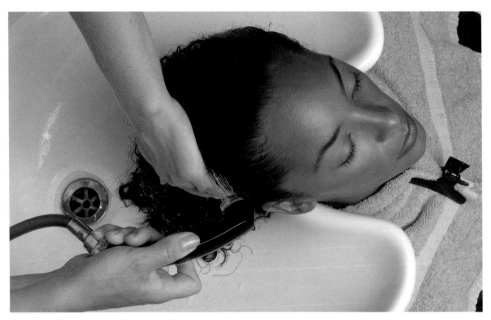

A backwash basin

Knowing shampoo products

Knowing the shampoo products in your salon is essential.

During the initial consultation with the client, you will have checked the condition of his or her hair and scalp. Generally, this will be:

- normal
- dry
- greasy
- dandruff-affected/flaky.

Check it out

List each shampoo in your salon and make a note of the following:

- its ingredients
- the hair and scalp type it should be used for
- the correct way to use it.

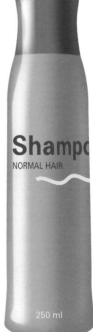

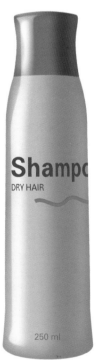

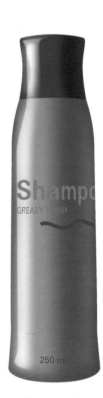

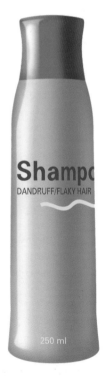

Normal hair   Dry hair   Greasy hair   Dandruff/ flaky scalp

You will then be able to choose the correct shampoo to suit the hair and scalp type. The general shampoo guide below will help you.

Shampoo	Hair/scalp type	Benefits
Coconut oil	Dry	Adds moisture
Almond oil	Dry	Adds moisture
Medicated	Dandruff	Relieves itchiness
Coal tar	Psoriasis	Releases scales; helps itchiness
Strawberry (fruit)	Normal	Cleanses
Lemon	Greasy	Removes grease
Egg and lemon	Greasy (sensitive scalp)	Removes grease; gentle on scalp
pH balanced	Damaged/after colour	Returns hair to natural pH
Protein	Damaged	Strengthens
Beer	Fine/limp	Adds body
TLS (soapless base, no additives)	All types	Pre-chemical process (e.g. before perm)
Lacquer removing/clarifying	Hair with product residue	Leaves no residue. Strips residue

General shampoo guide

The pH of a product is a measure of how acidic or how alkaline it is. A shampoo that is pH balanced will have a pH of 4.5–5.5, which is the same pH as the hair and skin. Because this pH is slightly acidic, pH-balanced products will automatically close the cuticle scales and produce shine and manageability.

Massage techniques for shampooing

The following massage techniques should be carried out using the pads of the fingers or the palms of the hands. Never use your nails as these could scratch the client's scalp and cause an infection. If the hair is long, you will need to adapt your massage movements as long hair can become tangled very easily. Remove one hand at a time if the hair lengths start to tangle. Always remember to keep contact with the scalp with at least one hand otherwise contact will be broken and the client may receive a jolt if they are very relaxed.

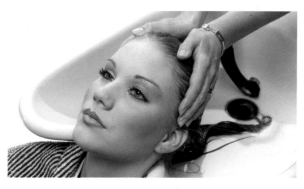

Effleurage
Using the palms of the hands:

- slow, smoothing, stroking movement
- spreads shampoo
- relaxes the client.

Effleurage massage

Remember
When you are shampooing your client's hair, you will be in very close contact. Make sure you are 'nice to be next to' by ensuring you do not have bad- or cigarette–smelling breath.

Rotary

Using the pads of the fingers:

- round, circular movements
- stimulates scalp
- removes dirt and grease.

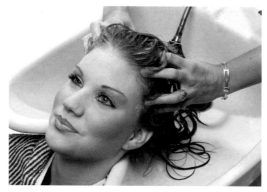

Rotary massage

Friction

Using pads of the fingers:

- lighter, quicker movements than rotary
- gently stimulates scalp.

Massage can be very beneficial to the client if it is carried out using the correct pressure. Always check with your client that the pressure you are using is comfortable, as some people's scalps are more sensitive than others.

Adapting shampoo massage techniques

There are certain circumstances when you may need to adapt your massage technique to suit your client's needs. This may be because of:

- hair length – long hair will only need rotary massage throughout the scalp. The lengths of the hair should only be massaged using effleurage as this will be effective at cleansing the hair but will not cause excessive knotting of the cuticle scales. Avoid tangling your fingers in long hair and avoid tugging the hair unnecessarily.
- hair density – hair density is a measurement of how much hair your client has per square cm. If there is a lot of hair per square cm, it may mean that you will need to use a firmer rotary massage technique in order for your client to feel any firmness of pressure.
- hair condition – hair that is very fragile, for example, highly bleached hair, should be massaged with caution as it is liable to break easily.
- scalp condition – scalps that are excessively oily should not be massaged vigorously using rotary shampoo massage movements. This will stimulate the sebaceous glands that produce our natural oil, sebum, to produce even more oil – not a good result for someone with an oil/grease problem.

Shampooing procedure

| Seat client comfortably. |

| Turn on water and test temperature before applying to client's scalp and wet hair thouroughly. |

| Apply appropriate shampoo, cost effectively, to the hair using effleurage, rotary and friction massage techniques. |

| Turn water on and check temperature before rinsing lather from first shampoo. |

| Apply second shampoo application using effleurage and continue with rotary and friction massage until hair lathers well and all the head has been covered. If hair does not lather well due to excessive build-up of product or grease, you may need to repeat with a third shampoo. |

| Turn water on and check temperature before rinsing second shampoo application thoroughly from the hair. |

| Apply a towel securely to avoid drips. |

In the salon

Mrs Ahmed is a regular client who suffers from psoriasis. During her consultation it is noticed that her psoriasis is very red and sore. On some parts of the scalp it appears to be open and weeping/bleeding. Mrs Ahmed is booked for a cut and blow-dry.

- Would you be able to shampoo Mrs Ahmed with psoriasis in this state?
- If not, what alternative service could you offer, if any?
- What advice would you give to Mrs Ahmed?

Shampooing procedure – ensuring client comfort

Step-by step shampooing procedure

Seat the client correctly at the basin and make sure he or she is comfortable. If using a backwash basin, make sure the client sits right back in the seat so that his or her neck fits the curve of the basin correctly without any gaps for the water to leak through. Make sure all the hair is in the basin.

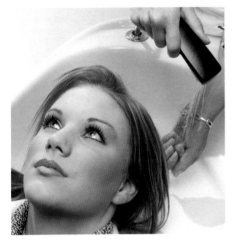

Turn on the taps and test the water temperature on the inside of your wrist before testing on the client.

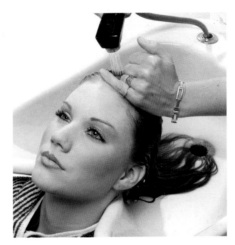

Check the temperature of the water with the client and then apply the water to thoroughly wet her hair and scalp, taking extra care around the hairline so that you don't wet her face. Turn off the water.

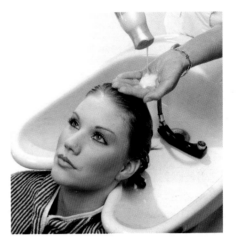

Dispense the correct amount of shampoo (about the size of a two-pence piece) into the palm of your hand and emulsify between both palms. Apply from hairline to nape of neck using effleurage massage technique.

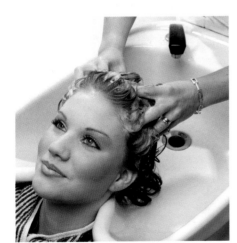

Start rotary massage technique from front hairline to nape, around side hairline and then through middle sections until the whole head has been covered. Repeat until the shampoo begins to lather.

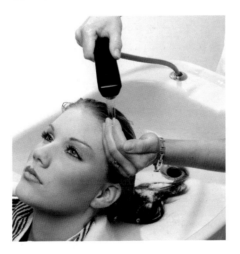

Turn water on and rinse thoroughly. Turn off the water. Repeat shampoo application and massage techniques. Turn water on and rinse until all shampoo has been removed.

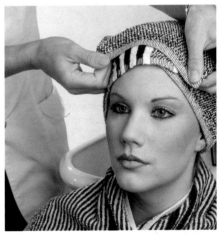

Turn off water, gently squeeze hair to remove excess water. Use a towel around the shoulders to stop any drips from the hair entering the eyes or face. The hair is now ready for the next hairdressing process.

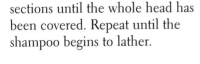

Condition hair and scalp

H9.3

Conditioning is a very beneficial part of a hairdressing treatment. It not only improves the visual appearance of the hair by making it shiny, but also improves the manageability, which aids all the other treatments. Conditioning treatments often sell themselves as clients are usually aware if their hair is out of condition and will often ask what they can do to improve its look and feel. It is your job to assess the condition of the hair and decide which sort of conditioner to use.

Conditioning products

> ### What you will learn
>
> - Preparing the hair for conditioning
> - Types of conditioning products
> - Massage techniques for conditioning
> - Conditioning procedures

Preparing the hair for conditioning

It is very important to carry out a thorough consultation before you begin to shampoo or condition the hair. This is because some conditioning treatments are carried out on dry hair (hot oil treatment, for example) and some conditioning treatment ranges include a two- or three-stage process using a shampoo, conditioner and scalp treatment, which should be used together for the best possible results. Once you have gowned the client (as for shampooing) and completed the consultation, you are ready to choose the correct products to suit the client's hair and scalp type.

Types of conditioning products

There are many different types of conditioners, but they fall into two main categories:

1 surface conditioners

2 penetrating and treatment conditioners.

Surface conditioners

Most modern surface conditioners usually come in cream form and work on the cuticle of the hair. They smooth and coat the cuticle region making the hair look shiny and manageable. They do not have the ability to go past the cuticle region and, therefore, cannot enter the cortex or re-strengthen the hair. Their function is very limited.

Where a surface conditioner is described as anti-oxy, it can also be used after chemical treatments when its function is threefold:

1 It stops the chemicals working any further (creeping oxidation).

2 It closes and smoothes the cuticle region of the hair shaft making the hair shiny.

3 It returns the hair to its natural pH value (4.4–5.5). Refer to 'Hair facts' for more information on the pH scale.

Smooths and coats cuticle scales

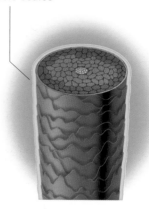

Action of surface conditioners

Types of surface conditioner include:

- hair aid or cream rinse
- herbal anti-oxy
- acid rinses, for example, lemon juice or vinegar
- pre-perm treatments – these are specifically designed to be used before perming to even out the porosity along the cuticle region of the hair to allow the perm to take evenly.

Penetrating and treatment conditioners

Penetrating conditioners work on the internal structure of the hair in the cortex because they have the ability to penetrate the cuticle region. Some have the ability to *temporarily* rebuild the bonds in the cortex region, which give the hair its strength and elasticity, and will also smooth and coat the cuticle. If the hair has become dry or chemically damaged, these conditioners will add moisture to help improve the overall look and feel of the hair.

There are two types of penetrating conditioners:

1　restructurant or protein conditioners – these will always state 'restructurant' on the packaging

2　moisturising conditioners, used to add moisture to dry hair and help scalp problems, for example, henna wax or olive oil.

If the hair is badly damaged, you may need to recommend a course of penetrating treatments, usually between six and twelve, over a period of weeks. As the treatments progress, you can analyse their effectiveness and decide if you have chosen the most appropriate one.

Scalp treatments

Treatment conditioners are usually two- or three-stage treatments involving a shampoo, conditioner and scalp treatment from a particular product range. They should be used together to provide the best possible conditioning results. Some scalp treatments claim to help regulate the production of sebum from the sebaceous glands, helping with excessive grease problems by halting the oil produced. They also claim to be successful when treating excessively dry scalp problems by helping to increase the production of oil from the sebaceous glands. You need to be familiar with the scalp treatment products in order to choose the correct product to treat your client's problem.

Dry scalps can also benefit from moisturising treatments such as hot oil treatments. Try to think of the skin on the scalp like the skin on your hands. If your hands are dry, you would use a moisturising cream. If your scalp is dry, you need to add moisture to it also.

Regular moisturising treatments will benefit a dry scalp and help to alleviate dandruff and some milder forms of psoriasis.

Massage techniques for conditioning

There are two main massage techniques used for conditioning hair. They are:

- effleurage
- petrissage.

Smoothes and coats cuticle scales and also penetrates the cortex to temporarily rebuild bands, helping improve hair strength and elasticity

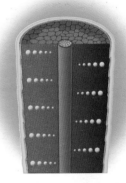

Action of penetrating conditioners

Reality check!

Always read and follow the manufacturer's instructions carefully so that the product provides the client with maximum benefit.

Remember

Always record the products used on the client's record card for future reference.

Effleurage

This is a smoothing, stroking movement, which starts and finishes the massage routine. It uses the complete palms of the hands to apply adequate pressure evenly across the whole head.

Start at the centre, front hairline and *slowly* work over the crown area towards the nape. Cover the whole head several times to ensure the client is used to your hands and the product is evenly distributed. It is important not to break contact with the scalp once the massage has started, so always keep one hand in contact with the scalp at all times. This is to ensure your client relaxes while you take the weight of his or her head in your hands – if you break contact with the head, the client may jolt his or her head back, which isn't pleasant or relaxing.

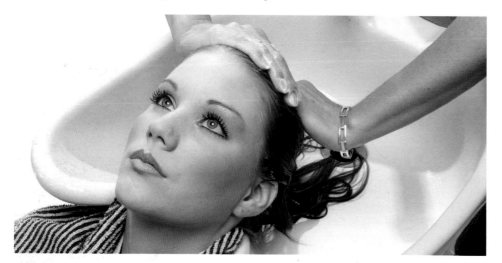

Effleurage

Petrissage

Petrissage is a deeper kneading movement, which stimulates the scalp. If carried out correctly, it stimulates:

- the sebaceous glands – to secrete sebum (the hair's natural moisture)
- the blood supply – to improve the healthy growth of the hair (it will not make hair grow faster, just keep it in better condition).

It also loosens a tight scalp by removing tension from the muscles, improves muscle tone, and ultimately relaxes the client thereby promoting a feeling of wellbeing.

When carrying out petrissage, you must use the pads of your fingers and keep your elbows out at a 90-degree angle from your body in order to produce an even amount of pressure over the whole head. Use a very slow, circular movement to pick up and knead the scalp (you will know whether you are doing this correctly if the client's scalp is moving). Start at the front hairline, knead towards the crown area and then gradually work towards the nape area. Continue massaging from the nape around the side hairlines to the temple areas and then through the centre spaces, over the occipital bone. Make sure the whole head is covered and repeat very slowly for ten minutes.

Do not massage the scalp if:

- the client feels unwell, has a temperature, or is feeling tender headed since massaging could become uncomfortable.
- the hair is greasy since massaging will only stimulate more sebum and make the problem worse.
- there are any cuts or abrasions on the scalp.
- there are any contraindications such as head lice or ringworm.

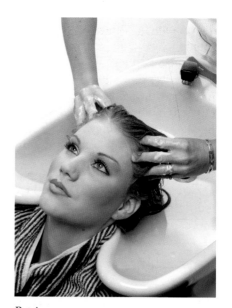

Petrissage

In the salon

While Sandra was carrying out a restructurant conditioning treatment on Mrs Barrett, Mrs Barrett fell asleep and started snoring loudly. Sandra was not sure whether to wake Mrs Barrett up or not so she decided to continue with the treatment and put her client under the steamer for ten minutes. When the time had elapsed and Sandra removed the steamer, she decided to finish the treatment with some lovely soothing effleurage massage movements. At this point, Mrs Barrett was awoken by her mobile phone ringing.

- Would you have woken Mrs Barrett if you had been the stylist?
- How can you judge if the treatment was successful?
- Discuss these points with your colleagues.

Conditioning procedures

Surface conditioners

These are applied at the basin after excess moisture is removed following shampooing. They should be applied using effleurage movements and worked through the hair thoroughly using petrissage movements and then combed through using a wide-toothed comb to make the best use of the conditioner. It is not necessary to leave the conditioner on the hair for a specified length of time, as its results are almost immediate. However, always read the manufacturer's instructions before using the product.

Penetrating and scalp treatment conditioners

These are usually applied using a bowl and brush method. This is a more cost-effective way of applying expensive products as you only dispense a small amount of product at a time and it ensures all the hair is adequately covered.

The client is protected with a gown, towel and plastic cape secured with a section clip (not too high under the chin). The hair is shampooed and towel-dried and the client seated at a workstation. The hair is then sectioned into four sections (hot-cross bun) and each section secured with a sectioning clip. On your trolley you will have prepared a tint bowl with a small amount of penetrating/treatment conditioner and a tint brush. Only dispense small amounts of conditioning product, as any excess cannot be put back into the original container because of the risk of cross contamination (your brush will have touched the client's scalp and the conditioner in the bowl).

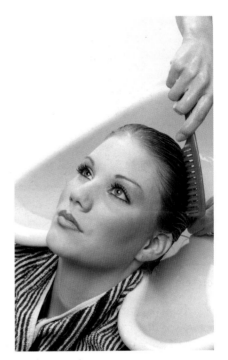

Surface conditioning

Remove a sectioning clip and apply the conditioner to a small sub-section of hair approximately 1.25 cm wide at the top of the section. Place the completed section away from the client's face and take a new section directly underneath. Continue this procedure until all the hair has been covered. You may only wish to apply to the ends of the hair or the roots, depending on the condition of the hair. When all the necessary hair has been covered, start the scalp massage routine using effleurage and petrissage as described previously.

When the scalp massage is complete, you may decide to use heat to aid the penetration of the conditioner. Heat swells the hair and raises the cuticle scales so the penetrating/conditioning treatment product penetrates into the cortex region more thoroughly. Moist heat is preferable as it is kinder to the hair.

Some scalp treatments come in tonic form and are applied to towel-dried hair directly after shampooing and conditioning. As they are the consistency of water, you must ensure your client keeps his or her head tipped as far back as possible to prevent the tonic entering the eyes, as this would be extremely painful. Once the scalp tonic has been applied to the whole scalp you are ready to continue drying the hair. Do not rinse out.

Types of heat used during conditioning

Steamer

A steamer produces moist heat through the evaporation of distilled water (tap water, especially from a hard water area, can make the steamer fur up – like a kettle). Safety checks, such as checking the water level is sufficient and checking the plug for frayed wires must be carried out before using the steamer.

Always dry your hands before plugging the steamer in to ensure the health and safety of yourself and the client.

A steamer takes a few minutes to warm up so it is best to switch it on before you start the application of the conditioner.

Hot towels

This is an alternative way to apply moist heat and especially useful if you do not have a steamer. You need at least three towels to carry out this procedure.

Step-by-step hot towel procedure

Fold towel lengthways, in half and then lengthways again. Thoroughly wet the towel with hot water at the basin. Carefully wring out the towel as much as possible (it should not be dripping with water).

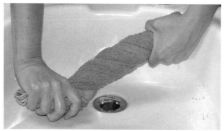

Check the temperature of the towel on your wrist before applying it to the client. As you apply the towel, ask the client if the temperature is satisfactory and, if so, wrap the towel on top of the head (the same as shampooing).

Leave the towel on the hair for approximately two minutes or until the towel has cooled (having a cold, wet towel on your head is not pleasant so remove it as soon as this happens). Remove cold towel and repeat the procedure with remaining towels.

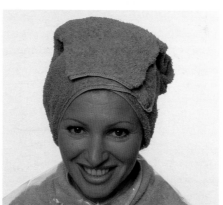

Hood dryers and accelerators

These produce dry heat, which is not always suitable to use during a conditioning treatment. If you are treating the hair because it is dry and damaged, never apply dry heat when it is not necessary. However, the manufacturer's instructions may state this is necessary to aid the penetration of the product.

Hot oil treatment

This treatment is carried out to moisturise severely dry scalps/hair. It is best to use good quality olive oil, as this is the most refined and purest oil with the most moisturising qualities.

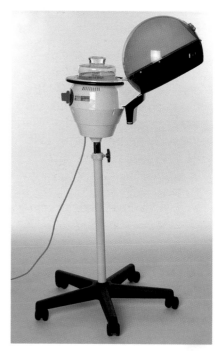

A steamer

> **Remember**
>
> Always use distilled water in a steamer.

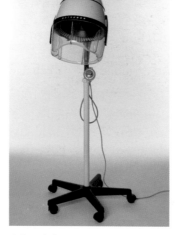

A hood dryer

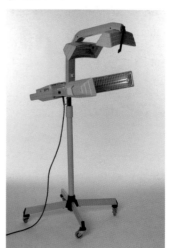

A climazone

Step-by-step hot oil treatment

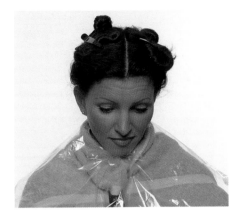

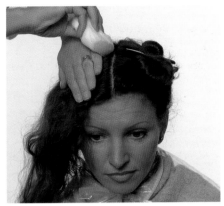

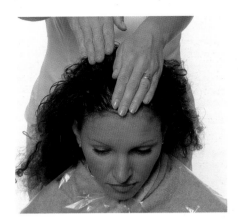

Protect the client with a gown, towel and plastic cape, divide the hair into four sections (hot-cross bun) and secure with sectioning clips.

Heat the oil by pouring it into a small plastic bowl, then place in a larger bowl filled with hot water.

Do not shampoo the hair – this procedure is carried out on dry hair. Roll a small length of cotton wool into a circular pad and test the temperature of the oil. Check the temperature with the client and apply the warm oil to the scalp/hair using the cotton wool pad (this is better than a tint brush as it makes the application of the oil less messy).

Place the completed section away from the client's face and take a new section directly underneath. Continue this procedure until all the hair has been covered.

Start the scalp massage routine using effleurage movements.

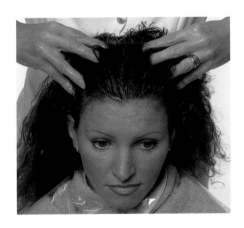

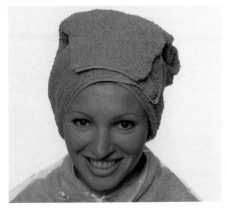

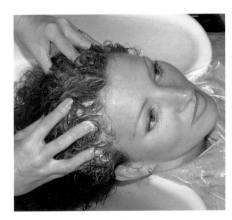

Continue massage routine using petrissage movements.

When the scalp massage is complete, you may decide to use heat to aid the penetration of the hot oil. The best moist heat to use for this treatment is the application of a few hot towels (see page 128).

Apply neat shampoo and massage using rotary movements to emulsify the oil thoroughly (until the shampoo turns white) before adding any water to the hair. Repeat shampooing process.

Your questions answered

Should I condition the hair before perming?
Not with a normal surface or penetrating conditioner on the same day as the perm. The hair could be given a conditioning treatment to improve the condition of the hair a few days before the perm. If necessary, a pre-perm treatment may be used immediately prior to perming, which would not interfere with the chemical action of the perming process.

Do restructurant conditioners improve the hair's condition?
Yes, they have an effect on the strength of the cortex but only temporarily.

Can you really stimulate the blood, sebaceous glands and nerve endings during conditioning?
Yes, if your petrissage massage movements are deep, they will stimulate these areas within the dermis of the scalp.

Are expensive shampoos and conditioners worth the money?
Expensive shampoos and conditioners often have the same ingredients as basic 'cheaper' products, but some are more costly due to extensive research and costly ingredients such as aromatherapy oils. The only way to decide if they are worth the money is to try them and come to your own conclusions.

Test your knowledge

1   What should you do to your hands after shampooing?

2   Which health and safety legislation covers the use of electrical equipment?

3   Why is it important to carry out a thorough consultation before shampooing?

4   Which health and safety legislation deals with the handling, storage and disposal of hairdressing products?

5   Why is it important to have a good knowledge of the shampooing and conditioning products used in your salon?

6   Which shampoo would you use before a perm in your salon?

7   What effect does a surface conditioner have on the hair?

8   What effect does a penetrating conditioner have on the hair?

9   Do you apply water first or neat shampoo to remove a hot oil treatment from the hair?

10   What types of heat are ideally used during conditioning treatments?

During conditioning

Apply conditioner cost effectively following manufacturer's instructions.

Start massage using effleurage technique.

Continue massage using petrissage movements for ten minutes.

Complete massage with some effleurage.

Rinse thoroughly to remove conditioner.

If using an oil conditioner, apply neat shampoo and massage before applying water.

Remove excess moisture from the hair.

Apply a towel securely to avoid drips.

Record products used, length of massage, and results of treatment on the client's record card for future reference.

Style, dress and finish hair using basic techniques

Unit H10

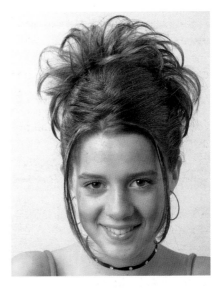

In this unit you will be looking at the different techniques that can be used to style and dress the hair. This unit is important because every stylist has to be able to present the client with a satisfactory finished result.

You will learn about the properties of the hair that enable you to manipulate and work the hair into different styles, how to blow-dry, set and dress long and short hair, and how to dress long hair to style. You will also find out about the products and tools you will be using to carry out treatments, while maintaining a high standard of health and safety as you work.

What you will learn
• Maintain effective and safe methods of working when styling hair H10.1 • Style hair H10.2 • Dress and finish hair H10.3 • Dress long hair H10.4

Maintain effective and safe methods of working when styling hair

H10.1

You must ensure the health and safety of your client and yourself at all times.

What you will learn
• Preparing your client for blow-drying, setting and dressing long hair • Choosing suitable products, equipment and tools • Following health and safety measures at work • Organising your working area and time effectively

Preparing your client for blow-drying, setting and dressing long hair

Gowning and positioning

Client comfort is always important. You must take care of your client when gowning and positioning her for a service.

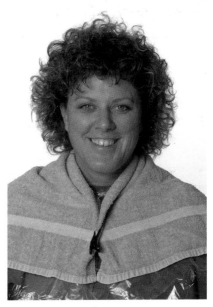

Make sure the client is gowned correctly

- Make sure you have not tied the gown too tightly around the client's neck – she still has to breathe!
- Always secure the towel with a clip so that it does not slide off the client.
- Remember when shampooing to use a disposable plastic cape on top of the towel for double protection.
- Make sure that the client is positioned correctly at the basin so that she is comfortable and the water cannot drip down her neck.
- Do not be afraid to re-position the client. If she is not sitting correctly, you cannot perform the treatment properly.
- Try not to let the client sit up in the chair before you towel dry her hair.
- Remove the plastic cape and allow the client to dry her neck and ears as she wishes.

When you seat your client in the chair at your workstation, it is important that the client is sitting squarely in front of the mirror with both feet flat on the floor or footrest. This is to enable you to move freely around your client and also to ensure that you get an even balance to the hairstyle.

Standing in the most comfortable and effective way

It is important to make sure that you position yourself correctly alongside your client as you are working. All your working positions should feel natural. The more comfortable you are, the less tired you will become.

Your work area

Your work area must be clean and tidy before you receive your client. This means putting away any electrical equipment that you will not be using and making sure that your work area is free from spillages, trailing wires, or anything else that might cause harm to you or your client.

Potential hazards include:

- products such as wax or serums, which may have dropped on the floor – mop them up immediately
- tongs and hot brushes which, if left on, may pose a risk to your client.

It is also important to keep your mirrors clean and wipe down working surfaces regularly. You need to be particularly careful if a client brings children into the salon.

Choosing suitable products, equipment and tools

Using products without being wasteful

For successful treatments, you need to know the effects of different products on all hair types. There is a wide range of products available, from those that protect the hair from the effects of atmospheric moisture, to products that make the hair easier to shape.

You need to know how, when and why you are using these products and the amount of product that you should be using. If you are wasteful when using products, you will be 'eating into' your salon's profits. It is always better to use a small amount and then apply a little more rather then squeezing too much of the bottle or tube and having to throw it away.

The following table will help you understand what the different types of products are used for.

Check it out

Each time you work, think about where you are standing in relation to the head of hair you are blow-drying and think about where you are going to move to when you come to blow-dry the next section of hair. If necessary, practise working with a friend.

Check it out

In groups, discuss and list as many ways that you can work that will help to reduce injury and fatigue.

Reality check!

Always follow the manufacturer's instructions. These give you all the information you need to use the product correctly.

Some styling, dressing and finishing products

Product	Application	Suitability	Comments
Gel (wet or dry look)	Apply to wet hair at the roots and spread through	Firm hold – gives support to short spiky styles	Ideal for short, textured styles
Mousse	Apply to wet hair and comb through evenly	Medium to firm hold – gives body and bounce to hair	Ideal for all hair types – not very thick hair
Glaze	Apply evenly to towel-dried hair	Firm hold – dries hard	Ideal for slicking back unruly hair
Dressing cream	Apply small amount evenly with hands	Light hold – large amounts will produce a slicked back look	Leaves hair sticky to touch
Setting lotion	Sprinkle or spray from bottle onto towel-dried hair	Light to firm hold – use with rollers for a firm result	Good for all hair types; can leave the hair a little hard to touch

Product	Application	Suitability	Comments
Blow-drying lotion	Apply before blow-drying	Gives hair a softer look and feel	Some contain chemicals that protect hair from heat
Hairspray	Apply sparingly onto styled hair from a distance of 20 cm	Holds finished style in place	Brushes out; will have drying effect on hair
Hair gloss	Apply small amounts on wet hair	Reduces frizz and increases shine	Ideal for African Caribbean hair
Moisturiser	Apply to hair before styling	Makes hair soft and shiny; loosens tangles	Useful for conditioning African Caribbean hair
Activators	Apply to wet or dry hair	Used to maintain curl or replace moisture in permanent or naturally curly hair	Defines curl; adds moisture and shine to hair

Correct equipment and tools for blow-drying and setting

When you blow-dry, the length of hair dictates the size of the brush that you choose in the same way the length of the hair dictates the size of the roller you use when setting. This is why stylists have a wide and varied range of brushes and rollers. To start with, you will need only a basic range of brushes and rollers. As you gain experience and master different techniques, you may wish to add to your equipment.

Tool		Effect	Suitability
Denman brush		Use for a smooth finish, e.g. a 'bob' style	Hair only requiring a slight curve or straight finish; curl cannot be achieved
Vent brush		Produces a soft, casual 'broken-up' effect	Good for quick casual result; not very suitable for curling
Circular brushes		Good for producing a curled effect. The smaller the brush, the tighter the curl	Large round brushes are ideal for long hair, smaller brushes for shorter hair. Any round brush can tangle in hair
Setting rollers for wet setting		Various sizes for different degrees of curl	Suitable for all hair types to produce soft to firm curls
Diffuser		Encourages curl into hair by scrunching the hair into the diffuser	Ideal for permed or naturally curly hair
Dressing-out combs		Use for backcombing and teasing style into hair	Use for all dressing-out techniques
African Caribbean and wide-tooth combs		Use to de-tangle hair	Suitable for straight and curly hair
Velcro rollers for dry setting		Good for body and bounce	Normally only suitable for dry setting; produces a very soft curl

Styling tools and techniques

Following health and safety measures at work

When you work in the salon, you are responsible for the health and safety of yourself and your client (see G1).

Information from manufacturers

All manufacturers of hair treatments and products must, by law, supply manufacturer's data sheets to comply with the Control of Substances Hazardous to Health (COSHH)

Regulations 2003. These sheets provide you with everything you need to know about the product you are using – the ingredients, the handling and storage of the product, and any disposal considerations.

The sheets will also tell you the first-aid measures to follow if the product comes into contact with the eyes, skin, or if it is swallowed. What would you do if you accidentally got some of the styling products that you were using in the client's eye? Ideally, you should call a first aider, but if one is not available immediately, then you need to take action. By following the first-aid measures stated on the manufacturer's data sheet, you will be able to deal with the problem until a first aider is available.

A manufacturer's data sheet

COSHH INFORMATION FOR:

HYDROGEN PEROXIDE

General Description
Stabilised acidic aqueous solutions or emulsions containing Hydrogen Peroxide of various strengths for use with:

- Permanent tints
- Bleach powder
- Permanent waves as neutralisers
- Hair lighteners
- Straighteners
- Dye remover

Hazardous Ingredients
- Hydrogen Peroxide up to 60 vol or 18%

Hazards
- Irritant to eyes and skin

Precautions when in use
- Always wear protective gloves
- Avoid contact with eyes and face
- Do not use on abraded or sensitive skin
- Always use non-metallic utensils, to avoid rapid decomposition of the product

Storage Precautions
- Store in a cool, dry place away from sunlight and other sources of heat
- Always store Hydrogen Peroxide in the container supplied
- It is particularly important that no contamination enters the container as this could lead to decomposition resulting in the liberation of heat and oxygen
- Replace cap immediately after use

Your responsibilities relating to legislation

As a stylist, you must be aware of your own responsibilities under the COSHH Regulations (see Unit G1.2, page 30).

All products used in hairdressing are covered by these regulations as they relate to:

- handling chemicals
- storing chemicals
- disposal of chemicals.

Risk assessment sheets

Every hairdressing product also has a risk assessment sheet. Usually, most salons keep these sheets together in a folder for easy access.

Risk assessment sheets contain the following information:

- chemical composition (ingredients) of the product
- personal protective equipment (PPE) needed when using the product
- storage instructions
- handling instructions
- the hazard under COSHH
- what the product is used for
- special safety measures to follow
- disposal instructions.

Check it out

In your salon or college/training institution, find out where the manufacturer's data sheets and risk assessment sheets are located. Select six products you commonly use and obtain copies of these for your portfolio.

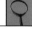

Check it out

Hairspray contains many chemicals. Some of these are flammable (easily catch fire). Find out and make a note of the following information for your portfolio:

- the safety considerations to be taken into account when using hairspray
- the correct procedure for storing a can of hairspray
- the correct procedure for disposing of an empty can of hairspray.

Compare your answers with your group and check with your tutor.

CONTROL OF SUBSTANCES HAZARDOUS TO HEALTH ASSESSMENT OF RISK

Expt. Title/No Substance Process		Year	
		Course	

Substance(s) used

Hazard(s) Please tick:

Irritant		Corrosive		Harmful		Very Toxic		
Oxidising		Explosive		Flammable				

Where used pleas tick:

Laboratory	Preparation Room	Chemical Store	Workshop	Other (specify)	

By whom please tick

Lecturer	Technician	Student	Other (specify)	

Document(s) outlining working method(s) e.g. Safety & Science Lecturers Guide etc.

Expected Hazardous By-Product(s)

	Tick	
		Irritant
		Corrosive
		Harmful
		(Very) Toxic
		Oxidising
		Explosive
		Flammable

Likely route(s) of entry

Inhalation	Mouth	Skin contact	Eyes	

Specified safety measures to be taken

Goggles	Fume cupboard	Apron/coat	Eye-wash bottle	Good ventilation	Safety screen	Wash hands	Gloves	Respirator	Dust mask

Specified procedures for dealing with:

First Aid ST or PH	Emergency Spillage SP	Fire	

Assessor_____ Date of Assessment _____

Head of Department _____ Date of Authorisation _____

A risk assessment sheet

Your responsibilities under the COSHH Regulations are to follow instructions given in:

- manufacturer's data sheets – read the instructions before using a product
- COSHH assessment sheets – where to store chemicals,

and to follow:

- salon requirements – use the correct PPE, notify a supervisor or manager if a problem arises.

Hazard warnings found on products and chemicals

Chemicals and products are considered hazardous if they can be:

- inhaled
- ingested (swallowed)
- in contact with the skin
- absorbed through the skin
- introduced into the body via cuts, and so on.

To alert everyone to a hazard, all chemicals that have some type of risk carry a safety symbol.

Reality check!

All products contain chemicals and are potentially dangerous. The more you are familiar with the products you use and what they contain (as well as what they do), the safer your practice will be.

Dust   Toxic   Flammable

Irritant   Corrosive   Oxidising agent

Hazard symbols

Sterilising

Sterilisation means the killing of all organisms such as bacteria, fungus and parasites. Disinfecting involves immersing equipment in a disinfectant solution such as barbicide for a certain length of time.

There are various methods for sterilising tools and equipment – see the chart below. Some are more effective than others and not all equipment can be sterilised in the same way. Your tools should be sterilised after every client so that you minimise the risk of cross-infection and infestation.

Remember
Disinfecting will kill germs only if you use a solution which is strong enough and leave the equipment immersed for the right amount of time. Always read the manufacturer's instructions for strength and duration.

Method	Comments	Tool/equipment
Boiling water (60° minimum) – the hot (boil) cycle on the washing machine should be used	Make sure that gowns can withstand high temperatures	Towels and gowns
Barbicide solution	Will not rust metal. Read manufacturer's instructions for quantities and the amount of time required to sterilise equipment	Metal equipment, combs, setting rollers, brushes (not wooden handled)
Ultra-violet cabinet	Odourless. Will only sterilise the part of the equipment that the ultra-violet rays reach. Equipment has to be turned over after 20–30 minutes	Combs, brushes, rollers, metal equipment
Autoclave	Only suitable for equipment that can withstand heat. Will not rust metal	Metal equipment only. Plastic will melt!
Sterilising wipes or sprays	Do not use near naked flame as they are inflammable	Clippers and clipper grades, scissors

Methods of sterilisation and disinfection

Organising your working area and time effectively

Organising yourself and your time at work is an important part of your role as a stylist. Every salon allows a set amount of time for every process that is carried out, from shampooing to colouring.

Organisation for blow-drying, setting and dressing long hair

You must have:

- a hairdryer and other electrical equipment such as electric tongs and a hot brush
- a good selection of brushes and combs for blow-drying and dressing out
- a wide range of setting rollers and a hair net
- pin curl clips, hair grips and fine hair pins for long hair
- a selection of styling products.

A good trolley layout with all the necessary equipment will allow you to spend more time with the client on the service.

Generally salons allocate the following timings to each service:

- shampoo and conditioning – five to ten minutes depending on the length of the hair
- blow-drying – 30–40 minutes
- setting – one hour for the complete process
- dressing long hair – 45 minutes maximum.

Safe working for you, your clients and colleagues

Clean equipment

As well as making sure that all of your equipment is sterilised, you need to make sure that it is clean from hair and products. If you are using your equipment regularly, you will find that hair builds up. You may also find that you get a build-up of product residue in between the teeth of brushes and combs. This needs to be removed before you can sterilise your equipment.

Personal hygiene

If you have overslept and not had time for a shower in the morning, not only are you going to feel uncomfortable but your work colleagues and clients might as well! Personal hygiene is as important as keeping your tools and equipment clean and sterilised, and you should have the same standards for yourself.

You should:

- make sure you wash your hands before each client, especially if you are a smoker!
- use mints or a breath freshener if you have had strong-smelling food the previous night, e.g. a curry.
- wear a minimal amount of jewellery
- ensure your uniform is freshly laundered and ironed
- wear your hair tied back if that is a salon requirement
- wear a small amount of make-up to portray a professional appearance
- wear shoes that are comfortable and that you can stand in for long periods of time
- use your common sense and think about the image you would like to see when you walk into a professional salon
- conduct yourself in a manner when using tools and equipment that will not put yourself or others at risk
- make regular checks on your equipment
- keep your work area clean and tidy and free of trailing wires, products or anything else that could cause harm or injury.

Consultation

For every hairdressing service, an in-depth consultation is the key to success. Without gathering the right kind of information from your client, you will not be able to fulfil her wishes.

Style books

Style books will also help you and your client agree together what kind of look is going to be achieved. Using style books as a basis of discussion also helps you to identify to the client what type of products have been used and what kind of aftercare would be needed at home.

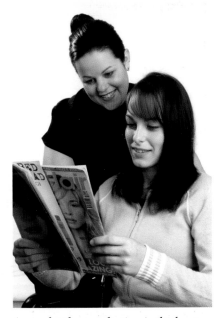

An in-depth consultation is the key to success

Remember

If you do not identify infestations before you shampoo, then you are obliged to complete the service.

Check it out

Working with a partner, carry out a consultation on each other and identify what size brushes and products you will need to use to achieve the desired effect and how the style is going to be maintained at home.

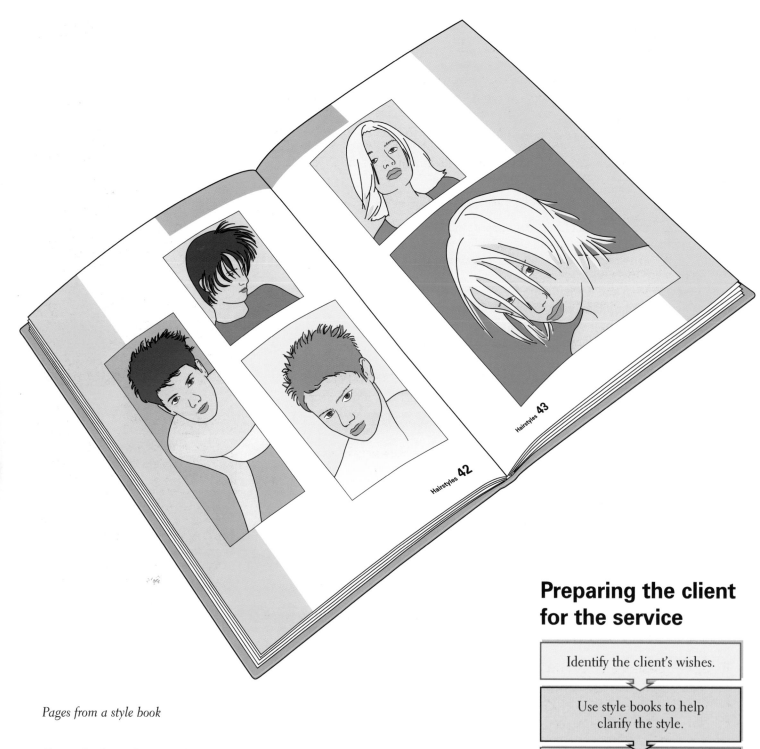

Pages from a style book

Completing the service within a commercially viable time

A salon will work out the timings of its services so that all time is used to its best advantage and that it sees enough clients to make a profit. As a stylist, you need to be aware of the timescale that you have to carry out various services.

Until you gain experience you will not be expected to work to these time constraints, but you need to aware of the times that you have to work towards to be financially viable for your salon.

Preparing the client for the service

Identify the client's wishes.

Use style books to help clarify the style.

Seat the client correctly.

Make sure you have all the relevant equipment.

Check client's comfort throughout the service.

Style hair

H10.2

Most hairstyles have been blow-dried or finished in some way. For daily wear, most people want styles that are easy to manage, but they may also want to have the option of dressing hair up for evening wear. In this element you will learn how to use current drying and finishing techniques to be able to produce these styles, taking into account different hair types and critical influencing factors. You will also be looking at the effect blow-drying and setting has on the hair's structure and the effect that moisture in the atmosphere has on the hair.

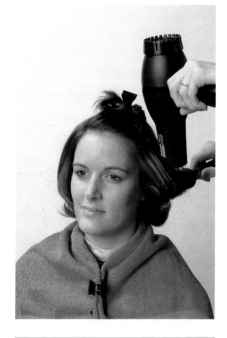

> ## What you will learn
>
> - Consulting and preparing before styling
> - Blow-drying hair using correct products and tools
> - Setting hair using correct products and tools
> - Critical influencing factors
> - Using styling techniques that ensure client comfort
> - Blow-drying
> - Wet and dry setting

Consulting and preparing before styling

Consulting the client

During the consultation, check:

- for anything that may not let you carry out the service such as infections and infestations
- the type of hair you are working on – look at the texture and density of hair as this will influence the choice of styling product
- any critical influencing factors that may influence the blow-dry such as head and face shape
- how the client is currently wearing her hair – if she wants the same style, you have an advantage by seeing her hair before it is shampooed
- how much natural movement there is in the hair – this will affect your product choice and the choice of brush size
- whether there are any natural partings – it is always better to allow the hair to fall into its natural partings as the style will last longer.

Types of questions to ask during the consultation

- Is the curl in your hair a perm or is it naturally curly (if relevant)?
- Would you like a styling product on your hair?
- How would you like your hair blow-dried? (Use style books to help.)
- Is it a daytime or an evening look?
- Do you get any problems with particular parts of the hair? (Let the client identify what she considers to be awkward areas.)

Questions to ask during the service

- Is the heat of the hairdryer comfortable for you?
- Is that enough body and height for you?
- Are you happy with the finished result?

It is important to check during the service that the client is happy with the way her hair is taking shape. This is the time to make any changes that either of you may feel are appropriate or necessary.

> ## Reality check!
>
> The consultation is the first communication that you have with the client. It is important to spend time questioning her on her requirements and expectations of the service. It is also the time when you need to complete a blow-drying analysis. It may be useful to prepare a checklist to help you.

Blow-drying hair using correct products and tools

When you have completed your client consultation using the checklist on page 139, you should have gathered enough information to help you decide on your choice of products, equipment and techniques that you are going to use. If you are unable to make all of these choices, then you have not completed a thorough consultation!

Controlling your styling tools

You need to be able to control your equipment and the hair as you blow-dry it. The way in which you manage the hair is very important, as this will affect the finished result. Here are some tips to help you.

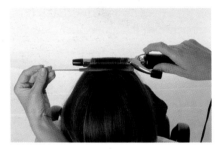

Hold the electric tongs in the correct position so as to avoid contact with the scalp

- Rough-dry excess moisture from the hair before you begin to style it.
- Take small sections to allow the heat of the hairdryer, electric tongs and heated brush to dry/penetrate the mesh of hair.
- The airflow from the hairdryer should flow over the cuticle in the direction of the hairstyle, not against it, otherwise this will roughen the cuticle scales making the hair look fluffy and dull.
- Try not to direct the heat from the hairdryer directly onto the scalp, as this will cause great discomfort to the client.
- When using electric tongs or other electrical equipment, do not allow the tongs to come into contact with the scalp – see the photo opposite.
- Do not overdry the hair. When a mesh of hair is dry you will not be able to alter its shape.
- Adjust the height that the client is sitting at to enable you to work around her effectively.
- Always warn the client if you are going to adjust the position of the seat.
- When blow-drying the nape of the hair, position the client's head downwards so that you can work freely in that area.
- Remember to change hands (with the dryer and brush) so that you can work effectively around the head.
- Section off the bulk of the hair that you are not working with so that you work in a controlled manner.

Reality check!

- When blow-drying, always work from roots to points, keeping the cuticle scale flat.
- Keep the dryer moving to prevent burning the hair or the scalp.
- Always lift the hair when removing the brush to prevent tangling.
- Keep an even tension on the hair but do not overstretch it by pulling too hard.

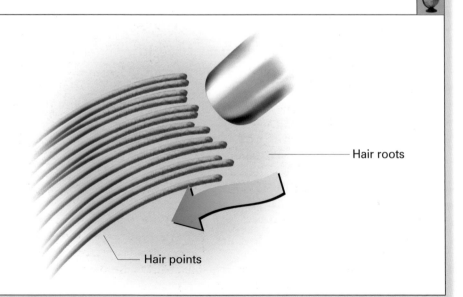

Hair roots

Hair points

Step-by-step blow-drying technique

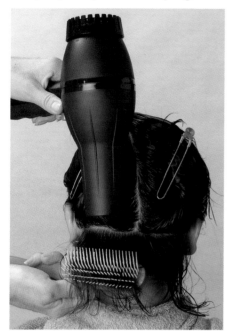

Section the hair into four and bring down a sub-section in the nape where you are going to begin blow-drying. Blow-dry the hair under to create root lift.

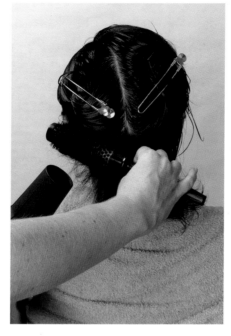

Choosing the correct size brush, begin to blow-dry the hair upwards making sure the airflow of the hairdryer is flowing over the hair in the correct direction.

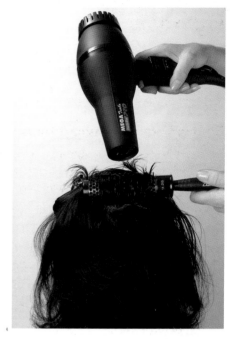

Work your way up towards the crown area, making sure each section is completely dry and falls in the desired direction.

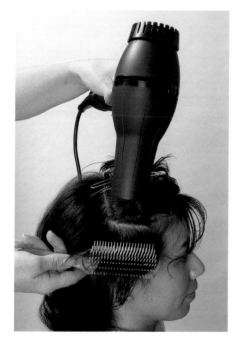

Take a section of hair at the sides and continue to blow-dry the hair so that it blends in with the back of the hair. Work your way towards the parting and repeat the same on the opposite side.

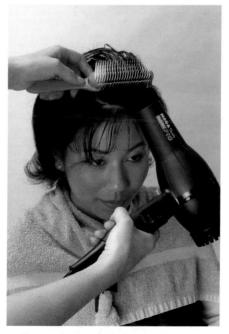

Move to the top and front sections of the hair, constantly moving the hairdryer so that you don't cause discomfort to the client.

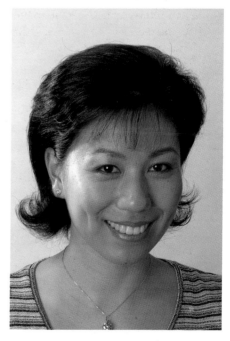

The finished result should be completed with the correct finishing products and the total look confirmed with the client.

Using the correct tension and meshes of hair to suit the styling tools and process

It is important, when blow-drying, setting or dressing out the hair, that you use the correct size of meshes. This is so that:

- the heat from the hairdryer can penetrate the hair mesh evenly enabling you to dry the hair evenly.
- when placing your rollers they will sit correctly on their own base without root drag.
- the mesh of hair suits the length and width of the brush/roller you have chosen so that hair does not get caught and tangled around the sides of either.
- heat from electrical appliances can penetrate the mesh of hair to achieve the result required.
- you work in a methodical manner covering the whole of the head, ensuring all of the hair is dry.

It is equally important that you keep tension even along the mesh of hair when you work so that:

- the curl you may be putting into the hair from either a roller, brush, tongs or hot brush, gives you an even result along the section of hair.
- if you are straightening the hair, you will ensure an even result.
- when winding the hair around a roller, tongs or hot brush, you will not get 'baggy' sides!

Setting hair using correct products and tools

Setting techniques

There are three key points that apply to both wet and dry setting techniques.

1   Sectioning – the section of hair that you take when placing rollers is very important. If the section of hair is too big, you will have 'baggy' ends that will produce an uneven curl result. If the section is too small, you will have 'overcrowding' of rollers and will run out of headspace! The section that you take should be slightly narrower than the length of the roller and no deeper than the width of the roller.

2   Tension – good even tension will distribute the hair evenly around the roller ensuring a uniformed curl result.

3   Angle – the angle at which you hold the hair when winding will determine the amount of root lift created. For good root lift the hair needs to be held at 90 degrees from the head. This position should be maintained while the roller is wound to the base. For fashion setting techniques you can drag the roots of the hair if little or no root lift is required.

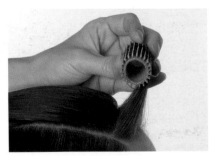

Take a section that is slightly narrower than the length of the roller and no deeper than the width of the roller

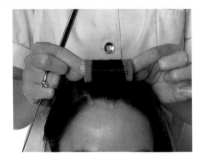

Good even tension is essential

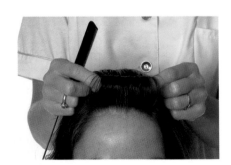

Poorly placed roller

Remember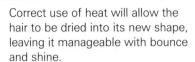

Correct use of heat will allow the hair to be dried into its new shape, leaving it manageable with bounce and shine.

Incorrect use of heat will dry out the hair, making it unmanageable by roughening the cuticle scale and leaving the hair in poor condition.

Reality check!

Practise holding the dryer in your left hand and using the brush with your right hand, and then change over. You must be able to work with the dryer using both hands.

Applying styling products to control the hair taking into account critical influencing factors

You have looked at the use of styling products (refer back to pages 132–3), at what they do and their suitability for different types of hair. Styling products can also be used to help you overcome or control some of the critical influencing factors that you may come across.

Styling and setting aids

Since the hair has the ability to absorb water (allowing you to shampoo it), it can also absorb atmospheric moisture. Atmospheric moisture is humidity (water) in the air (atmosphere) from rain, the shower and the bath. By using styling products you are putting a slight barrier on the hair, which will protect the hair from atmospheric moisture and will help to prevent your finished look from collapsing. Styling products also help to protect the hair from the effects of added heat when styling.

Sets and blow-dries may not last long, because as soon as the hair comes into contact with

atmospheric moisture

it will start to

drop.

The use of setting or styling products will help to produce a longer-lasting set or blow dry. There are several types of products but all modern products work in the same way.

They coat the outside of the hair shaft in a

plastic film.

This prevents

atmospheric moisture

penetrating the cuticle layer.

These modern products are made of plasticisers, e.g. Polyvinyl Pyrolidone, which is a clear film that dissolves in hot water and shampoo. It is therefore removed easily from the hair. The products soften the hair shaft allowing shapes to be formed readily and prevent the hair from becoming 'fly away' which makes it more

manageable

when it is dressed out.

They also

protect

the hair from

added heat.

Check it out

Gather together some styling products that you have in your salon or college/training institution. Draw up a chart using the column headings 'Hair type/style', 'Product(s)', 'Application' and 'Benefits to the hair'. Fill it in deciding which products are suitable for the hair types listed below.

Hair types:

- short and spiky
- curly/permed
- fine, flat hair
- African Caribbean hair
- dry, porous hair.

Remember

The golden rule when using products is: always read the manufacturer's instructions before you use the product.

Check it out

When using styling and finishing products, what type of moisture are you protecting the hair from?

Critical influencing factors

When choosing products, equipment and blow-drying techniques, you should consider:

- hair texture – very fine hair will need a product that gives it lift and volume
- haircut – the length of the layers and style will determine what size brush you will use and what type of product. If it is a very textured cut, you may need to use more than one product on the hair
- head and face shape – these influence your drying technique and how you style the hair
- hair growth patterns – you may need a 'firm hold' product to help you to style the hair to disguise a double crown or to hold down a fringe with a cowlick
- hair elasticity – this will influence your product choice and choice of equipment, for example, you would not use electric tongs or a heated brush on hair that had poor elasticity because you would be adding heat to already 'stressed hair'. You may choose to use a product that will help to improve the condition of the hair such as serum or a gloss
- hair length – if you are working on very long hair, you may need to use a product that is not too heavy and will weigh the hair down. You may want to opt for a light blow-drying lotion
- hair density – this will have an influence on your product choice. If the client has very thick hair, you will not want to use a product that will increase the volume in the hair, you will want to choose one that will reduce the bulk in the hair.

As well as using styling products to help you control critical influencing factors, you also need to be aware of what equipment and styling techniques can be used to help you with potential problems.

Dealing with critical influencing factors

Problem: Strong cowlick movement in the fringe area on straight hair.

Solution: Use a firm hold product at the roots, blow-dry the hair in the opposite direction to the way it wants to sit, finish with a firm hold spray.

Problem: Flat spot at the back of the head.

Solution: Use a root lift product, direct the heat of the hairdryer into the root to achieve maximum lift using a round brush (pick the size brush suitable for the length of hair you are working on).

Influencing factors for setting wet and dry hair

When deciding whether to set hair wet or dry, you should consider the following questions:

- How firm do you require the curl in the hair to be? Wet setting produces a firmer curl.
- How much time does your client have for the service? Dry setting or using heated rollers does not take as long as wet setting.
- What type of setting method would suit your client's hair type/texture? Straight hair would require a firmer set; naturally curly or permed hair will hold a curl better.
- How long does the client require the set to last? If it is for one evening, you can use fashion setting techniques. If it is to last a week, you may need to choose a more traditional method of setting that will last longer.
- What is the condition of the hair? If the hair is very dry and damaged, for example, you would not use heated styling tools, such as hair straighteners or heated rollers.

Check it out

What would you consider to be critical influencing factors? Working with a partner, make a list of as many points as you can that will affect the way in which you would work with the hair. Write a brief statement about how the factors you have identified would affect your treatment and how you would overcome some of the problems.

Using styling techniques that ensure client comfort

When you shampoo, you are not only removing dirt and grease from the hair but you are also changing the properties of the hair that make it possible to alter its shape temporarily by blow-drying or setting.

The hair has two properties, which allow us to do this.

1   Hair is hygroscopic – it is able to absorb water.

2   The hair has natural elasticity – it will stretch and return to its original shape.

Hair in its natural state is called alpha keratin. Hair in its stretched state is called beta keratin.

Naturally straight hair becomes curly, changing alpha to beta keratin

Naturally curly hair becomes straight, changing alpha to beta keratin

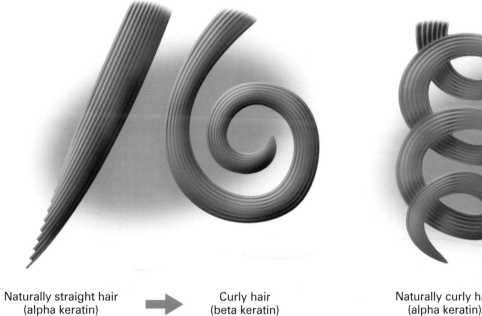

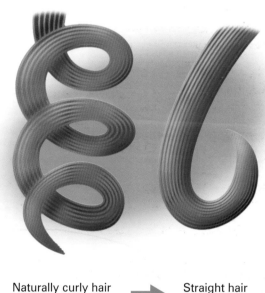

Naturally straight hair (alpha keratin) → Curly hair (beta keratin)

Naturally curly hair (alpha keratin) → Straight hair (beta keratin)

Without the hair's ability to absorb water and stretch and return to its original shape, you would not be able to alter its shape.

Straight and curly hair in natural and stretched states

When hair is shampooed, water is absorbed into the cortex. The water breaks down the hydrogen bonds (which are the weaker bonds in the hair) and allows the hair to be stretched. By applying heat to the hair in this stretched state, you can re-form the bonds into a new shape around either a brush or a roller (the hair is now in its beta keratin state). This is called a physical change because it is only temporary and the hair can be blow-dried or set as often as required.

Blow-drying

There are a number of different looks that you can achieve when blow-drying, from a very soft, casual look, to a firmer, more set-looking style. The tools and techniques that you use will help you to produce these looks (look back at pages 132–3 to remind yourself of the equipment available).

Blow-dry on straight, long, one-length hair

The bob is a classic style that when dried correctly will look smooth and sleek.

What you will need:

- client with straight, one-length hair
- Denman or medium to large round brush
- selection of styling and finishing products
- sectioning clips
- hairdryer (possibly straightening irons)
- dressing-out combs.

Step-by-step blow-dry of one-length hair (a bob)

Apply products.

Section the hair into four.

Drop a section of hair in the nape and begin blow-drying with the heat flowing over the section of hair.

Bring down the next section working towards the crown.

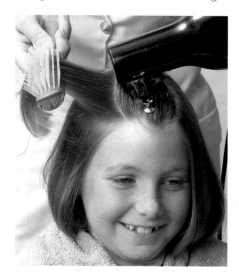

Take a section from the side of the hair and blow-dry in the same manner up to the natural parting.

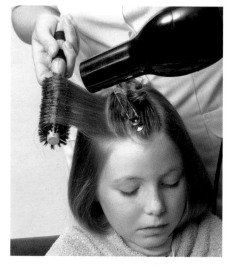

Use a large, round brush to curl the ends under. Repeat the same on the other side.

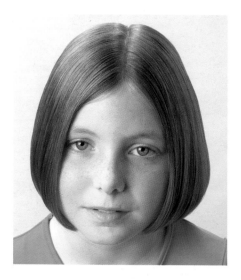

The finished style.

Blow-dry on short, straight or curly, layered hair

These are often referred to as 'back and bubbly' styles because they follow a specific design and require a small round brush for a firm hold. When you blow-dry the hair, you are trying to achieve little sausages over the head!

What you will need:

- client with short, layered hair
- hairdryer (possibly electric tongs or hot brush)
- selection of round brushes
- sectioning clips
- selection of styling and finishing products
- dressing-out combs.

Step-by-step blow-dry on short, straight or curly, layered hair

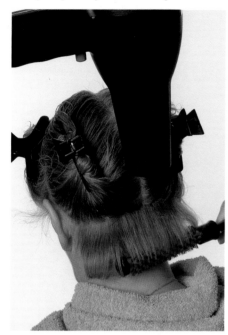

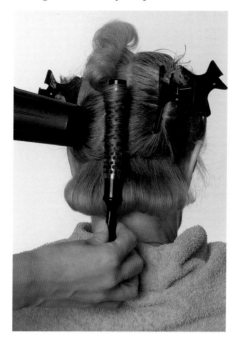

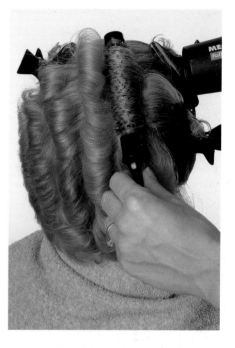

Divide the hair into four and bring down a sub-section of hair in the nape and blow-dry this section under.

Release one of the main back sections and begin to blow-dry the hair towards the centre of the head.

Continue to blow-dry the whole section of hair in this manner and repeat on the opposite side.

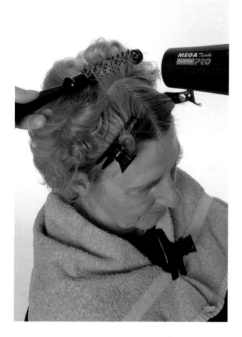

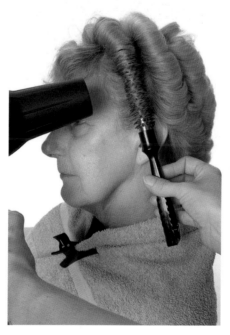

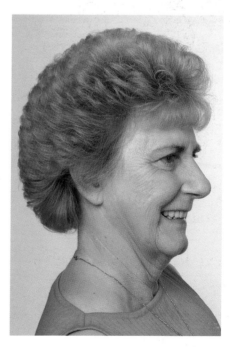

Go to the top of the crown area and begin to blow-dry the hair backwards over the crown.

From the top sections, continue to join the side sections to these to form 'sausages' over the head.

The finished result. The hair is blow-dried all over using a slightly cooler heat. Run your fingers through the hair to soften the 'sausages'. Apply appropriate finishing products to suit the hair type.

Finger dry on permed or naturally curly hair

Using this technique will encourage the curl into the hair. You want to control the hair so that the curl is well formed and does not appear frizzy.

What you will need:

- client with naturally curly or permed hair
- hairdryer with diffuser
- selection of styling and finishing products
- sectioning clips.

Step-by-step scrunch-dried hair

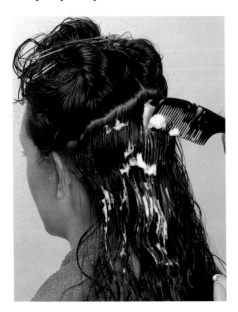

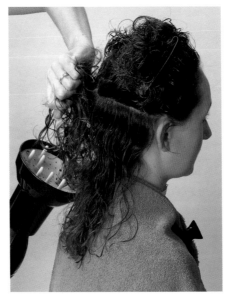

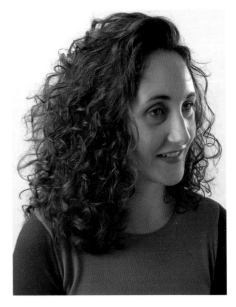

Apply styling products and section hair into four.

Take a section of hair in the nape area and scrunch the hair with your hand into the diffuser.

Continue taking sections down and dry in this way until you reach the crown area.

Drop the first side section and scrunch into the diffuser.

Repeat previous step until all the hair is dry.

The finished style.

Wet and dry setting

Carrying out wet and dry setting techniques safely

Wet setting the hair involves shampooing and you need to remember to gown your client correctly for this part of the service. After shampooing, towel-dry the hair to remove any excess moisture, comb the hair through, then apply the product you have chosen.

With dry setting you will not be shampooing the hair, but you still have to prepare the client and the hair for the treatment (for example, gowning). You should brush the hair through to remove any tangles and then apply a setting aid (product) if one is required.

Remember

Only apply products to towel-dried hair, otherwise you could find most of the product running down the client's face.

The different effects of wet and dry setting

Wetting the hair causes the hydrogen bonds in the hair to break down. This allows you to change the shape of the hair by blow-drying or setting. When you wind wet hair around a roller and add heat to the hair, the bonds re-form into their new shape around the roller – this is how we are able to style the hair time and time again.

Dry setting the hair does not break down the hydrogen bonds (except a few from your application of styling product). It involves 'baking' the hair into its new shape around the roller. Care has to be taken when doing this – you do not want to overdry the hair causing any damage. Dry setting is very useful for fashion setting techniques – it will produce a softer curl, ideal for preparing the hair for hair-up techniques.

Products for setting

Styling products coat the hair with a protective barrier that will help to prevent moisture getting through and causing the set to collapse. Look back at the chart on page 132–133 to remind yourself of the products available.

Coloured mousse and setting lotions clearly state in the manufacturer's instructions that they should be used on wet hair. You will not achieve an even distribution or colour result if applied to dry hair.

Wet setting

- Mousse – towel-dry the hair, comb through and section. Use a large-tooth comb and evenly comb the mousse from the roots to the ends of the hair.
- Coloured mousse – make sure that you have gowned your client correctly and you are wearing the correct protective clothing (gloves and apron). Repeat the procedure above.
- Setting lotion – can come in spray form or individual bottles. When using setting lotion from a bottle, place your forefinger slightly over the top of the bottle and sprinkle onto the hair, keeping the client's head back to avoid accidents.
- Coloured setting lotion – make sure that your client is correctly gowned and you are wearing protective clothing.

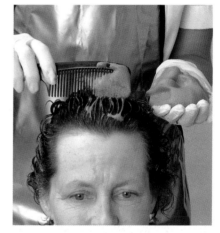

Applying coloured mousse

Dry setting

- Mousse (not coloured) – use the same method as for wet hair.
- Thermal setting lotions – these are sprayed onto dry hair and activated by applying heat.
- Setting lotions (not coloured) – use the same application method as for wet hair.

Tools and equipment for setting

What you will need:

- a pintail comb – this is used to section and comb through the mesh of hair
- a selection of rollers – the length of the hair and degree of curl required determines the size of the roller used
- setting pins – these are used to secure the rollers
- pin curl clips – these may be required for shorter hair that will not wind around a curler
- styling products – these will make the hair more pliable, add body, and protect it from atmospheric moisture
- water spray – the hair must not be allowed to dry out when wet setting
- hair net – this covers the rollers when placing the client under the dryer and stops any small hairs escaping from the rollers
- hood dryer – this supplies an even distribution of heat all around the head.

> **Remember**
>
> Always secure the lids on bottles before putting away.

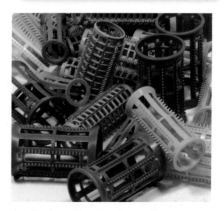

A selection of wet setting rollers

Setting techniques

There are various techniques that can be used to set the hair.

Channel

This type of setting technique is uniformed in its layout. Begin at the front hairline, directing the hair backwards and place a row of rollers in a channel down the centre of the head. Then move to the crown area and, still directing the hair downwards, place a section of rollers each side of the middle channel. Finish by placing another set of rollers at the sides of the head. All of the rollers should be seated in channels down the head.

Brickwork

Think of bricks in a wall, this is how you will be placing the rollers in the hair. Begin at the front hairline and place one roller, then move behind this roller and take a section from the middle of the first roller. Continue in this way working down the head, remembering that the head is round and not square so some alterations in your rollering position may be required.

Directional

As the name suggests, place the rollers in the direction that you want the hair to be dressed. Incorporate all of the setting techniques when completing a directional wind as long as the rollers are wound in the direction you wish the hair to sit.

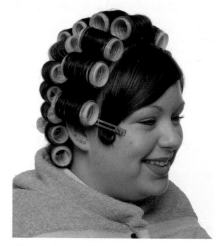

Channel technique

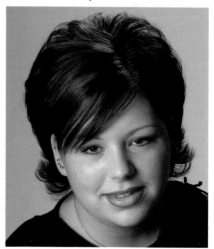

Rollers seated in channels down the head and the finished result

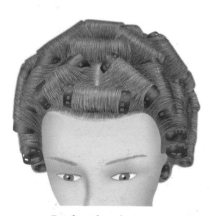

Brickwork technique

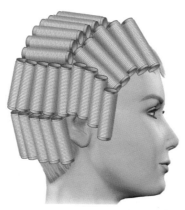

Directional winding

Pin curling techniques

Pin curling techniques are also used in setting, and are very useful for shorter hair that may not wind around a roller easily.

- Flat barrel – this will sit flat on the head with an open middle and produce a curl that is even from roots to points.
- Barrel – this creates lift from the root producing soft curls or waves and can be used in place of a roller.
- Clockspring – this will also sit flat on the head with a closed middle. It produces a curl that is looser at the root and gradually tighter towards the ends.

Finger waving

Finger waving offers a different type of look and works with the natural movement in the hair. To produce finger waves, work with the fingers laying outstretched on the hair, pressing down to form

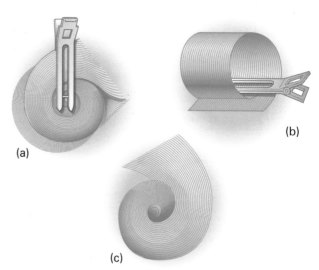

(a) Flat barrel, (b) barrel and (c) clockspring pin curls

deep crests and troughs. For the finished result you should have an 'S' formation working down the head.

Finger waving takes patience and a lot of practice, but it is a really worthwhile exercise as it will help you to work with, and understand, the natural growth patterns and fall of the hair. It will also improve your manual dexterity. Here are some tips to help you.

- Stand directly opposite the area that you are working on.
- Keep the hair thoroughly wet.
- Keep your elbows high.
- Keep the palms of your hands up and off the head. Just work with outstretched fingers.
- Work in a controlled state of relaxation.
- The first wave should follow the hair's natural fall. If not, it will not hold.
- Start the wave at the closed end of the wave.
- Add on wave at the open end.
- Check that your comb is in contact with the scalp when forming the wave.
- Waves are usually approximately 2.5 cm deep.
- The crests of the wave should be clearly defined.
- If spring clips or fine pins are used, they must be placed in the troughs, positioned into the wave, and must not twist the hair.

What you will need:

- styling combs
- styling aids
- towels
- water spray
- section clips.

Step-by-step finger waving

Prepare the client for styling. Apply setting gel and comb the hair evenly away from the natural parting.

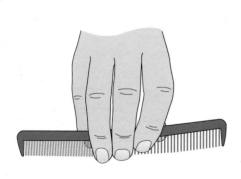

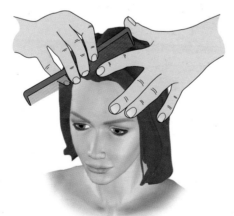

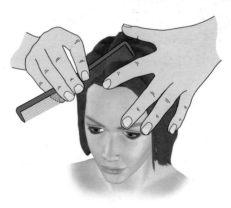

Hold comb with the thumb and little finger underneath, and three middle fingers on the top of the comb.

Form a semi-circle by combing the hair anti-clockwise across the head.

Place the index finger into the centre of the curve. Put the comb in at a 45°-angle and slide it to the right to form the first crest. Replace the index finger with the middle finger. Put the index finger on the comb and slide down to grip the crest between the fingers whilst changing the comb to the opposite angle of 135°. Comb through to the ends of the hair, making a curve in the opposite direction.

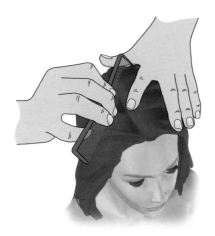

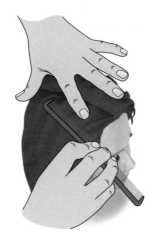

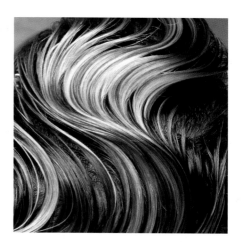

Repeat as before but taking the comb in the opposite direction.

Continue in this manner, working around the head.

The end result.

Although you may not have to carry out finger waving that often, it is a useful technique to learn for controlling hair.

Keeping the hair moist throughout the service

When styling the hair, it is important that the hair does not dry out before you have either placed your roller in the correct position or blow-dried the hair into the shape required. Use a water spray to dampen the hair slightly; you may find that this will be required more on finer hair as it has a tendency to dry out quicker than thicker hair.

If the hair does dry out and you do not re-dampen it, you will not achieve a smooth finish and the style will not last as long. This is because the hydrogen bonds will have re-formed into the hair's natural state and not taken on the shape of the roller or brush that you are using to style the hair.

Ensuring you achieve the volume, balance and curl required

Throughout any of the blow-drying services, always check with your client that:

- you are working towards the style desired by the client – check that the parting is in the right place
- you are achieving the correct amount of width and height that the client requires
- she is happy with the finished result – for example, have you used enough backcombing?

Choosing the correct products and techniques

| Complete in-depth consultation. |
| Identify suitable style for client. |
| Set the hair if required. |
| Choose suitable styling tools. |
| Use suitable products to set and dress the finished result. |

Dress and finish hair   H10.3

In this element you will be looking at how to use heated styling equipment, taking into account health and safety issues. You will be also looking at how to use backcombing and back brushing techniques and applying finishing products to complete the look required by the client.

What you will learn

- Leaving your client's hair free from sectioning marks
- Other considerations
- Using heated styling equipment
- Dressing-out techniques
- Applying finishing products, taking into account critical influencing factors
- Confirm the finished look with the client, giving the correct after-care advice

Leaving your client's hair free from sectioning marks

When you place your client under the dryer, either use a timer or check the time on your watch or a clock to make sure that the client is not left under the dryer unnecessarily. Check the temperature control of the dryer and remove any setting pins or pin curl clips that may cause discomfort. If there are any rollers seated on the clients' ears, place cotton wool underneath.

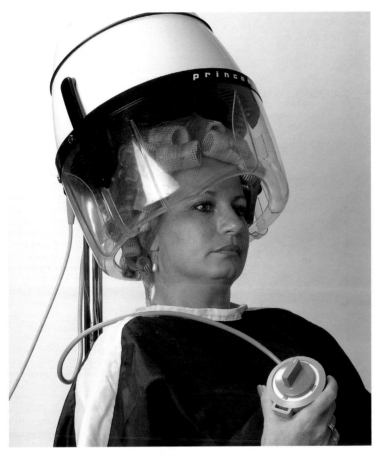

Placing the client under the dryer

Other considerations

- Keep even tension without pulling the hair from the scalp.
- When securing the roller with a pin, make sure the pin is not too tight or sitting on the client's head.
- Do not use electrical equipment with wet hands.
- Check that your client is comfortable and the dryer is not too hot for her.
- If using a portable hood dryer, make sure that trailing cables are not obstructing other clients or members of staff.

When removing the client from under the dryer, make sure that she is not caught up on anything and ease her gently away from the dryer. Unplug and remove the dryer.

- Seat the client at your dressing out unit, remove the hair net and check the hair is dry.
- Remove the setting pins before you take out any rollers. This gives the hair a chance to cool down, making the set firmer.
- Begin removing the rollers from the bottom of the hair first so that the rollers do not become tangled.

- Starting at the nape of the neck, use a Denman brush and a soft brush, and gently double brush the set through in the direction that you have set the hair. This will remove the sectioning marks from the set making all of the curls join up together ready to be dressed out.

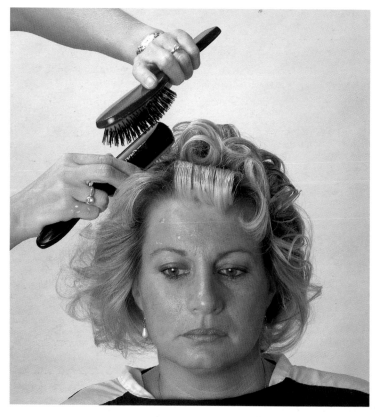

Double brushing the set

Note: If you are working on a fashion set and want to keep a crisper curl, you would gently run your fingers through the hair.

When you have completed a blow-dry, you will need to do the same and gently run your fingers through the hair to soften the look, especially if the client has had her hair blow-dried on a small round brush – you do not want to leave sausages in the hair!

Using heated styling equipment

Additional equipment

Other equipment you can use to help give extra support when you blow-dry or set the hair includes:

- electric (heated) tongs
- hot brush
- straightening irons
- crimping irons
- heated rollers.

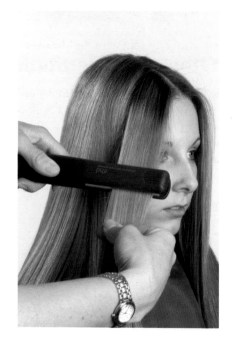

These are very useful pieces of equipment, but they should only be used to add support to the set or blow-dry that you have already completed. It is not appropriate to rough-dry a client's hair and then go back through with a set of tongs or hot brush to put curl into the hair. The chart on page 155 outlines the uses of each of these pieces of equipment.

Tool	Effect	Suitability	Comments
Electric (heated) tongs	Produces curls, waves and ringlets	Only to be used on dry hair; useful for all hair types but not very porous or damaged hair	Hair ends must be wound smoothly around barrel to prevent buckled ends
Hot brushes	Produces a softer curl	Only to be used on dry hair; finer sections need to be taken on thick hair	Easier to work with than electric tongs, but can become become tangled in hair. Make sure that you place a comb between the brush and scalp to prevent the brush from touching the scalp
Crimping irons	Creates volume in hair, producing a line of crimps	Only to be used on dry hair; not suitable for very short hair	The finer the sections of hair, the better the end result
Straightening irons	Temporarily straightens curly/wavy hair	Only to be used on dry hair; not suitable for very porous dry hair	Overuse dries out hair
Heated rollers	Adds soft curl and body to hair	Only to be used on dry hair	If sections taken are too large, the hair can become tangled and the heat won't be able to penetrate the mesh of hair

Electrical tools

Health and safety rules when working with electrical equipment

To minimise the risk of damage to your tools and to work safely you should:

- always check that the client is comfortable and not too hot when under a hood dryer
- never place tongs, hot brushes and crimpers directly on the scalp – this will cause serious burns to the client
- make sure the heat is not directed on one spot when using a nozzle attachment on a hairdryer
- always sit tongs and hot brushes on the stand so as not to scorch work surfaces
- always check the heat setting and speed controls before you start blow-drying or setting
- regularly clean the air intake grille at the back of hairdryers to remove dust and fluff to prevent hairdryers from overheating
- put away equipment when not in use
- avoid winding flexes of electrical equipment too tightly when storing
- never store tongs, hot brushes or other electrical equipment until they have cooled down.

You should regularly carry out the following safety checks.

- Make sure all plugs are wired correctly.
- Make sure the dryer cable is safe. (Look for frayed flexes and loose plug tops.)

By law, all electrical equipment should be checked by a qualified electrician every six months.

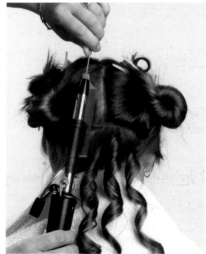

Never place tongs directly on the scalp

Remember
Never use electrical equipment near a water supply or when your hands are wet.

In the salon

Mrs Sanjay always brings her young daughter Poona into the salon with her. Mrs Sanjay usually has a wash and blow-dry, which does not take long, and Poona is happy to sit on her mother's knee while the blow-dry is taking place. Poona is happily swinging her feet watching the hairdresser doing her mother's hair. The styist noticed that this might create a hazard and asked one of the assistants to bring a chair and a book for Poona. Poona sat quietly reading the book whilst the stylist finished her mother's hair.

- In your group, discuss the potential environmental hazards that had been avoided in this situation.

Dressing-out techniques

Dressing out a blow-dry

Only dress out a blow-dry if the hair is completely dry. Even if the hair is only slightly damp, it will go back to its original shape, lose its springiness and then you will not achieve the style you want. To dress out a blow-dry:

1   make sure the hair is completely dry

2   tong or hot brush if more movement is required

3   loosen the blow-dry by running your fingers through the hair

4   apply backcombing if required

5   use a dressing-out comb to lift, smooth and shape the hair

6   check the balance of the style by using your mirror and turning the client's head to view the style from different angles.

Reality check!

Avoid changing from the style you planned, otherwise you are doomed to fail.

Backcombing and teasing

If you want to add height and width to a set or blow-dry when dressing, backcomb the hair. If you do not want to add too much height, but want to remove roller marks from the hair, tease the hair into shape.

If the hair is very thick, section off the hair so that you begin at the nape area. Take a section of hair and hold between the first two fingers and thumb, place your dressing comb into the hair about halfway up and push the hair back towards the roots. The amount of times you do this on a mesh of hair will determine how much backcombing you put into the hair.

When teasing the hair, use the prongs on a dressing out comb. Since these prongs are far apart they will allow some of the hair to fall through without being affected. Again, if the hair is very thick, section the hair off and begin at the nape area working upwards towards the crown.

Always consult with your client about how firm they require the end result and confirm the finished look by using the back mirror to show them all angles of the style.

Back brushing

Back brushing is carried out in the same way as backcombing only you are swapping the comb for a brush. It is best to use a flat bristle brush as this will not tear or damage the hair. Again, if the hair is very thick, section the hair off and work in

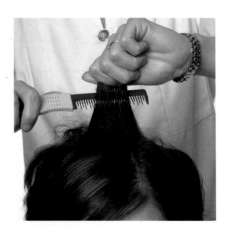

Backcombing

sections. By choosing to back brush instead of backcombing you can cover a greater area of hair and it produces a slightly softer effect.

Applying finishing products, taking into account critical influencing factors

You have looked at the different types of styling products that are available to you (refer to pages 132–133). What you need to consider at this stage is what products you will use to help you to achieve the finished result.

Most products can be used on wet or dry hair and will give very different effects on both.

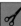

In the salon

Mandi came into the salon to have her hair trimmed into the short, textured, crop that she usually has. During the consultation she explained that she has difficulty in achieving the same look that she leaves the salon with. She has tried using wax to get the texture in her hair but always ends up putting too much on.

- What other products could you recommend to her that she might find easier to use that would achieve the same result?

Finishing products are:

- dressing creams
- wax
- oils
- gel.
- sprays

Finishing products can also be used to help hide any critical influencing factors (see page 144).

If a client has very fine hair, use a product to give the appearance of thickness and bulk to her hair. If the client has dry, fluffy or coarse hair, a finishing cream or oil will give the hair shine and lustre.

Some critical influencing factors cannot always be hidden with styling or products. When they cannot be hidden with styling or products make sure that you adapt your styling (end result) so that you work with the problems. For example, if you have a client who has very fine, straight hair, you would find it difficult to achieve a really textured look.

Confirm the finished look with the client, giving the correct after-care advice

Throughout the service you should be communicating constantly with your client.

- Confirm the style before you begin.
- Check the client is comfortable under the dryer (if relevant).
- Check that you have achieved the intended shape, direction and amount of volume required.
- Is there enough hairspray on the hair?

Finally, the most important question – ask your client whether she likes the end result! The client may have a few suggestions and it is important to listen to and respect her wishes. If, however, you strongly disagree, explain why and come to a compromise.

Check it out

Make a list of the products you have available to you in the salon and look at the instructions on the packaging to see when and how the different styling products can be used. How many of the products can be used on either wet or dry hair, or both?

Remember

It is important to look at your client's hair both before and after you have shampooed the hair so that you can identify any potential problems and address them with your products and styling techniques.

Remember

Before using any of these products you need to read manufacturer's instructions for application and the amount to use.

Check it out

In your group, think of how your different products can be used to help hide any critical influencing factors. You will need to make a list of the factors that you have to consider and then how you would overcome them with your product.

After-care advice

Giving your client after-care advice is an important part of the overall service. You do not want to produce something in the salon that the client will never be able to achieve again – that will only dishearten her!

Explain to the client what you are doing throughout the service. What tools and equipment you are using and why you are using them. Show her the correct angle at which to hold the hairdryer and brush. Explain what products you are using why you are using them, and what you hope to achieve by using them. Show the client the amount of product you are using and the benefits of the product.

If you give good after-care advice, your client is more likely to purchase the products that you have recommended from your salon.

Client care

Check the client is comfortable.

Check heat settings on dryer.

Make sure no pins or grips are marking the client's skin.

Make sure you time how long the client is under the dryer for

Dress long hair

H10.4

Dressing long hair is all about controlling the hair, sectioning off the hair not required at various stages, and secure pinning.

Dressing long hair can be as easy or as complicated as you wish to make it! Some of the simpler hair-up styles can look very effective, for example, the scalp plait. You could use added ornamentation to dress up the plait. Other hair-up techniques may look more complicated, but if you break them into simple step-by-step stages and work in a methodical manner, you will be able to reproduce all of the styles shown in this element.

What you will learn	

- Preparing your client for dressing long hair
- Choosing products and equipment suitable for dressing long hair
- Critical influencing factors
- Controlling and securing long hair
- Checking and confirming the balance of the style to the client's satisfaction

Preparing your client for dressing long hair

When consulting with your client prior to the service, follow the consultation checklist shown on page 139. Other questions that you need to consider are:
- Does the hair need to be set to achieve the desired result?
- Can I achieve the amount of curl needed by dry setting the hair?
- How much time does the client have?
- How long is the style expected to last?
- Is there enough hair (length and thickness) to enable me to achieve the end result?
- Will the chosen style suit the client's face and personality?

If your client has straight hair and would like it up with some curls on the top, you would need to set the hair. If a client wanted a straight, sleek style, then you would not need to set the hair prior to dressing.

It is always useful to have a style book showing long hair styles so that you can confirm the required look with your client.

It is also important to check with the client while you are putting her hair up that she is happy with what you are doing and it is how she expected her hair to look. It is no good waiting until the end and then discovering that it is not going to suit the dress she is wearing or is not going to be appropriate for the occasion that she is going to.

Choosing products and equipment suitable for dressing long hair

What you will need:

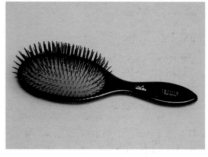

- a wide, flat bristle brush (Isinis or paddle brush) for smoothing over the hair
- hair grips for securing the hair
- fine pins – useful for creating a smooth finish, tucking in ends, and so on
- covered bands – for securing plaits without damaging the hair
- tail comb and dressing comb for creating final finish
- mousse or gels – can be used if the hair is wet and then dried to give a firm hold
- dressing cream – will help produce a sleek appearance on dry hair
- shine spray – for evening hair-up looks it puts a soft shine on to the hair
- hairspray – a light-hold hairspray will aid in the dressing out of the style
- gel spray – for a firmer hold when the style is completed, also good for producing spiky finishes.

An Isinis or paddle brush

Remember

Always read the manufacturer's instructions when using styling products. These will instruct you on how much product to use and if you are to apply the product to wet or dry hair.

Critical influencing factors

When deciding on which style to dress the client's hair, take into account the following factors.

- Density or thickness of the hair – very fine hair may look 'gappy' if the wrong style is chosen; very thick hair may look too bulky to put up into a vertical roll.
- Hair texture – if the hair is very coarse in texture, depending on the style required, the hair might have to be straightened to smooth or set to form soft curls.
- Hair length – if the client has long hair which is layered, you may find that short pieces of hair will fall out from the plait.
- Head and face shape – if the client has a high forehead, don't scrape the hair back too severely from the face. If the client has a long face shape, do not give her a style with too much height which makes the face look even longer.

When considering head and face shapes, your aim is to achieve balance. The idea is to draw the eye away from the least flattering point and towards the balance of the style. Look at the four face shapes below.

Oval face shape

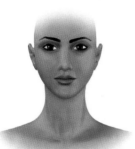

Round face shape

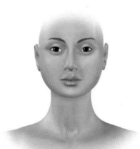

Square face shape

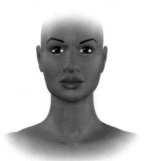

Oblong face shape

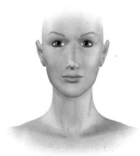

Think about how the hairstyles shown compliment each of the face shapes.

Oval face shape

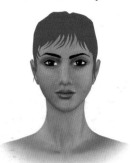

Will suit any hairstyle

Round face shape

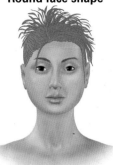

Lots of height, half fringe and soft tendrils to hide roundness at jaw line

Square face shape

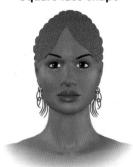

Corners need to be 'cut off' when dressing the hair i.e. fringe and soft tendrils to soften the squareness

Oblong face shape

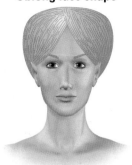

Width required to balance out the length no extra height, as this will elongate the face

Controlling and securing long hair

Dressing long hair requires secure pinning of the hair in such a way that the grips are not visible to anyone looking at the hair. The grips should not be so firm as to cause discomfort to your client, but should be firm enough for the style to hold.

The secret to dressing long hair is not to be afraid of the amount of hair that you are working with and using the right tools and equipment for the job.

It is a good idea to practise your long hair techniques on a block first so that you get used to handling long hair, working with your equipment and learning to secure the hair firmly without causing discomfort to the client.

With most long haired work it is a good idea to secure all the hair that you are not working on out of the way. This will allow you to see where you are working and you will not be trying to hold fistfuls of hair in one go (unless you have very large hands!).

> **Reality check!**
>
> It is unhygienic to put pins in your mouth while dressing long hair. By using your teeth to open pins you could break your teeth! Pins also harbour germs – every time you put a pin in your mouth you are also putting hundreds of germs into your mouth.

You will need to make sure that you have all of your equipment to hand so that you are not halfway through pinning up your client's hair to discover you have run out of grips or other equipment.

You will need to check with the client that her hair feels secure but that none of the grips or pins are uncomfortable. You will also need to grip the hair so that you can't see any of the grips and bands unless they are meant to be part of the finished look.

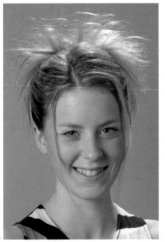
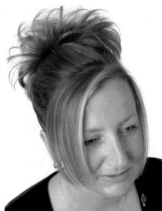
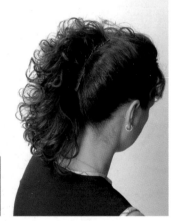

Vertical roll (French pleat)

The vertical roll is a versatile way in which to dress the hair. When you have secured the roll, the ends of the hair may be protruding from the top of the head. You can tuck these ends in, producing a very formal roll, or curl or straighten them to produce a more fashionable, casual look. The hair will require a lot of back brushing (done with a bristle brush) for volume, which is then smoothed over to produce a sleek finish.

Step-by-step French pleat (Vertical roll)

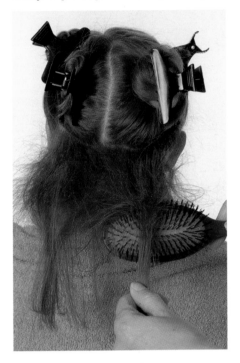

Section the bulk of the hair away and begin to back brush the hair gently from the nape area.

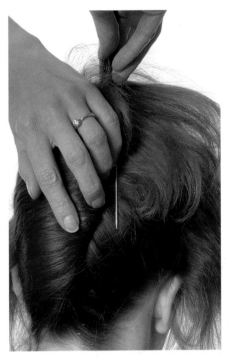

Smooth the hair over to one side and secure slightly off-centre, crossing the hairgrips over one another for firmness.

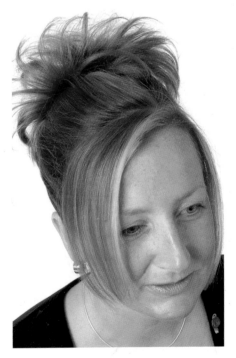

Sweep the hair over from the opposite side and wrap the ends into the pleat.

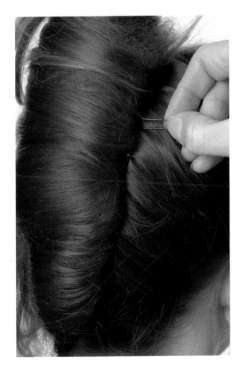

Secure the roll, making sure you anchor the roll to the rest of the hair. Do this by slightly opening the pins before placing into the hair.

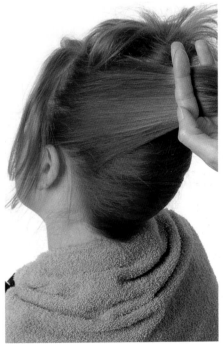

Any shorter sections of the hair can be added into the pleat by smoothing out the back brushing and securing the hair into the pleat.

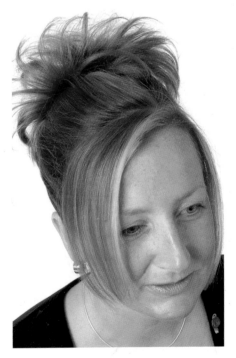

The finished result is then dressed using wax and spray gel.

Scalp plait (French plait)

This way of dressing the hair is frequently used for bridesmaids. The plait can be left plain or you could weave ribbon through to dress up the look.

What you will need:

- tail comb
- brush
- band, ribbon or clip for securing ends.

Step-by-step French plait

A scalp plait

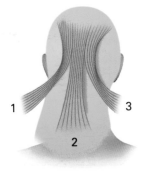

Beginning at the front of the head, take a small triangle of hair and split into three equal strands.

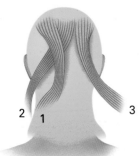

Cross the left strand (1) over the centre one (2) so that the left strand becomes the new centre strand.

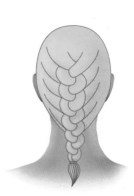

Cross the right strand (3) over the centre strand (1). It is important to keep the tension equal in each strand so that the finished braid will be even.

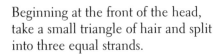

Extra hair here

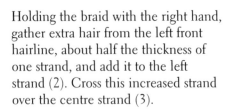

Holding the braid with the right hand, gather extra hair from the left front hairline, about half the thickness of one strand, and add it to the left strand (2). Cross this increased strand over the centre strand (3).

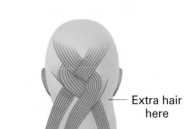

Extra hair here

Repeat the previous step but hold the braid with the left hand and gather the extra hair from the right. Add it to the right strand (1) and pass this new increased strand over the centre strand (2).

Repeat these two steps until there is no loose hair at the hairline. Plait the remainder of the three strands and secure the ends with a clip or band.

Applying products

When you have dressed the hair into a style, you may need to use finishing products to enhance the style, smooth or add texture to your finished look.

In the salon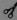

Aisha had completed a lovely vertical roll on Mrs Johnson and had a few stray ends to tuck in. Mrs Johnson had very fine hair and Aisha had done a good job of making the hair look thicker and fuller. She had come to the end of her appointment time so grabbed the nearest product that came to hand, which was gel. When she had applied the gel she realised that it made the hair look 'wet' and had separated the hair so it ended up looking gappy!

- What would have been a better product for Aisha to have chosen in this instance?

If you are using sprays, protect your client's face. Either use your hand to stop any of the product coming into contact with the client's face or use a clear plastic face shield if your salon has one.

Checking and confirming the balance of the style to the client's satisfaction

When you have completed your hair-up design, check that you have achieved the intended shape and balance and that the client is happy with the end result. To do this you will need to check the shape and balance of the 'hair-up' design from all angles. It is important to do this as other people and the client will not just be looking at the hair from one direction. Check that you have not left any flat spots or gaps in the hair. You will need to use a back mirror to show the client her hair from all angles.

When showing the client her hair, you should show both profiles (sides), the back and crown of the style. By doing this you can get her to confirm that she is happy with the end result and she will know that her hair looks as good from the back as it does from the front.

General after-care advice

As part of the complete service give your client the correct after-care advice on her hair. Hair-up styles are usually meant for one night only. However, some clients like to keep their hair up longer if they can and other clients may have their hair put up once a week and have a comb out to tidy up their hair in between visits.

After-care advice for a one-off, hair-up style

If you have put the client's hair up early on in the day and it has to last right through to the evening, give her the following advice.

- Re-tong any tendrils that may lose their curl by the end of the day.
- Use a small prong comb to lift, tease or gently backcomb any areas that may require it (demonstrate the techniques to the client).

- Re-apply hairspray in the evening to ensure the style will last.
- Advise the client to stay away from moisture (hot baths), as this will make the hair drop.
- You might like to give the client a few extra grips, just in case! She should not need them if the hair is secured correctly, but it will give her a comfort zone and show thoughtfulness on your part.

After-care advice for regular weekly clients

Some clients (usually older) may only have their hair washed and set once a week and have a comb out in between each visit.

- When using hairspray, advise clients to spray the hair from a good distance so that there is no build-up of hairspray on their hair.
- Use a prong comb to lift, tease or gently backcomb any flat spots.
- They shouldn't have very hot baths and should protect their hair when in the shower as the moisture will make the style collapse.
- When they do have their hair taken down for shampooing, it will require a thorough brush through to remove all of the loose natural hair fall that cannot escape when the hair is up.
- Explain to them about the amount of hair a person loses on average per day, so they will not worry that they are losing too much hair. Explain that the hair gets caught up and cannot fall away because of the way they wear their hair. This means that when it is taken down there will be a lot of natural hair fall in one go.
- Offer advice on the best types of products for them to use during the week to keep the shine and lustre of the hair.
- You can offer advice about the best brushes and combs to use for their hair.
- You can suggest the types of clips, pins and grips that are best to secure their hair with and that will not cause any damage.

All of this advice and any other top tips that you might have are all part of offering a complete service to your client.

Your questions answered

If I have begun a styling treatment with a client and halfway through realise that I am using the wrong product, what should I do?
If you have used the wrong product and it is going to have an adverse effect on the client's hair, take her to the basin and wash the product out of the hair. Alternatively, you may find that the product works well with the client's hair. You will have to read the manufacturer's instructions to work out whether you think you can use the product on the client's hair.

If I have a client with very fine hair and she does not like styling products on her hair, what can I do to achieve volume and body in her hair?
You will have to adapt your styling techniques to take this into account. Make sure you use the right brushes to help you to achieve maximum lift in the hair. Instead of offering a blow-dry, you could suggest a wet or dry set to achieve the extra volume.

Test your knowledge

1   Identify four safety considerations when using hairspray.

2   What is a manufacturer's risk assessment sheet?

3   Describe three health and safety considerations when using electrical equipment.

4   What does 'COSHH' stand for?

5   What range of protective equipment should be available for clients?

6   Why is it important to have good posture when working on a client?

7   Why it is important to keep your work area clean and tidy?

8   Name three methods of sterilisation and explain what equipment they can be used on.

9   What effect does humidity have on the hair?

10 Why should the hair be allowed to cool prior to dressing out?

11 How can critical influencing factors have an effect on your work?

12 List three potential critical influencing factors.

13 Why is it important to read manufacturer's instructions when using products?

14 What are the three main types of setting techniques used?

15 Why is the direction of the airflow important when drying the hair?

Cut hair using basic techniques

Unit H6

This unit is the core of your hairdressing qualification. It will guide you through the skills you will need to learn to be able to cut hair. You must master these skills before you can become a professional hairdresser.

The unit looks at the different cutting tools, their uses and effects. It also covers safety, hair-cutting techniques and the cutting of wet and dry hair. You will also consider critical influencing factors – hair textures, hair growth patterns, and head and face shapes.

What you will learn

- Maintain effective and safe methods of working when cutting hair H6.1
- Cut hair to achieve a variety of looks H6.2

Maintain effective and safe methods of working when cutting hair

H6.1

It is essential that you work safely and effectively when cutting hair. One of the requirements of this element is that you ensure your work standards meet health and safety laws and regulations for both the client and yourself. By following these laws and regulations you will help to minimise the risk of cross-infection and infestation.

You should be able to organise yourself and your equipment so that your tools are suitable to achieve the desired look and your work methods minimise the risk of damage to tools and equipment. Time spent on the preparation of the client and the duration of the treatment must be within the timescale required by the salon.

What you will learn

- Client care during a cutting service
- Health and safety issues
- Choosing the right tools and using them correctly
- Good organisation and time management
- Health, hygiene and sterilisation

Client care during a cutting service

Gowning

Throughout the hairdressing service, it is your responsibility to make sure that your client remains comfortable: having hair cut and styled is a pleasurable experience. As part of this service, you must make sure that you gown your client correctly so that hair cuttings do not go onto the client's clothing or cause her any irritation.

Some stylists prefer to gown the client after the consultation so that they can see how the client dresses, which gives the stylist an idea of style suitability.

When you are ready to begin the service, you are then ready to gown the client.

- For a cut on wet hair, first use a normal cutting gown. Over this place a towel then a plastic disposable cape on top (this double protection will ensure the client does not get wet). When you have completed the shampoo, towel-dry the client's hair and replace the plastic cape with a cutting collar.
- When cutting dry hair, you should use a cutting gown and then place a cutting collar around the client's neck. Using a neck brush, gently brush in downwards strokes to remove the hair cuttings from the client's face and neck. You must make sure that you clean your neck brush on a regular basis to prevent any cross-infection or infestation between clients.

Positioning the client

The positioning of the client is very important as it can affect the line and balance of the haircut.

Once the client is seated and you are ready to cut, check that she is comfortable and is sitting correctly. If the client has her legs crossed, this will encourage her to lean to one side – with one shoulder up and one shoulder down – and this will throw you off line when cutting, resulting in an uneven finish.

The client should be sitting with the small of her back against the back of the chair and with both feet on the floor or on a footrest. This will ensure that she is sitting squarely in the chair and not lopsided.

Reality check!

If hair cuttings are sticking to the client's skin and are difficult to remove, you can use a small amount of talc.

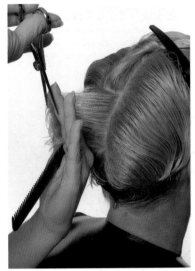

Plastic cape and towel replaced by a cutting collar

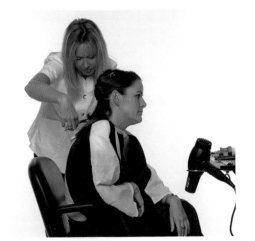

Incorrect sitting position

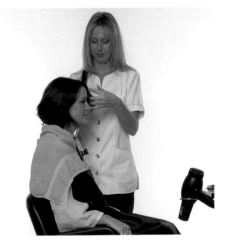

Correctly seated

Positioning – you the stylist

You also need to consider your own posture and position when you are working at your workstation.

Some salons may have their workstations situated close together. You then have a trolley alongside you, which will take up space. If you work on a client without bending your knees, you may find that you will be bumping into your work colleague. It will also put a strain on your back if you are not standing in the correct position and could result in spinal problems and fatigue.

Check it out

Discuss with your colleagues the correct and incorrect ways of positioning yourself and your client so that you reduce the risk of possible injury and fatigue while you are working.

Health and safety issues

Every client must be treated with care and attention from the beginning to the end of her treatment. Good health and safety practices must apply to all clients.

It is essential to keep your work area clean, tidy, and free of waste. Hair cuttings should be swept away and disposed of in a bin, not piled up in the corner of the room. Tea, coffee and magazines should be removed from your workstation in preparation to receive your next client. Remove any used product packaging and dispose of in the relevant place. Make sure equipment is allowed to cool and is correctly stored.

Spillages

All spillages should be mopped up immediately and not left for others. It is your responsibility under the Health and Safety at Work Act to ensure the environment is safe for colleagues and clients.

Hazards chart

Hazard	Ways to avoid it	When referral may be necessary
Spillages	Take care when mixing products. Mop up any excess water after shampooing	If the spillage is corrosive or an irritant
Slippery floors	Sweep up hair immediately after cutting. Mop up any spillages from products	When grease, wax or polish is spilt
Tools or equipment	Store equipment correctly. Allow electrical equipment to cool before storing, making sure there are no trailing wires	When something is broken or defective
Obstructions to access and egress (exit)	Store equipment and products in their correct place after use. Do not obstruct walkways with bags, boxes, etc.	When the object is too heavy to be moved

In the salon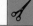

Jenni was putting her client under the hood dryer when she saw that the fittings on the wall were slightly loose. She was in a hurry and forgot to report it to her boss. On her day off, another stylist used the same dryer and as she moved the dryer to put her client under it, the whole unit came away from the wall. Luckily, both the client and the stylist managed to move away in time so they were unhurt.

- What should Jenni have done when she spotted the loose fittings?
- Who should she have reported it to?

Potential hazards in the salon

Other hazards that you may come across in the day-to-day running of a salon include:

- hair cuttings not swept up from previous client
- trailing leads from electrical equipment
- client incorrectly gowned for a service

- bags or coats left on the floor
- spillages from previous treatments, for example, a water spray used during a cut might have left the floor wet.

Choosing the right tools and using them correctly

You will need a variety of tools and equipment to help you complete a haircut successfully. You need to understand their uses, the methods of sterilisation for them, and how to use them safely.

Scissors

The most important piece of equipment for a hairdresser. Scissors vary in design, size and price. The best way to find out if a pair of scissors suits you is to pick them up and see if they are comfortable to hold. Hands and fingers vary in size, so holding them is the only way to tell if they suit you.

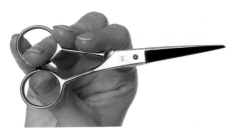
Standard haircutting scissors

The cutting comb

This is an essential piece of equipment. Combs are available in different sizes to suit your needs and the type of hair you are working with. If you are using clippers, you will require a cutting comb that is more flexible than the normal straight, rigid cutting comb. The flexibility of the comb used for clipper work or a scissor-over-comb cut allows you to work closely and follow the client's head shape.

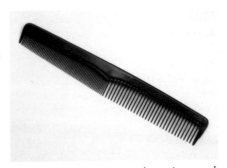
A cutting comb

Thinning scissors

The purpose of thinning scissors is to remove bulk from the hair without removing length. There are two main types: those that have two notched (serrated) blades and those that have one ordinary blade and one notched blade. The spaces between the notches vary in size and determine the amount of hair that is removed.

Scissors with two notched blades will take off more hair than thinning scissors with one notched blade and one ordinary blade. Notched scissors with wide spaces between them will remove more hair than thinning scissors with smaller spaces between them.

Thinning scissors are also called:

- texturising scissors
- serrated scissors
- notched scissors.

They should be looked after in the same way as standard scissors.

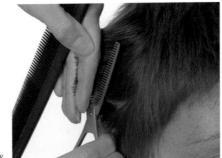

Thinning scissors

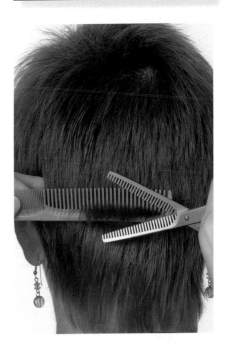

Razors

The most commonly used razors are open or cut-throat razors, shapers or safety razors.

The more modern razor has a disposable blade and a guard over it so only a small amount of the hair is cut. This also gives added protection and helps prevent cutting the client's skin.

The disposable razor is easy to use. Once the blade becomes blunt it can be replaced quickly and easily ensuring you do not tear the client's hair.

Razoring is always carried out on wet hair as this reduces the friction on the hair and is less painful for the client. (Razoring dry hair pulls and is very uncomfortable!)

Look after razors in the same way as scissors, making sure that you dispose of used blades – known as sharps – in a sharps bin (see page 173).

Electric and rechargeable clippers

Clippers are generally used for short, graduated styles. They are used on dry hair only. They can give the effect of a scissor-over-comb cut and are used in both men's and ladies' hairdressing.

Clippers work by the bottom blade remaining fixed whilst the top blade moves at a very high speed. You can add clipper attachments to vary/alter the length of the cut, depending on the size of the grade that you attach – the higher the number is on the grade, the longer the hair will be; the lower the number on the grade, the shorter the hair will be.

Rechargeable clippers are generally smaller than electric clippers and give a closer haircut. They can be used to trim behind the backs of the ears or other hard-to-reach areas. Different heads are available for these clippers for use in hair sculpting. After use they should be replaced on their stand for recharging.

You should oil both types of clippers after every use to maintain them and to make sure that they run smoothly. This will help to prolong their life.

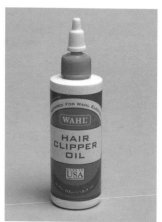

Use clipper oil after each use of the clippers

Neck brush, water spray and sectioning clips

You will require these items when cutting.

- Neck brush – removes cuttings from the client. You should use this throughout the haircut. To maintain good health and hygiene standards and care for your equipment, you will need to wash your neck brush in warm soapy water on a regular basis.
- Water spray – used to damp down hair that dries too quickly. If the hair is allowed to dry out halfway through, you will not achieve even tension. You should empty the water from your water spray on a regular basis. This will help to prevent the water becoming stagnant or leaking onto other tools and equipment.
- Sectioning clips – divide/section large quantities of hair. These can be sterilised by immersing them in barbicide solution for the manufacturer's recommended time.

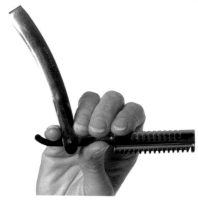

> **Reality check!**
>
> Razors must be kept sharp at all times – if the blade becomes blunt this will tear the hair and cause discomfort to the client.

Razor

> **Reality check!**
>
> - Check your clippers regularly to make sure that they have not been knocked out of alignment. (If the moveable top blade is above the bottom still blade, this will cut the client.)
> - If your clippers are out of line, check the manufacturer's instructions to re-set them.
> - Special sterilising sprays should be used on your clippers after every use.
> - Do not use clippers with broken teeth, as they can pull, tear or cut the scalp.

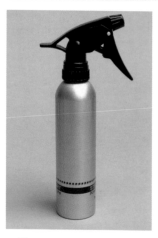

Use a water spray to ensure that you keep the hair damp as you cut

Using tools that are safe and fit for their purpose

It may help you to have a daily ritual, either when you get your equipment out or when you pack it away, or a quick checklist to ensure that you do not overlook any safety issues.

Equipment that you are using should not be damaged or broken in any way. You need to make sure that teeth are not missing from combs, hairbrushes should be free of any loose hairs, and all equipment should be sterilised on a regular basis.

You will also need to check that electrical equipment is safe to use by checking that the cables and plugs do not have frayed wires. You will need to check the water levels on steamers and temperature controls on other electrical equipment.

Using equipment safely to minimise the risk of damage to tools

When working with electrical equipment, you need to make sure that you follow good codes of practice. To ensure that you are working safely, use the following list. (This list is not exhaustive.)

- Do not use electrical equipment with wet hands.
- Check plugs and wires are not loose/damaged before use.
- Use the correct piece of equipment for the job you want to do.
- Replace equipment carefully after use, ensuring it is clean and in good working order.
- Switch off electrical items when not in use and unplug to avoid trailing wires.
- When putting away electrical equipment, avoid folding flexes too tightly as this will cause them to short circuit if they get damaged.

In accordance with the Electricity at Work Regulations 1989, all electrical equipment should be checked every six months by a qualified electrician, who should then place a sticker on the equipment to show that it is safe to use. The salon should keep a record of the visit for future reference.

Check it out

Make a list of what you think are the important safety issues relating to your equipment that you would need to check on a daily basis.

Check it out

What would you do if you accidentally cut a client? Discuss this together before you read on.

In the salon

Vaz was using an extremely old set of clippers on his client. He forgot to make sure that the clipper blades were in alignment and as a result cut his client's neck. This not only caused pain and discomfort to his client, it also put him at risk from cross infection.

- How would you deal with this sort of accident?
- Where should you record the details of this accident?

What to do if you accidentally cut a client

- Put on protective gloves.
- Apply a small amount of pressure to stem the blood flow, either with a pad or towel.
- Call for a first aider.
- Remain calm while the first aider is coming and speak reassuringly to your client.
- Fill in an accident report form – this ensures that you have a record of what happened should this be required for future reference. You should also inform the salon manager or your trainer.

Protecting yourself

For your own health and safety, you need to be aware of potential hazards to yourself, for example, the possibility of cross-infection of Hepatitis and the HIV virus from exposure to blood.

Prevention is better than cure. You can have a vaccination for Hepatitis A and B if you are in a high-risk group, of which hairdressing could be considered one. You are at risk because of the potential of cuts from scissors and sharps – this increases the risk of exposure to blood. The use of protective gloves may be necessary as a preventative measure.

If you have an open cut, make sure that it is covered with a dressing so that if you accidentally cut a client you will not be at risk from cross-infection of blood.

Good organisation and time management

You need to be prepared for every client, which means you must have the right tools available to cover every aspect of the hairdressing services that your salon offers.

Good organisation means:

- a full trolley layout
- all equipment is clean and sterilised
- record cards, style books and shade charts are at hand ready for the consultation
- a tidy working area that is free of excess waste (cut hair), has no slippery surfaces or potential hazards. Remove any equipment not needed, for example, free-standing climazones.

Using your time effectively

You should always be organised and ready for the client's arrival. Each salon has its own time allocation for services offered, for example, most experienced stylists will allow only 20 minutes for a dry cut and a maximum of 45 minutes for a cut and blow-dry. As a trainee, you should be aware of the time it takes you to cut a client's hair. It is expected that you will take longer than an experienced stylist for your first cuts.

It is important to have all of the relevant equipment ready to hand before you receive your client. This will also help you to use your time effectively.

Before you receive your client, you will need to get out the relevant record card and look at the appointment page to see what service the client is having. By doing this you will then be able to 'set' yourself up to receive the client with all of the equipment that you are going to need.

Working within a commercially viable time

You will have researched how long your salon or training establishment allows for the services that it offers and this will be the timeframe that you will be trying to work within.

By breaking the service down into fragments, it should show you how much time you will have to spend on each stage and give you a timescale to work towards. What you do not want to do is watch the clock. This will not only get you flustered but will also make the client feel uncomfortable. All you need to do is be aware if you are on track and not running over on one part of the service, which will have a knock-on effect on the rest of the day's services.

Reality Check!

When cutting children's hair, you need to be aware that they may not be able to sit as still as you would like. Their attention span may be shorter and their movements sudden. Try to give children something to occupy them, such as a book or toy. This will help to keep them sitting for a little longer and prevent any cuts or injuries to yourself or the child.

Check it out

Find out how long your salon allows for the following services:

- wet cut
- cut and blow-dry
- dry trim
- highlights
- perm.

Check it out

Pick one of the services that your salon offers and write down the time that is allocated for this service. Make a list of all the things you will need to do to complete this service from beginning to end. Remember to take into account your time for consultation and shampooing.

Health, hygiene and sterilisation

You have looked at how to prevent cross-infection of blood by covering any open cuts when working. Tools must be sterilised to ensure that you minimise any risk of cross-infection or infestation that can be passed on by your equipment. The table below shows the best methods of sterilising tools used in cutting.

Tool/equipment		Method of cleaning/sterilisation
Neck brush		Wash bristles in soapy water and then immerse in barbicide solution for specified time (20 minutes) and allow to dry
Water spray		Wash out bottle with barbicide solution. Rinse well before use
Sectioning clips		Wash regularly in soapy water and immerse in barbicide solution for specified time (20 minutes)
Cutting comb		Wash in hot, soapy water to remove dirt and grease. Ultra-violet cabinet, barbicide solution
Scissors		Ultra-violet cabinet, autoclave, alcohol/sterile wipes or sprays
Thinning scissors		Ultra-violet cabinet, autoclave, alcohol/sterile wipes or sprays
Razor		Ultra-violet cabinet, autoclave, alcohol/sterile wipes or sprays (except blades)
Clippers and attachments		Remove loose hair cuttings and then spray blades with sterilising clipper spray

Disposal of used sharps

'Sharps' is the term used in hairdressing to describe the blades used in safety razors.

Salons should supply a yellow sharps bin for the disposal of blades. It is a hard plastic bin that cannot be pierced and is collected by the local health authority to be incinerated. If you put a disposable blade from your razor/hair shaper in an ordinary black bin liner, the person emptying the bin may cut themselves.

Check it out

Investigate the sharps bin in your salon or training institution.

- Where is it kept?
- What colour is it?
- Who collects it for emptying and how often is it collected?

Personal hygiene

As well as looking after your tools and equipment, you must also make sure that you take your own personal hygiene into account to minimise the risk of cross-infection and infestation.

You may be required to wear a uniform in many establishments. This may be so that you follow the college's or salon's health and safety policies, which will have taken into account safety and hygiene points.

Some hygiene requirements that should be expected:

*   long hair to be worn up to cut down on the risk of cross-infection
*   minimum amount of jewellery to be worn so that water and hair cuttings will not become trapped underneath causing bacteria to grow
*   flat enclosed shoes to be worn for health and safety purposes
*   sterilise all tools and equipment after each client
*   make sure your personal presentation and hygiene are of a very high standard
*   make sure you use a breath freshening spray if you smoke or have had strong-flavoured food (e.g. curry, garlic or chilli) the night before
*   wear cotton tops in the summer and use a good deodorant
*   always wash your hands after every client and after a trip to the bathroom
*   always keep cuts and open wounds covered with a plaster.

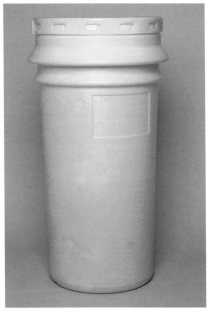

Sharps bin

Cut hair to achieve a variety of looks   H6.2

In this element you will be looking at how to complete a thorough consultation, the different cutting techniques and factors that you have to take into consideration to complete a successful haircut, and giving the correct after-care advice to a client.

What you will learn
• Consultation   • Critical influencing factors   • Preparing for cutting   • Cutting techniques   • Step-by-step guides to the one-length look   • Step-by-step guides to layered looks   • Adapting your cutting techniques to take into account critical influencing factors   • Client satisfaction   • After-care advice

Consultation

Before cutting the client's hair, you should carry out a thorough consultation with her. There are a number of important factors to consider before the service can take place and these can be addressed by completing a consultation cutting checklist before you begin. A suggested checklist is given on page 175.

You will be checking the hair and scalp for any infections or infestations (see table on pages 92–4 in Unit G7) that may not allow you to carry out the service. You will also be looking at the hair growth patterns, hair texture, density, the shape of the client's face and the elasticity of the hair, as these are critical influencing factors that you will need to identify.

When you carry out the consultation, it is a good idea not to gown up your client straightaway. Seeing the way she dresses will help you to determine the personality

Check it out

Find several different formats of consultation card. Some may be in electronic form. What are the particular features that occur each time? Make a note of these for your portfolio.

and the type of lifestyle she may lead, for example, a client who is conservatively dressed may not appreciate bright pink hair!

The use of style books will help to give both you and the client a clear picture of the end result that you hope to achieve.

Consultation checklist

Client's name: _____ Tel. no: _____

Address: _____ _____

Date: _____ Stylist: _____

Factors to consider

Client requirements:
What are your client's wishes? _____
Their expectations of the haircut? _____

Face shape: Square ☐ Round ☐ Oval ☐ Oblong ☐
Body proportions
Hair type/movement
Has the hair got a wave/curl in it? _____

European ☐ Asian ☐ African Caribbean ☐

Hair texture
Very fine? Very coarse? _____

Abundance of hair
How much hair do you have to work with? _____

Natural growth patterns
Double crown, widow's peak, and so on _____

Hair condition
Porosity and elasticity _____

Client personality/dress/lifestyle _____

Client limitations
Check whether the client will be able to maintain the style at home _____

Suggested style
Use the information gathered above to suggest or guide your client towards a style that you both feel suits his or her needs
_____

Cutting techniques and reasons
List the techniques you are going to use and your reasons for using them. Make sure that the chosen cutting techniques, for example, razoring, suit the hair's condition. (This will also act as a record card of your consultation and the cut for future reference.) _____
_____

Critical influencing factors

A critical influencing factor is anything that you may have to take into account that will have an effect on the end result that you hope to achieve.

Hair density

When you talk about the hair's density, you are referring to the amount of hair that an individual client has per square inch on their head. On some heads of hair you can see the scalp through the hair, which means that the client does not have very dense hair. On other heads, there may be a lot of hair per square inch, meaning the client has very dense hair.

It is sometimes easy to get density and thickness of hair confused. You will need to remember that density refers to the amount of hair on the head and thickness refers to the texture of an individual hair, not the amount of hair the client has.

Hair texture

You should examine the hair's texture very carefully during your consultation with the client because this may affect the cutting technique that you choose to use. If you decide on a particular cutting technique because of the hair's texture, you will have identified a 'critical influencing factor'. For example, if the client has very fine hair, you may choose the club cutting method to increase bulk in the hair. On the other hand, you would not want to increase bulk in thick hair (also a critical influencing factor), so you might choose a thinning technique for this hair texture.

You can identify the texture of the hair by separating a few strands of hair and placing them across the palm of your hand. The texture of the hair usually falls into three categories: fine, medium and thick. You will need to look at the hair closely and decide which one of these categories the hair falls into to determine the hair's texture.

Head and face shapes

When consulting with the client, before deciding on the length of the cut, you should take into consideration the client's head and face shape because these can become critical influencing factors in your choice of length for the cut.

You should be able to see that careful consideration needs to be taken when choosing a style to suit a particular face shape. If you made the wrong choice, you could end up enhancing a feature that the client wants to detract from and not emphasise.

Hair growth patterns

This means the way in which the direction of the hair grows from the roots. On some heads of hair, growth patterns are very apparent. For example, if the client has a cowlick in the middle of her fringe and the fringe has 'jumped up', this will be obvious to you. In another case, the client may have blow-dried her hair so well that she has disguised a double crown or strong hair growth movement.

To identify hair growth patterns, you will need to take fine meshes of hair down around the hairline and secure the rest of the hair out of the way, then look closely at the direction in which the hair is growing. Some hairlines may sit perfectly in the direction that you want them to; others may push in the opposite direction, making it difficult for you to carry out a particular haircut.

You need to look very closely at potential problem areas when the hair is dry and take a second look as a safeguard if you wet the hair. By deciding to leave length because of the client's hair growth patterns, you will be identifying a critical influencing factor.

Check it out

Gather together some current hair-styling books or magazines and cut out pictures of hairstyles that you think would be appropriate for clients in the following age bands:

- 20–30 years
- 31–40 years
- 41–50 years
- 51+

Note how the hairstyles that you have chosen for the 20–30 years age group would not be suitable for the clients in the 51+ age group. Discuss this in your group.

Check it out

In pairs, look closely at your partner's hair and determine whether your partner has fine, medium or thick textured hair.

Check it out

On a piece of paper, draw the four most common face shapes (round, square, oblong and oval). For each shape, draw the length of cut (including fringes if appropriate) that you feel would best suit that face shape.

Check it out

Working in pairs, look at each other's hair growth patterns and try to identify any critical influencing factors.

Imagine that you are going to cut the hair into a one-length look. How would any of the critical influencing factors you have identified affect the cut?

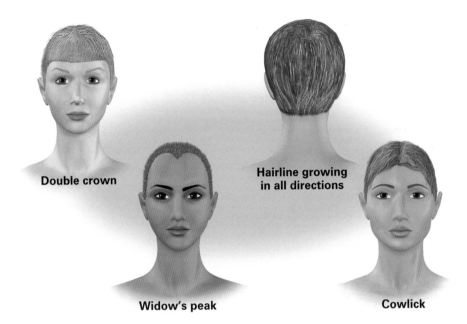

Hair growth patterns to consider and how to overcome them

- The nape hairline grows unevenly – the hair should not be cut above the hairline.
- There is a cowlick in the fringe area – the fringe needs to be made heavier to keep weight to help the hair stay down.
- There is a double crown – the parting may have to be changed to distribute the hair more evenly either side of the head to disguise the double crown.

Elasticity

We test the elasticity of the hair to see how good the internal strength of the hair is. (Remember, porosity testing is to determine the condition of the outside of the hair shaft.) Refer to Unit G7 for hair tests. If the hair was in bad condition, you may not choose to use razoring techniques on the hair. This is because if the hair was very fragile, it may not be able to withstand this method of cutting as it can put extra stress on the hair.

Preparing for cutting

Before you receive clients, check:

- your work area is clean and tidy
- all equipment is to hand and sterile
- client record cards, style books and consultation checklists are ready.

When you receive clients:

- carry out a consultation – complete a cutting checklist to help you to achieve the desired result (see page 175)
- gown them up (see page 166)
- prepare their hair for cutting.

> **Remember**
>
> You need to be aware of the salon's legal requirements when cutting hair and using electrical equipment, for example, the Electricity at Work Regulations.

Hair preparation

During the consultation, it is important to consider whether you are going to complete the cut on wet or dry hair. There are a number of factors you need to take into account when deciding this.

- Cost – in most salons it is usually more expensive for a client to have a wet cut. This is to cover the cost of water, shampoo, conditioners and the extra time taken by the stylist.
- Time – if the client has come in in her lunch hour, she may not have the time to have a cut and blow-dry.
- Influencing factors – some heads of hair may have very awkward hairlines or growth patterns. By wetting the client's hair, it becomes more difficult to identify these growth patterns, as wet hair can be manipulated in any direction. When the hair is dry, the growth patterns are more apparent and you can adapt the cut as necessary.
- Techniques – some cutting techniques require you to cut the hair when wet, for example, razoring, while others such as clippering must be carried out on dry hair.

Advantages and disadvantages of cutting both wet and dry hair

Wet hair		Dry hair	
Advantages	Disadvantages	Advantages	Disadvantages
More precise lines	Client may be uncomfortable if salon temperature is too cool	Hair will be same length when finished	Hair flies everywhere (client comfort)
Hair is easier to manage and control	Unable to see bulk/weight lines in hair (especially permed/naturally curly hair	Easier to see the bulk to be removed from hair	Cut can be uneven
Hair can be manipulated into style during cutting		Easier to identify and remove split ends	Hair can be hard to control and hard to keep even tension
			Client may have greasy/dirty hair

Accurately establishing and following cutting guidelines

When you are ready to begin your cut on the client, you need to make sure that you work in a methodical manner. You will be working through the haircut by dividing the hair into small workable sections.

Firstly, you will need to decide where you are going to begin your haircut. If you are beginning in the nape area, you will need to comb down a fine mesh of hair, this is classed as a section of hair. As you work through the haircut, you will continue to bring down new sections of hair, making sure they are neat and level.

Hair that you are not working on will need to be secured out of the way. The sections of hair should be no more than half an inch deep; this will enable you to see your previous guideline through each section of hair.

By following these guidelines, you will be able to work around the head, using your time to the maximum benefit and ensuring you achieve the desired result.

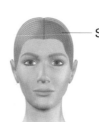 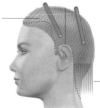

Sectioned hair

Mesh to cut

Correct sectioning
Hair is divided into 4 and secured, an even mesh of hair is taken at the nape, combed smooth ready to cut

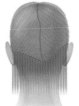 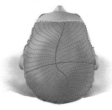

Incorrect sectioning
Uneven sectioning, hair taken from either side, no precise lines, no methodical working method!

Cutting techniques

Club cutting

This method leaves the ends of the hair blunt and level. It is sometimes called the blunt cut. The technique is the most commonly used one for removing length from the hair and is ideal for fine hair, as it gives the appearance of increasing bulk. It can also help to reduce the tendency of the hair to curl.

Club cutting is very suitable for straight and curly hair. Sections are combed through and held with tension, ensuring that the ends of the hair are blunt and level. This technique can be used on hair that is either above or below the shoulders.

Freehand cutting

This technique is mainly used on straight hair when cutting a one-length look. This is because curly hair will not sit in one place; the curl in the hair means it will lift and not remain stationary to allow it to be cut free hand.

As the name of the technique suggests, you do not hold the hair with tension – the hair is combed into place and cut free hand. The freehand technique gives you a truer indication of where the hair will sit when dried because you will not have used tension by pulling the hair down. This is an ideal method to use on fringes as they have a tendency to 'jump up' when dried and is also better suited to one-length looks that are cut above the collar. Cutting hair above the collar length requires a very blunt even line – by combing the hair down flat on to the neck and cutting free hand, you will be able to achieve this precise line.

Step-by-step freehand cutting

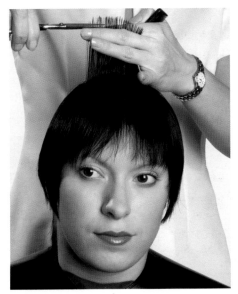

Club cutting

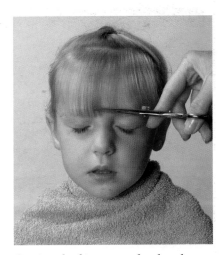

Reality check!

When club cutting, sections taken must be combed through so that the hair is smooth and held with even tension to ensure an even result.

Cutting the fringe area free hand.

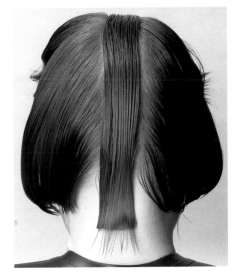

Hair is combed down flat into the nape of the neck.

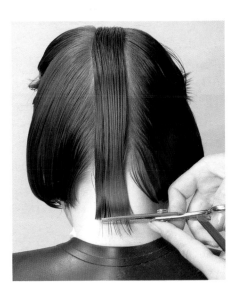

The hair is cut free hand without picking up the section or using tension on the mesh of hair.

Scissor-over-comb

This technique is used to cut hair very short following the natural contours of the head. It is most frequently used in the nape area or around the ears and is often used in men's hairdressing to taper the hair into the hairline.

The technique can be used on wet or dry hair, although you will achieve a better result on dry hair, as the cutting line is clearer.

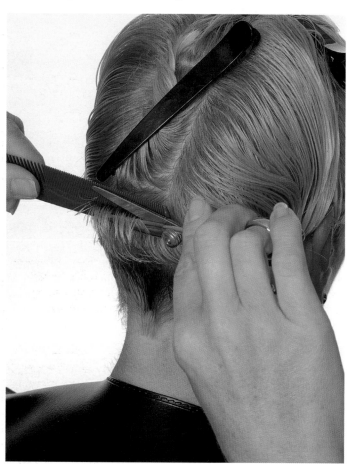

Scissor-over-comb technique

Clipper-over-comb technique

Clipper-over-comb

With clipper-over-comb, clippers are used instead of scissors to give a similar effect to scissor-over-comb. Both techniques allow you to cut the hair shorter than if you were holding the hair between your fingers.

Thinning

There are various cutting techniques that can be used to thin the hair as well as using thinning scissors and razoring techniques (for information on tools, see page 169).

Some of the thinning techniques that you will be using are also referred to as texturising techniques. The thinning method of cutting removes bulk from the hair without removing the overall length. Thinning can be carried out on wet or dry hair. On dry hair, it is more obvious where the bulk/weight is in a haircut (the only exception is when using a razor).

Remember

Only use clippers on dry hair.

Reality check!

You should sterilise and oil your clippers after every client.

Technique		Suitability	Benefit
Weave cutting		Not for the whole head because of size of the meshes of hair. Can be used on wet or dry, long, short, straight or curly hair	Shorter pieces of hair will stand up supporting the remaining hair, creating lift
Pointing/chipping		Ideal for straight hair	Breaks up hard lines in the hair, creating a textured look
Castle cutting		Can be used on wet or dry hair	Breaks up hard lines in the hair
Razoring		Only to be used on wet hair. Not recommended for very fine hair. Ideal for thinning large areas of hair, curly or straight hair	Will encourage the hair to curl. Removes a lot of bulk, leaving the ends soft and feathered
Thinning scissors		Not recommended for very short or very fine hair. Ideal for medium to long hair and for large areas of thinning. Suitable for straight or curly hair	Removes bulk without removing length. Overuse will result in the ends becoming wispy

Thinning techniques

Avoid using thinning techniques on front hairlines, natural partings or the crown area. This may produce unwanted spiky effects.

Step-by step guides to the one-length look

When asked to describe a one-length cut, most people would point to a bob cut on straight hair. However, a one-length cut can be carried out on curly hair (either permed or naturally curl), which would look totally different although it is the same cut. You need to remember that different factors have to be taken into account for every head of hair that you cut. Each client and head of hair is unique. The main purpose of a one-length cut is to keep maximum weight in the hair.

Cutting techniques for a one-length look

There are two main types of techniques to achieve a one-length cut:

- club cutting
- freehand cutting.

Both types of cut can be used on either wet or dry hair.

Step-by-step cutting for straight hair

Section the hair into four (hot-cross bun).

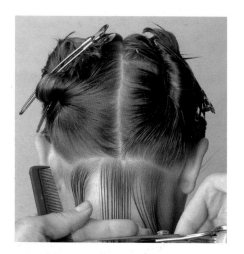

Take a small horizontal section of hair in the nape approximately 1.25 cm wide and cut to the desired length (your guideline).

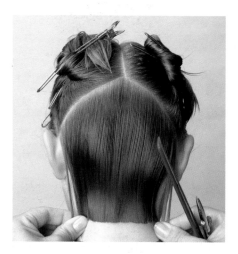

Drop a small sub-section of the hair and cut the new section of hair to the same length using the original guideline. Continue in this way up to the crown area.

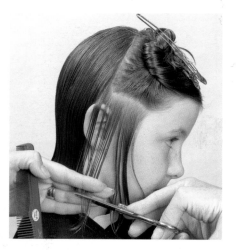

Take a small section from the side and connect it to the back, allowing for the hair to spring up over the ear (slacken off the tension).

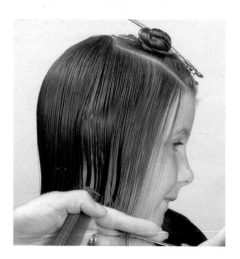

Take a sub-section of 1.25 cm and cut to your guideline. Continue up to the natural parting. Repeat this step.

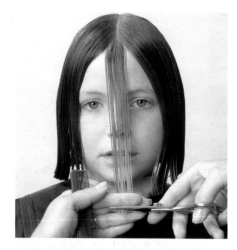

Section the front area and secure unwanted hair. Trim fringe if required or blend the front sections with the rest of the cut.

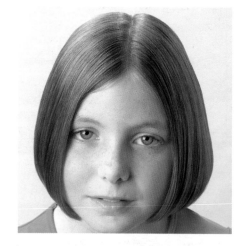

Confirm with the client that the finished style suits her requirements.

Important factors to consider when cutting one-length hair

- Tilt the head forward when cutting the back sections – to prevent unwanted graduation.
- Section evenly – for an accurate cut.
- Keep tension even – for an accurate cut.
- The hairline at the sides is finer than the nape hairline – allow for this hair to 'jump up'.
- Make sure there is no hair caught behind the ear when cutting the sides.

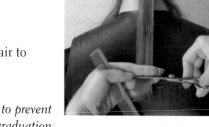

Tilt the head forward to prevent unwanted graduation

Step-by-step cutting of curly hair

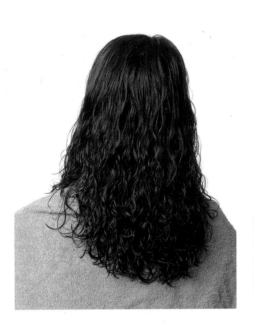

Comb the hair through and look for the amount of natural curl in the hair. Section the hair into four (hot-cross bun).

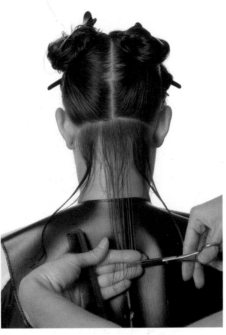

Take a horizontal section and cut to the desired length, remembering the hair will bounce up when dried.

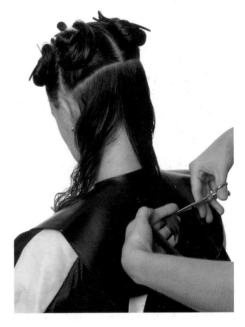

Take a sub-section of hair (1.25 cm) and cut to your guideline. Continue taking sections horizontally to the crown area.

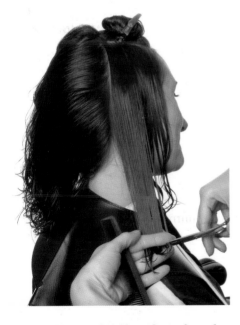

Drop a fine mesh of hair from the side and connect this to the back section.

Repeat the last two steps on the opposite side of the head.

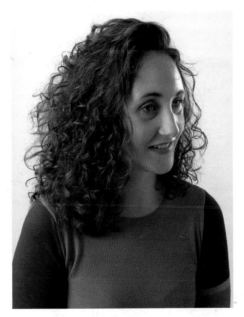

Confirm the finished cut with the client.

Important factors to consider when cutting curly one-length hair

- Allow for the hair to get shorter as the curls dry.
- Apply more tension to your sections to achieve an accurate cut.

Step-by-step guides to layered looks

Uniform layer cut

This technique involves putting layers into the hair following the natural shape of the head. Imagine a client with a crash helmet on – think about how the shape of the helmet follows the shape of the head. In a uniform layer cut, the layers are cut to the same length all over the head, hence its name.

Step-by-step uniform layer cut

Section hair into four (hot cross-bun).

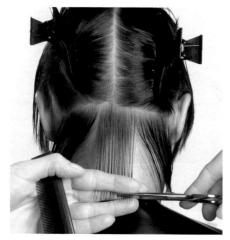

Drop a fine mesh of hair in the nape and cut the baseline to the desired length.

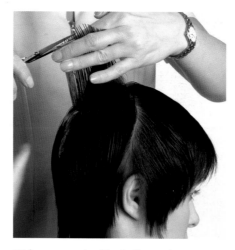

Take a panel of hair from the crown down the middle of the head to the nape baseline. Cut the hair, beginning at the crown at an angle of 90 degrees to the head.

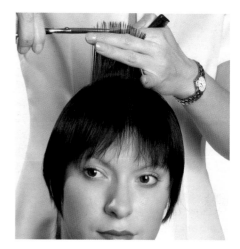

After working in orange sections through the back, go back to the top crown hair and pull up a section of hair 90 degrees to the head and continue to remove the appropriate length.

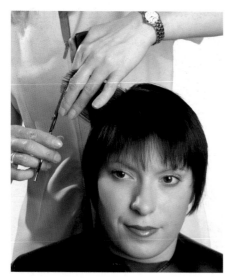

Following the head shape round, continue to cut the hair either side of this section, working towards the front hairline.

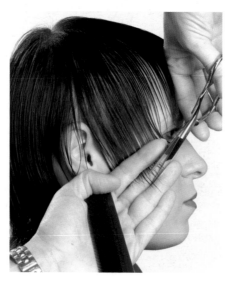

When all inner layers have been cut 90 degrees to the head, go back to the perimeter length and remove any unwanted hair to ensure a clean even shape.

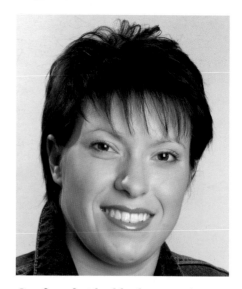

Confirm finished look meets the client's satisfaction.

Graduated layer cut

This technique involves changing the angle of the layers that you are cutting. The angles can be anywhere between 45 and 180 degrees. Increasing or decreasing the amount of angle of the layers will determine the amount of weight left in the hair.

Step-by-step graduated layer cut

Section the hair into four.

Reality check!

- Clean and even sectioning will ensure an accurate cut.
- The steeper the angle you choose to cut at, the more weight/bulk you will add into the hair.

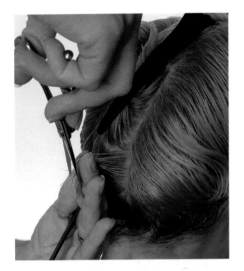

Drop a section of hair in the nape and cut to desired length, at the desired angle, to achieve the graduation required (45 degrees in this instance).

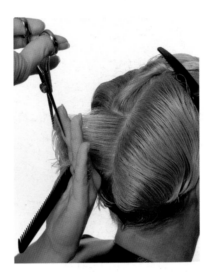

Working in panels, follow this section up the head, maintaining the correct angle to achieve desired graduation.

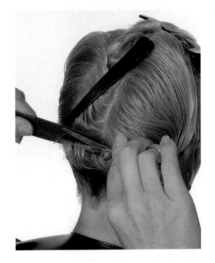

To take the graduated look in 'tighter', scissor-over-comb techniques can be used in the nape area.

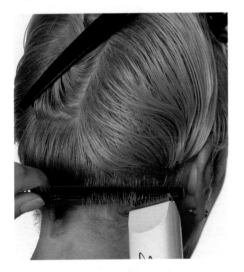

Clipper-over-comb techniques can also be used to remove unwanted length and stray neck hairs to give a shorter, tapered graduated look.

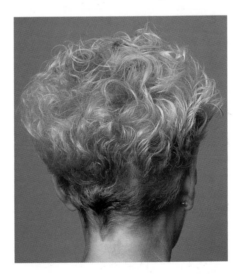

Finished back shape. Check for balance and even distribution of weight.

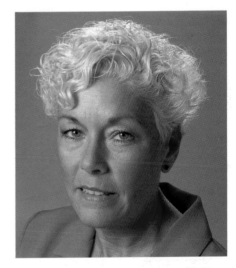

Confirm the finished look with the client.

Step-by-step long-layer cut

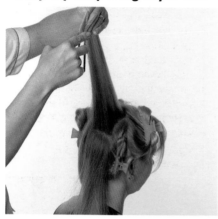

Begin at the centre crown section, holding the hair up at 90 degrees to the head and remove unwanted length.

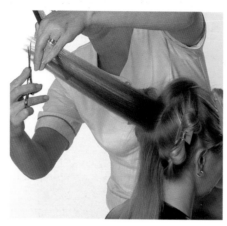

Working in sections down the head, continue to bring sections up to your original section, looking to maintain maximum length through the perimeter of the cut.

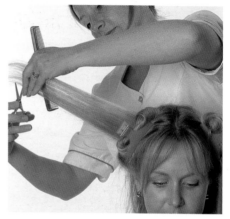

Continue to work through the sides of the cut, pulling the hair up and cutting to blend with the original guideline.

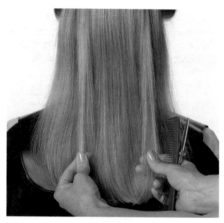

Check the lengths on either side of the head, making sure you have balance and even distribution of weight.

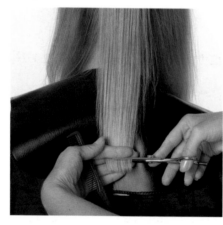

Remove any unwanted length to neaten up the perimeter shape.

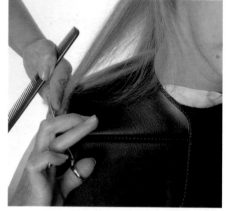

Continue to follow the perimeter length through to the side sections. Tilt the client's head to prevent unwanted graduation.

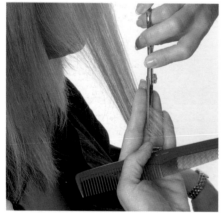

To add shape around the front sections, pull the hair down and forward. Pick a starting point (no higher than the mouth) and blend through to the longer back section.

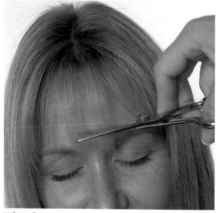

The fringe area can be cut free hand to take into account cowlicks that may make the fringe 'jump up'.

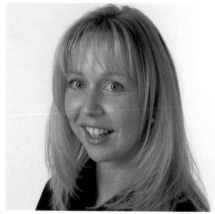

Confirm the finished result with the client.

Adapting your cutting techniques to take into account critical influencing factors

You have looked at cutting methods/techniques and critical influencing factors, now you need to put the two together.

When you are going to carry out a hair cutting service on a client, you will need to establish during your consultation what critical influencing factors (if any) that you have to consider.

It is important to check through the client's hair before and after you shampoo the hair. This is because not all critical influencing factors are apparent on either wet or dry hair. If a client has straightened her hair and you have carried out your consultation on straight hair, when you take her to the basin and wash the hair, you may discover that she has a very strong natural wave in her hair which means that you may need to use a different cutting method to the one you had discussed.

It is important to carry out your consultation on dry hair and then re-check the hair when it is shampooed to make sure you have identified all the potential critical influencing factors.

Client satisfaction

Consulting, checking and confirming the client's satisfaction with the finished cut

As you are progressing through your cut, you will need to adjust the position in which you work around the head.

If you think about a tennis player, he does not stand in one position on the court and stretch to reach the ball; he moves around the court and adjusts his positioning so that he achieves his end result to win the game.

Although heads come in different shapes and sizes, they are all round. If you stand 'square on' to a head of hair and try to cut the hair in this position, you will not achieve a balanced shape.

You will need to move around the head as you work so that you are covering all angles of the haircut. This will help you to achieve an accurate cut, ensuring that you have even distribution of weight and balance throughout the style.

Crosschecking your haircut as you work is another factor that will help you to achieve even distribution and weight throughout the style.

To crosscheck a haircut, you will need to take sections/meshes of hair in the opposite direction to the way in which you have carried out your haircut. You still hold them at the same angle as you did for the original haircut and should continue to work in small methodical sections so that you are covering the whole of the haircut.

Your mirror is another good tool to use to check the shape, weight and balance of a haircut. If you stand directly behind your client and lift sections of hair, you will be able to use the mirror to confirm that they are of the same length, that you have used the same angle on both sides, and have achieved a balanced result.

When you have gained experience, you can also carry out this process without using your mirror. You will be able to check sections through by feel, looking to see if the hair is 'sitting' in the style you have cut, seeing if the weight left in the hair is working, giving you the effect both you and the client wanted to achieve.

Check it out

In pairs, discuss any potential problems that you may come across, such as double crowns, very fine hair, strong nape growth patterns and thick naturally curly hair. For each of the problems that you identify, make a list of the cutting methods and techniques that you would use to minimise the effects of the problems identified.

Hair is held up and cut at 90° for the main haircut. To cross check, the hair is combed and a section taken in the opposite direction, still held at 90° and checked.

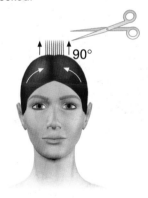

Section taken along the head to crosscheck the cut

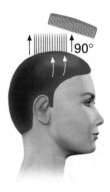

Crosschecking a haircut

By crosschecking and using your mirror to check the weight and angles of your cut, you are giving yourself and your client the opportunity to make any changes to the haircut before you get to the drying stage. It is important to check with your client that she is happy with what you have done and is ready for you to dry her hair into the finished result.

After-care advice

Giving after-care advice is important as part of the whole service. You would not expect to go to a hi-fi shop and purchase a stereo system and not receive information or instructions on how to use the equipment that you have bought. The same applies to giving information to your client following any service given in the salon.

The types of information on aftercare that you should be giving your client include:

1   How often she should come back into the salon for a trim to maintain the look.

2   Which products are best suited to her hair type and will help her to re-create the look you have achieved.

3   Which tools (for example, correct size of brushes) and equipment are best for achieving the look.

Basically, you are trying to give information that will aid the client to maintain her hair and achieve the desired effect.

You can talk to her about the use of products and drying techniques during the service and give her information on how much the average head of hair grows each month so that she will have a better understanding of why it is important to come into the salon for regular trims.

In the salon

Beenal completed a fantastic re-style on Mrs Watson who was very pleased. Beenal gave Mrs Watson some good tips so that she could maintain the style at home. Mrs Watson was so pleased that she booked her next appointment with Beenal.

- What are the benefits of good after-care advice?

Your questions answered

What do I do if I am halfway through a haircut and discover that my client has head lice?
You will need to tactfully inform the client of the problem and advise her of the best way to treat her hair. You are required to complete the haircut and then sterilise all tools and equipment that has come into contact with the infestation.

Is it always better to cut hair wet rather than dry?
It depends on the individual head of hair that you are dealing with at the time. For example, thick, naturally curly hair would be easier to control when cut wet, whereas fine hair that may have strong growth patterns (double crown, for example) would be better suited for a dry cut.

Check it out

In your groups, discuss the types of questions that you can use to confirm with the client that she is happy with the desired look.

Remember to think about using open questions rather than closed questions, which will help to gain more of a response from your client.

Client satisfaction

Gown the client in the appropriate manner for the service that is to be carried out.

Ensure good client care throughout the service by removing any hair cuttings as you work.

Use a back mirror to check and confirm that the client is happy with the cut.

Does it matter if you share your haircutting scissors with another stylist?
Yes, because you will find over a period of time that your scissors will adjust to your style of cutting. If you are sharing scissors, you may find that they become too loose for your technique.

What would I do if a client asked for a style that was not suitable for her hair?
You would need to explain to the client why the particular style she had chosen was not suitable for her texture (type) of hair. The use of style books may help you to explain your reasoning.

What would I do if I came across damaged or faulty equipment?
You would need to report the faulty equipment to the person in charge. This may be your tutor, technician or manager/manageress. You may need to document your findings to ensure all relevant parties are kept informed.

Who is responsible for health and safety at work?
Everyone has a duty to ensure a safe working environment for members of the public and staff.

What do I do if a client turns up late for her appointment and it is going to make me run over the allocated time?
You will need to explain to the client that you have another customer after her, so are restricted with time. Depending on the service that the client was booked for, you may be able to offer a smaller alternative treatment. If the client is unhappy with this, you could check to see if another member of staff is available to carry out her treatment or offer her another appointment.

Test your knowledge

1   List as many critical influencing factors as you can that you may come across when working on a head of hair.

2   What is the difference between a uniform layered cut and a graduated layered cut?

3   List three methods of sterilisation.

4   What safety checks do you need to carry out before using electrical clippers?

5   List two advantages of cutting wet hair.

6   What are you referring to when talking about the hair's density?

7   What is an acceptable time allocation to complete a cut and blow-dry?

8   Why is it important to maintain the correct posture whilst cutting a client's hair?

9   Where do you dispose of used sharps?

10   Why is it important to keep your working area clean and tidy and free of hazards?

11   What is meant by the term 'hazard'?

12   Why is it important to keep your sectioning neat, tidy and accurate when cutting?

13   Why is it important to give your client after-care advice?

14   What is the purpose of thinning scissors?

15   What should you do in order to maintain the good working condition of your tools and equipment?

Perm and neutralise hair using basic techniques (including African Caribbean hair)

Unit H12/H16

Perming and neutralising are permanent chemical processes that change the structure of the hair (perming comes from the old-fashioned term 'permanent wave'). They can be damaging to the hair if you do not understand what effect the chemicals have on the hair structure. Anyone can buy a home perm from the chemist, but if you do not know what the chemicals in the perm and neutraliser are capable of doing to the hair and scalp, the results can be disastrous. Therefore, it is very important to understand the hair structure, especially the cortex region where the chemical changes take place during both perming and neutralising, in order to achieve a professional result. The correct use of after-care products such as restructurants is also extremely important. This unit contains all the information you will need to know about perming and neutralising for both units H12 and H16. (Before you begin this unit, look back at the section 'Facts about hair and skin' for a reminder of the hair's structure).

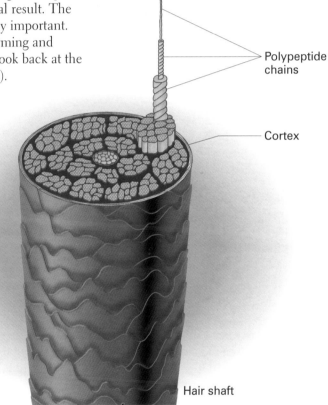

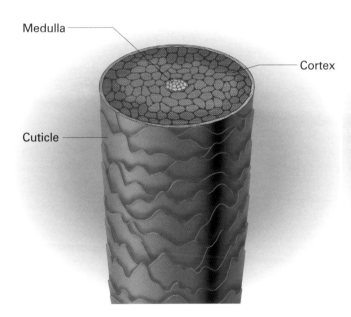

What are perming and neutralising?

Perming is the process of curling hair by chemically altering its physical structure.

Neutralising is the chemical process that fixes the hair in a new position after it has been altered by the action of perm lotion.

What you will learn

- Maintain effective and safe methods of working when perming and neutralising hair H12.1 and H16.1
- Prepare for perming and neutralising H12.2 and H16.2
- Perm and neutralise hair H12.3 and H16.3

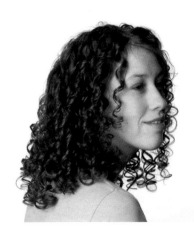

Maintain effective and safe methods of working when perming and neutralising hair

H12.1/H16.1

It is vital that you follow all health and safety rules and regulations during the perming and neutralising process to ensure the highest level of client care possible. This will also ensure you reach a high standard of work, as health and safety is an essential part of every process you carry out as a professional stylist.

What you will learn

- How perms work
- Preparing your client
- Health and safety issues
- Organisation and stock control
- Commercial timing
- Maintaining a record card system

How perms work

Perming involves three stages:

1   softening   2   moulding   3   fixing.

The softening stage

Perm lotion opens and swells the cuticle, so that it can enter the cortex. Some acid perm lotions need added heat to help open the cuticle scales – remember the pH scale from 'Facts about hair and skin'. Mildly acid products *close* the cuticle scales. You may need to use a hood dryer when using acid perm lotions – always read and follow the manufacturer's instructions.

The moulding stage

The perm lotion enters the cortex where it deposits hydrogen. The hydrogen attaches itself to the disulphide bonds and breaks them apart into sulphur bonds. (Not all disulphide bonds are broken during perming.) The hair, which has been softened, is now able to take on the shape of the perm rod. This is known as moulding.

The fixing stage

Neutralising removes the hydrogen from the cortex by adding oxygen (a process of oxidation). This process joins together the sulphur bonds to re-form disulphide bonds in a new position, which permanently fixes the curl.

Neutraliser is added and oxygen is released. Oxygen joins with the hydrogen to make H_2O (water)

Perm lotion opens and swells cuticle scales

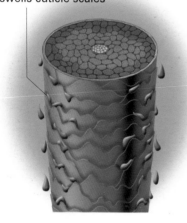

The softening stage

The hydrogen attaches itself to the disulphide bonds and breaks them into single sulphur bonds

Before perming, disulphide bonds intact

Perm lotion is added and releases hydrogen

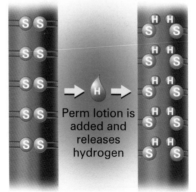

The moulding stage

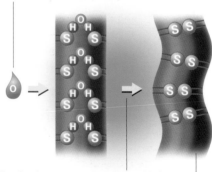

$2 \times$ hydrogen + oxygen = H_2O, which is rinsed from the hair

Sulphur bonds re-form to make disulphide bonds in a newly curled formation, which permanently fixes curl

The fixing stage

Preparing your client

Gowning

The chemicals used in perm lotion and neutralisers can cause a colour change in some fabrics. It is important to ensure the client's clothes are fully protected with a towel, chemical gown (this is plastic coated and will stop any liquid penetrating through it), second towel for extra protection, and plastic cape.

Consultation

A thorough consultation is an essential start to a successful perming result. In addition to the normal areas to assess such as hair texture and porosity, you need to ask the client some specific questions relating to the perm.

- Do you have any perm or colour on your hair?
- What size curl do you require?
- How do you manage your hair at home – do you set, blow-dry, leave to dry naturally?
- Do you have any problem areas that do not perm very well?
- Is your skin sensitive to perm lotion?
- Are you on any long-term medication? This could have affected the internal quality of the hair, which may lead to the hair becoming too fragile for the perming process. In the worst cases, the hair can break, so this is an important question to ask.

Once you have the answers to these questions you can decide:

- if any hair tests are necessary
- what size perm rods and winding technique to use
- which perm lotion and application technique to use.

Health and safety issues

Perming and neutralising involves the use of chemicals and you have to know and understand your responsibilities when using these products. You must always read and follow the manufacturer's instructions for the particular product you are using. If you decide, for whatever reason, that you no longer need to read the instructions, you will be showing a complete disregard for the safety and wellbeing of your client and going against the professional standards of the hairdressing industry.

Personal protective equipment (PPE)

When applying perm lotion and neutraliser it is important to protect yourself from the possible effects of the chemicals. You must wear an apron to protect yourself from any splashes of perm or neutraliser. As mentioned above, these chemicals can discolour fabrics.

It is also very important to protect yourself from the occupational hazard of the skin complaint dermatitis, which has caused such severe skin problems for some hairdressers that they have had to change careers. If you always wear gloves when applying perm lotion and neutraliser to avoid contact with these chemicals, you will minimise the risk of this happening to you.

Under the Personal Protective Equipment at Work Regulations, your employer has a responsibility to provide protective materials and gloves for you to use and you have a responsibility to wear them.

Check it out

Compare two different manufacturer's instruction leaflets for two different perm lotions. Write down and compare the:

- ingredients
- processing times
- neutralising times
- rinsing times.

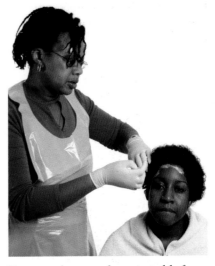

You must be properly protected before applying perm lotion, relaxer and neutraliser

Control of Substances Hazardous to Health Regulations (COSHH) 2003

Under the Control of Substances Hazardous to Health Regulations (COSHH) 2003, you must read the data sheets provided by the manufacturer of the perm so that you know how to handle, store and dispose of the chemicals used in the product.

Generally, perms should be stored in a cool, dry place away from bright sunlight. They should be used in a well-ventilated area and the manufacturer's instructions must be followed. When disposing of any leftover perm lotion or neutraliser, you should dilute the chemicals by flushing them down the sink with plenty of water.

Effective working methods

As a salon employee or college trainee, you will be expected to use all products carefully and effectively. Safe and effective working methods will include:

- minimising the wastage of products – always use the right amount of product for the individual client's hair. Never overload the hair with perm lotion or neutraliser as the excess will drip off the hair onto the client and the floor causing potential health and safety risks. Wastage of product is not cost effective to the salon and will mean salon profits will decline.
- minimising the risk of cross-infection – during the consultation you will need to evaluate the condition of your client's hair and scalp prior to perming. If you find any risk of cross-infection to yourself, your colleagues and other clients, you must not continue with the perm. These would be classed as contraindications (see page 92 'Hair facts'). Remember, contraindications are things that prevent you carrying out the treatment, for example, skin sensitivities, history of previous allergic reaction to colour products, known allergies, skin disorders, incompatible products or medical advice, or instructions not to have this treatment.
- making effective use of your working time – you should always make the best use of your time in the salon. If you were an employer paying an hourly rate, would you pay someone for wasting time? If you do not make the most effective use of your working day, you will not be deemed competent for your Level 2 qualification and a salon owner with a business to run will not want to employ you.
- ensuring the use of clean resources – would you like to sit in a dirty salon or have dirty brushes or towels used on you? All clients have the right to know that the salon tools, equipment and resources used on them are totally clean and sterilised if necessary. A dirty salon will not attract or keep clientele.
- minimising the risk of harm or injury to yourself and your clients – you and your salon have an obligation to your clients and visitors to ensure their safety. Your salon also has an obligation to you as an employee to ensure your safety while you are at work. All members of the salon team must make sure they know how to work safely to avoid accidents happening in the salon. This can be done by following all of the salon's health and safety rules and regulations.

Working area

Your working area must be kept clean and tidy at all times to prevent hazards and potential accidents. Always wipe up any spillages of water, perm lotion or neutraliser immediately to avoid slippery patches on the floor. Once you have finished with a piece of equipment, always put it away so you have as much space as possible to work in. Used towels should be placed immediately in a towel bin so that it is obvious to staff and clients that they are ready for washing. Discard soaked cotton wool, used end papers and plastic caps in appropriate waste bins – not on your trolley!

Check it out

What would you consider to be contraindications to perming? List five, explain why, and keep as evidence in your portfolio.

Check it out

How might wastage happen in your salon? How can you help to minimise wastage? Write down three methods and keep in your portfolio for evidence.

A clean and tidy working area helps you work efficiently and promotes a good professional image to your client.

You must also make sure your posture is good whilst working, as hairdressers stand for long periods of time and poor posture can lead to fatigue and more permanent risks of bodily injury.

Organisation and stock control

It is important to build into your working day time to organise yourself for your client's service before she arrives. When perming, this means organising your perm trolley to include:

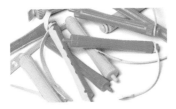

- perm rods in different sizes

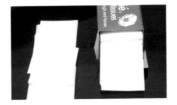

- end papers

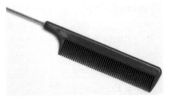

- pintail comb

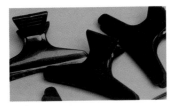

- sectioning clips

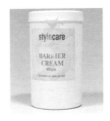

- barrier cream

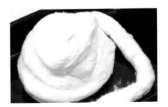

- cotton wool

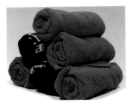

- towels

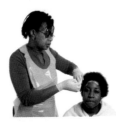

- gloves and apron

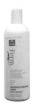

- perm lotion (if you know which one the client requires)

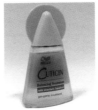

- pre-perm spray or lotion.

If you do not organise yourself in readiness for the perm, you will be wasting valuable time. Your employer will want you to use all of your time at work effectively and your clients will not want to be kept waiting.

Check it out

Work out how long these sundries last in your salon:

- a bag of neck strip cotton wool
- a box of gloves
- a pack of plastic head caps.

Remember, these all cost money and must be included in the cost the client pays for her perm.

Stock control

In order for the salon to function effectively, you are required to follow stock control procedures. This will ensure that all perming products such as cotton wool, end papers and gloves are re-ordered when necessary and are available for use as and when required. A salon may lose business if the perm the client usually has is out of stock. There may not be another perm suitable to use on the client's hair and she may get the impression of a disorganised salon that does not care about its clients.

Perming sundries such as neck strip cotton wool, end papers and gloves need to be replenished regularly.

Commercial timing

It takes skill and accuracy to wind a perm perfectly and you will need a great deal of practice before you can perm a client's hair competently. As a Level 2 Hairdressing student, you have performance criteria (PCs) for perming and neutralising to meet before your assessor can be sure you are competent. In addition to these PCs, you also need to prove you can wind a perm accurately in a commercially acceptable time.

Timing for perm winding techniques (winding only)
- Pre-damping (applying perm lotion before perm rods) = 35 minutes
- Post-damping (applying perm lotion after perm rods are wound) = 45 minutes

The above timings are targets for you to work to and aim for. Remember you should always follow manufacturer's instructions. Try not to be disappointed if you cannot achieve them instantly: put all your energy into producing an accurate perm winding result and your timing will improve with practice.

Try perm winding on a practice block head if you have one, or ask someone patient to be your model. Ask your trainer or an experienced stylist to show you:

- how to section the block head into nine sections. This sectioning technique is helpful when learning how to place the perm rods correctly over a whole head of hair.
- how to practise winding a section at the nape area first, by taking sections of hair as wide and nearly as long as the perm rods you are using. Pull the sections out at a 90 degree angle and try to keep hold with good tension so that the hair stays straight and looks tidy. Then put a perming end paper at about the middle of the section of the hair and try not to bunch the hair together in the paper. Once the end paper is in place, you can place the perm rod in the middle of the end paper and, still holding with good tension, slide the perm rod and the end paper up to the ends of the hair. Make sure the ends of the hair go past the perm rod slightly (otherwise they will buckle and will look frizzy) and then fold the end paper around the perm rod and keep winding around until all the hair is wound down to the scalp. Ask your trainer to check.

Maintaining a record card system

It is especially important to keep your clients' records up to date when perming. Record cards should contain all the relevant information such as date of the perm, products used, size of perm rods used, amount of processing time needed, whether heat was used during processing, perm result, price of perm, and any other information you feel is necessary to record.

The record card needs to be filled in accurately so write the information in while the client is processing or immediately after she has left the salon, otherwise you will forget how long the processing time was – never guess at how long you think it took.

Check it out

Make a note of your salon's stock control procedures, including:

- the person(s) responsible for re-ordering stock
- how *you* are required to report shortages of sundries and products
- the telephone number of your nearest hairdressing wholesaler or established representative
- how the salon keeps a check on the stock it has.

Place your findings in your portfolio as evidence of your research.

Reality check!

An uneven, messy perm wind will produce a poor perm result. Perfect your winding skills first and then practise speed winding to become commercially competent.

Remember

The Data Protection Act states that all record card information should be accurate, up to date, kept for as long as the client is still attending the salon, must be accessible to the client and kept securely.

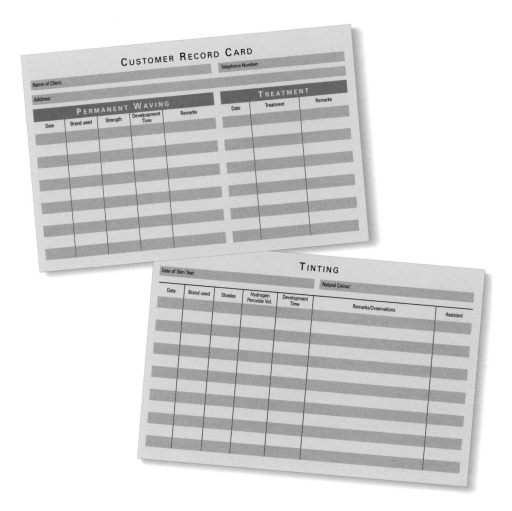

Health and safety

Gown client effectively to stop any chemicals staining clothes.

Carry out a thorough consultation and any hair tests necessary.

Always read the manufacturer's instructions for the products chosen.

Be organised and keep your area tidy as you work to avoid accidents happening.

Wear the correct personal protective equipment: gloves and apron.

Work efficiently throughout the perm – avoid wastage of products and sundries, minimise cross-infection by checking for any contraindications, and by working safely with clean tools.

Use your time effectively throughout the perm (time is money in the salon) and make sure all your resources are clean, minimising the risk of harm and injury to yourself and your client (remember the Health and Safety at Work Act from Unit G1).

Make sure you maintain a good level of stock.

Always record fully the perm lotion used, rod size used, processing time, and final curl result for future reference.

In the salon

Venetia has been working as a junior stylist in The Hair Parlour for nine months since gaining her NVQ Level 2 Hairdressing qualification. Miss Mumberson is a new client who is booked in for a perm. When the client arrives, Venetia gowns her and conducts a thorough consultation, which enables her to choose the correct products. The subsequent perm and neutraliser produce a lovely perm result, which the client is satisfied with. However, when Miss Mumberson is ready to leave and the gown is removed, Venetia notices slight discoloration to the collar and back of her blouse.

- Should Venetia tell her client about the staining?
- How could this situation have happened?
- What could be the result of this situation?

Prepare for perming and neutralising

H12.2/H16.2

In this element you will be taken through the steps and information needed to ensure you have the understanding to prepare your client fully for perming and neutralising processes. Once you have prepared a client thoroughly in readiness for perming and neutralising, you will realise that everything you do during preparation has an effect on the subsequent perm and is very important to the perming and neutralising process.

What you will learn	

- Questioning your client about contraindications and recording responses
- Hair tests for perming and neutralising
- When not to perm
- Seeking assistance about contraindications and test results
- Perming and neutralising products
- Preparing and protecting your client

Questioning your client about contraindications and recording responses

Remember, a contraindication is something that prevents you carrying out the treatment. It is vital that you ask your client if she suffers from any contraindications to establish whether it is safe to carry out the perm. Perming lotion can irritate sensitive or allergic skin and can be very painful if applied to skin with disorders such as psoriasis.

It is important to record your client's responses to the questions you ask about contraindications in order to have proof that she was asked before the treatment in case of any problems which may occur during or after the perm. A good way of making sure that this is standard procedure in your salon is to have some standard contraindication questions printed on your client's record card, which can be ticked when they have been asked. You should also ask your client to sign the record card to validate that the questions were asked and their responses were accurately recorded.

Hair tests for perming and neutralising

You should always explain the importance of tests to your client so she is aware that you are checking to see whether the hair can withstand the chemical process you are going to carry out.

Elasticity test

This is to test the internal strength of the hair (the cortex). Hair that has been damaged due to chemical treatments may have lost much of its natural strength. This type of hair may stretch over two-thirds of its original length and may even break off. It is important to carry out this test before perming. Hair that is in good condition will stretch and then return to its original length.

Take one strand of hair and hold each end firmly between the thumb and forefinger of each hand and gently pull. If the hair stretches more than half of its original length then it is over elastic and may snap or break during chemical processing.

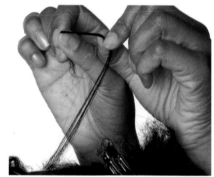

The elasticity test

Porosity test

This tests the condition of the outer layer of the hair shaft – the cuticle. If the cuticle is damaged, it becomes porous. Perming chemicals added to porous hair will be absorbed unevenly and may produce uneven curl results. This is why special perm lotions for tinted and highlighted hair are used. They are weaker in strength and are less likely to over process the hair and give a poor result.

Take a strand of hair and hold it by the points (where the hair has been cut) between the thumb and forefinger of one hand. Run the forefinger and thumb of your other hand from the root (where the hair grows from) down to the point. If the hair feels rough and bumpy, the cuticle scales are raised and open and this is an indication of porous hair. If the hair feels smooth, the cuticle is flat and closed and the hair's cuticle region is in good condition.

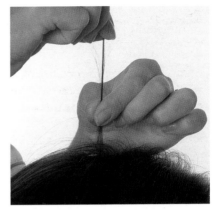

The porosity test

Incompatibility test

Some chemicals do not work well together (they are incompatible) and may have a bad reaction if one is used over the top of another. Some colours, for example, contain metallic salts, which are incompatible with other chemicals. You should carry out an incompatibility test before perming if you are unsure of the colouring products already on the hair or if the hair has a doubtful history.

- Mix together (preferably in a glass bowl) 10 ml of hydrogen peroxide and 10 ml of alkaline perm lotion.
- Place a small cutting of hair in the solution and wait. If heat is given off, the lotion fizzes and the hair breaks, dissolves or changes colour, then this is a positive reaction and the hair should NOT be permed or coloured with a product containing hydrogen peroxide. The hair contains metallic salts.

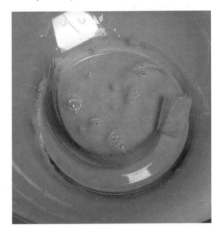

The incompatibilty test

Pre-perm test curl

When handling fragile, porous hair or hair with a doubtful history, it is advisable to wind, process and neutralise one or more small sections of hair. The results will be a guide to the best rod size, processing time and lotion strength to use. This test will also give a good indication of the condition after the perming process and will determine whether the hair is suitable for this treatment.

It is not always suitable or possible to carry out a test curl on the head, so a cutting of hair may be taken and tested separately, but remember, there will be no scalp heat to help the processing.

- Wind two or three rods of your chosen size in the hair.
- Apply perm lotion suitable for hair condition and leave to process for the manufacturer's specified time.
- Carry out a development test curl to see whether processing is sufficient. If so, rinse, neutralise for the time specified by the manufacturer, remove rods and evaluate curl result.

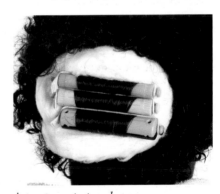

A pre-perm test curl

Development test curl

This test is carried out during the processing of the perm to check whether the desired development has been reached. Always wear gloves to carry out this test.

- Hold perm rod and undo rubber fastener.
- Unwind the curler one and a half turns or until you see the start of the perm paper, holding firmly.
- Push the hair up and then in towards the scalp, allowing it to relax into an 'S' shape movement. Be careful not to pull the hair as it is in a very fragile state.

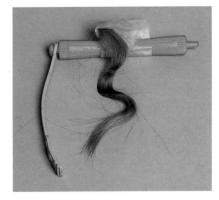

A pre-perm test curl tested seperately

- When the size of the 'S' shape corresponds to the size of the curler, the processing is complete and the hair should be rinsed with warm water to avoid over processing and neutralised following manufacturer's instructions.

Always take test curls on different areas of the head as one area may be ready before another and this would cause an uneven curl result. The temperature of the salon will make a difference. Perms will process quicker on warm days than on cold days.

Once you have carried out the necessary tests and you are satisfied with the results, continue with the service.

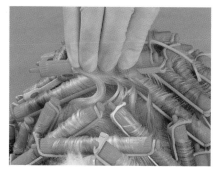

A development test curl

When not to perm

- When the scalp is damaged or the skin broken/damaged.
- When the hair is in poor condition.
- When the overall porosity of the hair is too high – over-bleached.
- In the presence of metallic salts, for example, Grecian 2000.
- When the hair has poor elasticity.

Reality check!

Always test the hair to check that it is safe to carry out perming.

Seeking assistance about contraindications and test results

We have discussed contraindications and the hair tests that may be necessary before a perm is carried out if you are doubtful about the hair or skin for any reason. Once you have identified a contraindication or have a problem test result, you need to know who you can ask for assistance from in your salon. It is important that this person knows how to assess both contraindications and hair test results and will normally be a more senior member of your salon team. If you are unsure what to do when you have one of the listed problems, you can ask this colleague to help you decide what action to take with your client.

Perming and neutralising products

Acid perm lotion

Acid perm lotion has been developed as a kinder alternative to the original alkaline perm lotion. Fewer bonds are broken in the cortex of the hair by acid perms and they are gentler to use on damaged hair or hair that processes very quickly (for example, porous hair).

Acid perms have activators that are added to them immediately before use. They rely on heat to open up the cuticle scales so that they can penetrate the cortex region. They generally have an acid pH of 6–7 and are made of a chemical called glycerol monothioglycollate.

Once an acid perm is mixed with its activator it only has a short life span and, consequently, any remaining lotion should be discarded. This makes pre-perm testing with acid perm lotions difficult, as you would not want to mix up a whole bottle of perm lotion to test one small piece of hair – this would not be cost effective for the salon.

Alkaline perm lotion

Alkaline perm lotion is generally stronger than acid perm lotion and comes in different strengths for different hair types. It has a pH of approximately 9.5, which opens up the cuticle scales and allows the perm lotion to enter the cortex region of the hair. The higher the pH of the perm lotion, the more damaging it is to the hair (see 'Facts about hair and skin', page 19). This is why alkaline perms have conditioning agents added to

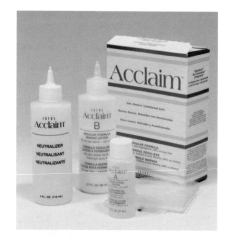

Acid perm lotion

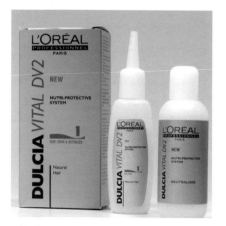

Alkaline perm lotion

them and acid perms are becoming increasingly popular. The chemical ingredient in alkaline perm lotion is ammonium thioglycollate.

Exothermic perms

Exothermic perms have the benefit of producing their own heat. Once the activator has been mixed with the perm lotion, you will be able to feel the lotion getting warm as you hold the bottle. Because they are self-heating, no added heat is necessary to open the cuticle or help the perm during processing.

Exothermic perms are generally made for use on all types of hair; however, you may need to leave them for less time on porous hair – always check the manufacturer's instructions. They can be a mixture of acid and alkaline or acid/alkaline depending on the manufacturer. The only way to check is to look at the chemical ingredients on the packaging and compare to the acid or alkaline perm chemical ingredients.

Dual action perm

These are used when perming African Caribbean hair and are more commonly used as they are kinder on the hair than single action perms. The active chemical found in most perm lotions for African Caribbean hair is ammonium thioglycollate. It is a two-step process: first, the curly hair is chemically softened using an ammonium thioglycollate cream to reduce the natural curl; secondly, a curl gel or winding lotion (a weaker solution of ammonium thioglycollate) is applied and the hair wound around perm rods and processed. This permanent treatment allows the hair to be formed into new looser curls after neutralising has taken place. Curly perms produce a tighter, more traditional curl, while a body perm will produce a softer wave or curl for a more modern finish.

Single action perm

Again, this perm uses the chemical ammonium thioglycollate, but only one application of the perm lotion is applied and remains on the hair (during smoothing and straightening and when the hair is wound around the perm rods) until processing is complete. Remember, you must always wear gloves when winding hair that has had perm lotion applied to it.

Perm and curly perm lotions come ready to use in different strengths for different hair types – see the chart on page 202.

Neutralisers

Neutralisers come in many different forms. Some are ready to use out of the bottle, some need to be mixed with warm water, some need to be foamed up in a bowl and applied with a sponge, and some neutralisers are instant. The chemical ingredient in neutralisers may be either hydrogen peroxide or sodium bromate, both of which can lighten or fade hair colour.

Most neutralisers used on African Caribbean perms usually contain sodium bromate as this has a much gentler action on the hair than hydrogen peroxide. This is why the neutralising process differs with African Caribbean hair, as the rods are left in the hair throughout the neutralising process because the gentler action takes longer to process. Sodium bromate also has less hair lightening properties than hydrogen peroxide.

Check it out

What are the active ingredients used in African Caribbean perm lotions? How do these differ from other perm lotions?

Reality check!

You should always recommend that your client has her perm before colouring treatment, as the neutraliser is likely to fade or lighten the colour.

Perm lotion	Hair type
Normal	Virgin hair that has not been treated with chemicals
Resistant	White or greying hair, or very tight compact cuticle scales
Tinted	Hair that has been treated with permanent colours
Bleached	Bleached or high-lift tinted hair including highlights (perm with great care if at all)
Porous	Dry, porous hair that has a poor cuticle area (perm with great care if at all)
Curly perm lotion	
Super	Resistant hair
Regular	Normal hair
Mild	Porous/coloured hair

Suitability of perm lotions for different hair types

Check it out

Find out about the perming products available in your salon. This will give you confidence when having to choose a perm lotion for your client's particular hair type. Keep this information in your portfolio of evidence.

Preparing and protecting your client

It is vital to the wellbeing of your client that you follow your salon's rules for preparing and protecting your client during the perming and neutralising processes. You must always consider the effects of the chemicals you are using and their potential for harming your client. This will help you evaluate any risks and prevent accidents happening.

Preparing the hair for perming

Begin by correctly gowning your client. Next, prepare the hair ready for perming by shampooing, using a soapless base shampoo with no additives, to ensure no residue is left on the hair as a barrier between the perm lotion and the hair.

When shampooing before a perm, use only cool/tepid water and do not massage vigorously to avoid over stimulation of the scalp, as this can lead to sensitivity during the chemical process.

Barrier cream

This is a thick protective cream that should be applied all the way around the client's hairline before applying perm lotion (including nape area) to avoid irritation of the skin. Care must be taken to avoid putting the cream on to the hair as this will cause a barrier between the perm lotion and the hair and will result in straight areas. Clients with sensitive skin will be more likely to have a skin reaction from the perm lotion so always take the utmost care to avoid this happening.

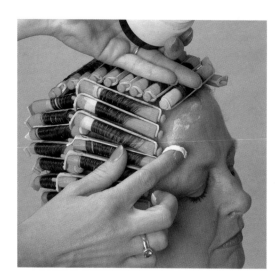

Reality check!

Some clients use a lot of styling products that can leave white deposits on the hair even after shampooing. This build-up could cause a barrier between the perm lotion and the hair and should be removed with a lacquer-removing/clarifying shampoo and then a second shampoo using TLS should be carried out.

Applying barrier cream

In the salon

Jonny is a junior at Jake's Hair Studio and is assisting Gill with a perm on Mrs Thomas. Jonny is asked to apply barrier cream and cotton wool before the perm lotion is applied. He absent-mindedly forgets the barrier cream and only applies cotton wool around the hairline. Later, Mrs Thomas complains of a sore neck and forehead during processing and Gill discovers chemical burn marks all around her hairline. Gill removes the soaked cotton wool and immediately soothes the affected areas with cool water while Jonny calls Charlie, the salon's first aider.

Have a group discussion on the possible consequences of this situation. Also discuss who is responsible for Mrs Thomas's hairline burns. What should be completed before Mrs Thomas leaves the salon?

Pre-perm treatments

Pre-perm treatments are applied to the hair after shampooing and before the perm rods are used. They are used to:

- even out the porosity along the hair shaft to help the perm lotion absorb at an even rate, which results in an even curl along the hair
- form a protective barrier along the cuticle region and close any cuticle scales that are raised
- make the hair more pliable when winding the perm rods into the hair.

Pre-perm treatments come in either individual bottles or sprays and are applied to shampooed, towel-dried hair.

Some companies make in-perm additives that are mixed with the perm lotion immediately before application to the hair. These types of products contain oils, which lubricate and strengthen the hair.

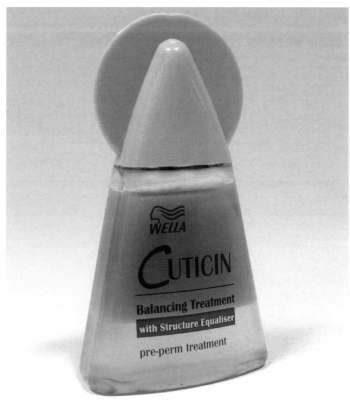

Pre-perm treatment

Preparing for perming and neutralising

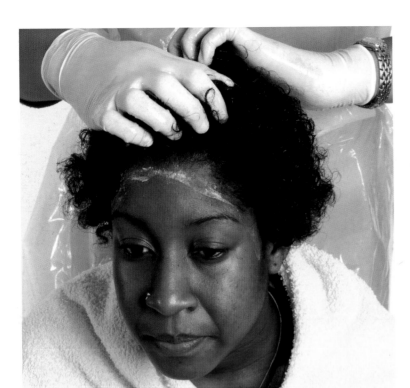

Applying pre-perm treatment

Post-perm conditioners

Special anti-oxidant surface conditioners are produced for use after perming. They have special properties.

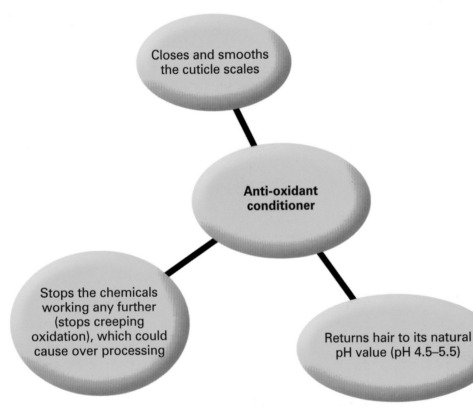

- Closes and smooths the cuticle scales
- **Anti-oxidant conditioner**
- Stops the chemicals working any further (stops creeping oxidation), which could cause over processing
- Returns hair to its natural pH value (pH 4.5–5.5)

Question your client about any contraindications to perming and neutralising and record her responses.

Carry out any hair tests you feel are necessary from your consultation.

Choose your perm lotion and neutraliser from the results of your consultation.

Prepare your client thoroughly and make sure you prepare the hair ready for perming by using the correct shampoo. Towel dry the hair to remove excess water.

Apply a pre-perm treatment if necessary from the results of your consultation.

Apply barrier cream around the hairline before applying perm lotion and neutraliser to stop hairline irritation.

Apply an anti-oxidant conditioner after neutralising to stop the chemicals working any further (always read the manufacturer's instructions to check if this is recommended).

Perm and neutralise hair

H12.3/H16.3

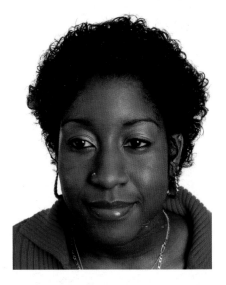

In this element you will be learning how to carry out a perm from the beginning right through to the end, curled result.

Perming is one of the technical units of the NVQ, which requires you to practise in order to improve your winding technique, correct placing of perm rods and timing. Once you have practised and developed these areas, you will be ready to perm a client's hair, while remembering and putting into practice all that you have learned from Elements H12.1 and H12.2.

Perming is one of the most rewarding hairdressing treatments, as you can achieve dramatically different results on a client's hair. For example, by perming, you can add large, subtle curls to give root lift and support to styles, or you can turn long, straight hair into tumbling, curled tresses. You can also completely change the shape of a hairstyle by adding curls.

What you will learn
• Preparing the hair for perming • Factors influencing the service • The perming procedure • The neutralising procedure • Coping with perming and neutralising problems

Preparing the hair for perming

Begin by correctly gowning your client (see page 166). Next, prepare the hair ready for perming by shampooing, using a soapless base shampoo, to ensure no residue is left on the hair, which could act as a barrier between the perm lotion and the hair.

Factors influencing the service

These are sometimes known as critical influencing factors and are anything that could affect the perming process, for example, hair condition. They must be taken into account for each individual client during the initial consultation before the perm is attempted.

You have already learned what needs to be assessed during a consultation for perming, but how can you be sure that you understand the curl size the client requires? Only by taking the time to discuss thoroughly the required results of the perm can you be certain you have gathered all the necessary information. Often a client will come in with a style book or picture of permed hair asking for the same result. You should explain that you can do something similar, but the model in the picture may have more or thicker hair, so the results will be slightly different.

Other critical influencing factors you need to take into account are:

- temperature of the salon
- direction and size of the curl required
- hair condition
- previous chemical treatments
- hair texture
- haircut
- hair length
- hair density.

Once you have considered the above, you will have the necessary information to choose the correct strength perm lotion, correct size perm rods, correct winding technique, application of perm lotion technique, and whether it is necessary to use added heat to aid processing.

Remember

When shampooing before a perm, use only cool/tepid water and do not massage vigorously to avoid over stimulation of the scalp. This could open the skin's pores and hair follicles, which, when perm lotion is added, may cause scalp irritation.

The perming procedure

Sectioning and perm-winding techniques

There are three basic sectioning and perm-winding techniques that you need to master for your NVQ. They are:

- brick winding – this is done to avoid any partings resulting from the perm and is ideal for fine hair
- directional winding – this is carried out when the hair needs perming in a specific direction and is ideal for clients requiring a parting within the perm
- nine-section winding – this is the most commonly used perm wind when training as it is easy to learn how to fit all the rods onto the head using this technique.

<table>
<tr><td>

Remember

When perm winding, you are trying to place straight perm rods onto a round head shape. This is not easy and takes practice – sectioning the hair first will help.

</td></tr>
</table>

Step-by-step brick winding

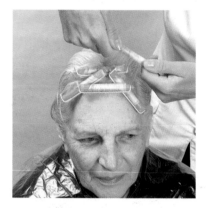

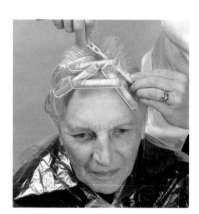

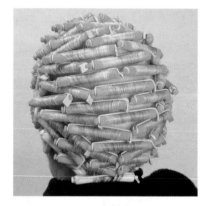

Start at the front hairline taking a section of hair as wide as the perm rod but not longer than the rod (this will prevent 'baggy' ends) and wind to the scalp.

Now start the brick effect by sectioning underneath the perm rod, in the centre, to stop a channel line appearing. Wind another perm rod the other side and the brick wall effect will start to appear.

Try to angle slightly the section of hair to be wound, as this will help the straight rods fit into the rounded shape of the head. Once all the hair is wound, check the rods are comfortable for your client.

Directional perm winding

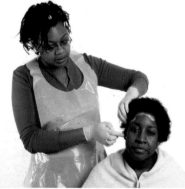

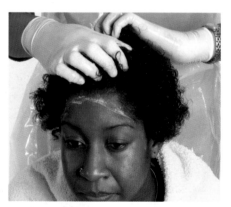

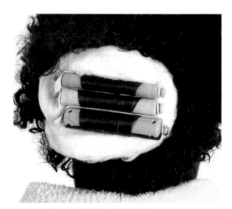

Apply barrier cream to the area just below the hairline, taking care not to apply it to the hair.

Apply a pre-perm treatment to the hair to protect any hair that has been chemically treated.

Using three curlers of various sizes, process the hair and evaluate the results.

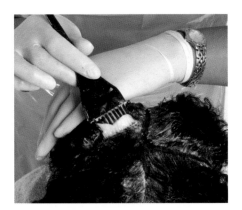

Apply re-arranger to re-growth area only (if hair has been chemically treated). Apply to all the hair if not. Crosscheck to ensure an even application. Allow to process.

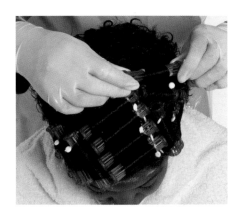

Rinse thoroughly to remove the re-arranger and towel dry the hair. Apply curl lotion (pre-damping) to the areas that have been permed and wind the curlers into the direction of the required style.

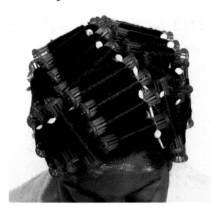

Allow the perm to process (following manufacturer's instructions)

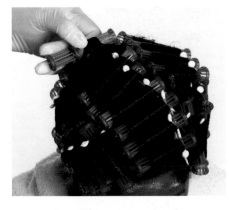

Unwind a curler approximately one-and-a-half turns and push the hair forward towards the scalp allowing it to relax into an 'S' shape. Test the hair in different areas.

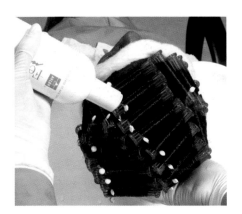

Rinse thoroughly according to manufacturer's instructions to remove the perm lotion. Remove excess water by blotting dry using either a towel or cotton wool. Apply neutraliser to each curler and allow to process according to manufacturer's instructions.

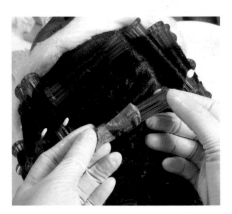

Remove curlers taking care not to overstretch the hair. Rinse thoroughly to remove all traces of neutraliser and apply conditioner. Apply after-care products to moisturise hair and activate curls. Style as required.

Nine-section perm winding

This involves dividing the hair into nine neat sections (see below) in readiness for perm winding. You should copy this technique on a head of hair using a perm rod to measure each section and checking that a perm rod will fit in each section across the whole head. Once this is complete, you can start to wind each section. When training, it is easier to start winding the perm rods from the nape area, beginning in the central section and then winding left and right nape sections.

When sectioning, you need to follow the same principle as for roller setting by taking the same size section as the length and width of the perm rod. The section of hair should then be held at a 90 degree angle (straight out) from the head, the end paper placed on the hair and, keeping good, even tension on the hair, use both hands to wind the perm rod towards the scalp. Secure the perm rod close to the scalp by placing the perm rubber securely over the end of the rod.

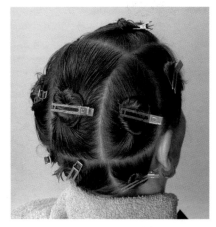

Nine sections

Continue winding the centre crown section and then the left and right crown sections. Lastly, wind the centre top section and then both left and right side sections.

It is important to check whether any of the perm rods are too tight as this can cause a pull burn, which, if scratched, can become infected and result in folliculitis (see page 93). This can be done by visual checking and asking the client if any rods are pulling.

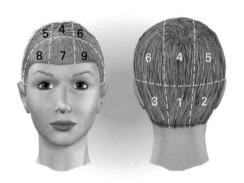

Correct method | **Incorrect method**

Perm rods/curlers should be at a 90° angle from the head, i.e. straight out

Wrong curler position on scalp

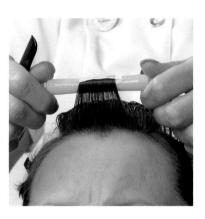

How to section

How to position perm rods correctly

Placing a perm rod

Application of perm lotion

Protecting technique

This involves either applying pre-perm lotion to the hair to protect any porous areas from over processing or applying barrier cream to protect the scalp and hairline from any possible chemical burns from the perm lotion.

Post-damping technique

This is where you apply perm lotion to hair that has been sectioned and wound around perm rods. When you are training and taking more than half an hour to wind a whole head of perm rods, this is the safest way of applying your perm lotion and will ensure that all areas of the head process evenly.

Pre-damping technique

Pre-damping technique involves applying perm lotion to hair that is resistant before sectioning or winding the perm rods. This technique is often used in salons where the stylist or perming technician is competent and able to wind a whole head of perm rods in a very short space of time. It is not recommended that you carry out a whole head of pre-damping technique while you are learning to perm hair, as you will find it takes longer to wind the whole head than it does for the perm to be processed. This would result in an over-processed head of frizzy hair. Protective gloves should always be worn when pre-damping.

When applying the perm lotion to the hair, always have a piece of cotton wool in your other hand to remove any splashes. Keep the bottle close to the hair and always apply to the top and bottom of each wound rod. Start your application at the most resistant

Book-end paper wrap

Slide paper down past hair ends

Applying end papers

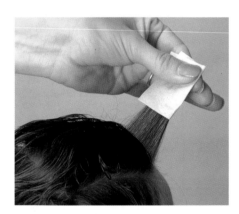

End papers are specially designed absorbent papers, which make winding easier and help to prevent fish hooks or buckled ends

Reality check!

After applying barrier cream and before applying perm lotion, always remember to place a strip of cotton wool securely around the client's hairline. The cotton wool will stick to the barrier cream and will fully protect the client from perm lotion entering the eyes or running into the ears or down the face.

For your own protection, you must always wear gloves to apply perm lotion to avoid the risk of dermatitis.

area and continue in a methodical manner until all the rods are covered. Be careful not to overload the hair so that the perm lotion soaks your client. Once the application is complete, remove the soiled cotton wool and replace with fresh cotton wool to avoid hairline irritation and burning. Read the manufacturer's instructions to see whether you need to cover the rods with a plastic cap whilst the perm is processing.

Monitoring curl development during processing

Heat speeds the development of the perming process and should only be used if advised by the manufacturer's instructions.

There are two types of heat:

- body heat – trapped by a plastic cap which will retain heat lost from the head
- hairdryers and climazones – can be used to speed up the processing time (usually by halving the time). Check the manufacturer's instructions. Because these use dry heat, you may need to use a plastic cap as well to prevent the perm lotion from drying out and subsequently not processing (check manufacturer's instructions).

> **Remember**
>
> A perm will process more quickly in a warm salon (summer) than in a cold salon (winter).

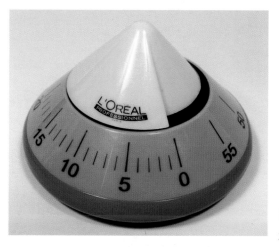

Use a timer to ensure that processing time is accurate

The processing time is very important and can be monitored accurately by using a timer. You must refer to the manufacturer's instructions to work out the length of processing time needed. This will also be dependent on the client's hair type, texture and condition. When it is necessary to check the development of the perm, carefully unwind a couple of perm rods from different areas over the head. Be careful not to disturb the curl too much as the hair is in a very fragile state. When the perm has processed sufficiently, it will look 'S' shaped and resemble the size of the rod being used when gently pushed towards the scalp (see page 199 for the development test).

The neutralising procedure

Neutralising is a permanent process that re-joins the sulphur bonds into their new curled position. If neutralising is *not* carried out correctly, the perm will be unsuccessful and the client will be disappointed.

Preparing for neutralising

Always read the manufacturer's instructions before beginning to neutralise hair. You must comply with the Personal Protective Equipment at Work Regulations by wearing an apron and gloves.

It is advisable to check the client's gown and towels before beginning to neutralise in case they need replacing.

Water temperature and flow

You must wear gloves when rinsing the perm lotion from the hair, so it is therefore important that you keep checking with the client that the water temperature is comfortable. It is easier to rinse the hair free of perm lotion if the water flow is not too strong, as too great a flow will soak both you and the client. Always rinse with warm/cool water, as the scalp may be tender and the hair delicate.

Why rinse thoroughly?

It is vital to the success of the perm that you rinse all the perm lotion from the hair. If any lotion is left in the hair, it will stop the sulphur bonds from re-forming fully and will result in a looser curl than expected that could even drop to completely straight.

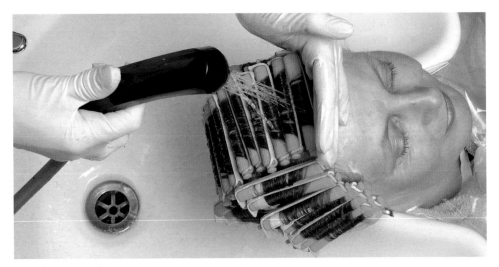

Rinse the perm for at least five minutes

After rinsing for about five minutes, use a perm indicator towel to test for any residue of perm lotion (the towel will change colour if any lotion is left). When you have rinsed sufficiently to remove all traces of perm lotion, blot the hair gently with a towel. This will allow you to sit the client up at the basin and apply a fresh strip of cotton wool around the hairline for protection. Use a pad of cotton wool to further blot any excess moisture from the hair, which could dilute the strength of the neutraliser. You are now ready to apply the neutraliser.

Applying neutraliser

After reading the manufacturer's instructions, you will know whether to apply the neutraliser straight from the bottle (the same technique as applying perm lotion) or if it is necessary to tip the neutraliser into a bowl, foam up and apply to the hair using a neutralising sponge.

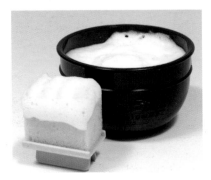

A neutralising sponge and bowl

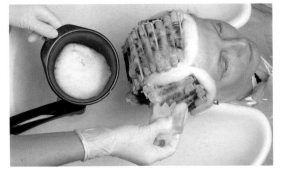

Applying neutraliser

Remember

Some neutralisers need mixing with water before use. Always read the manufacturer's instructions. Apply the neutraliser to each perm rod so that you are confident all the rods have been covered. If even one rod is missed, it will result in a straight section of hair, which will look very obvious.

Eye care when neutralising

If neutraliser sponges are too soaked, the product may drip down the client's face and go into her eyes. If this happens, you should rinse the eyes carefully with cold water and seek the help of a first aider. If there are further problems, advise the client to see her GP. You will need to fill in an accident report sheet. You will also need to notify your salon manager and make a note on the client's record card.

The importance of accurate timing

Once the first application of neutraliser is complete, you should start accurately timing the development. This timing will be dependent upon the manufacturer's instructions but is usually about five minutes. Since this is when the chemicals in the neutraliser (either hydrogen peroxide or sodium bromate) are re-joining the sulphur bonds to their new partners, it is important the chemicals are given sufficient time to function. If you rush the neutraliser, not all the bonds will re-join and the hair may be left weak and straight looking. If the neutraliser is left on too long, this could result in over processing the hair into a straight frizz.

Removing perm rods correctly

The removal of the perm rods is the next step once the time for the first application of neutraliser has elapsed. You should then gently unwind each perm rod removing the end paper as you work. When all the rods have been removed, apply a second application of neutraliser to the hair paying particular attention to the ends of the hair, which may not have been fully covered whilst wound around the rod. This is a more common problem when neutralising long hair. Once again, timing is important and you must be guided by the manufacturer's instructions.

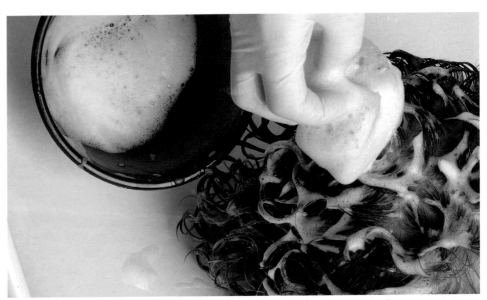

Once all the rods have been removed, apply a second application of neutraliser

Removing all neutraliser

When the time for the second application of neutraliser has elapsed, rinse the neutraliser thoroughly from the hair. Again, it is important to make sure all traces of the neutraliser are removed as the chemical ingredients may carry on working if left in the hair. This is called creeping oxidation and can affect the success of the perm. To avoid this happening, a surface conditioner containing anti-oxidant properties (herbal anti-oxy) is commonly applied, gently massaged into the hair and then removed by rinsing.

A successful perm

> **Remember**
>
> Make sure you apply the neutraliser with care to avoid any accidents.

> **Reality check!**
>
> Never treat the hair vigorously at this stage of the process – this could weaken the curl result as the bonds have only just re-formed into their new shape.

> **Check it out**
>
> What are the three functions of anti-oxidant conditioners? (If you need a reminder, look back at page 204.)

In the salon

Mrs Pearlman is a new client and has booked in for a perm with senior stylist Joy. During the consultation Joy asks what sort of colour Mrs Pearlman has on her hair. Mrs Pearlman tells her that it was a box colour from the local chemist. Joy therefore chooses a perm for coloured hair and proceeds with the perming process.

The hair processes very quickly and once neutralising is complete Joy starts to carefully remove the perm rods. As the rods are removed some of Mrs Pearlman's hair starts to fall out as well. Joy is horrified and when all the rods are removed she can see that the condition of the hair is like fluffy cotton wool. After conditioning with anti-oxy conditioner the hair is softer but still very damaged and stretchy. Joy explains to Mrs Pearlman and says that the only other time she has seen this sort of perm result was on a client with a full head of highly bleached hair. Mrs Pearlman explains that she used to have a full head bleach before she coloured over it a few weeks ago. The hair is beyond repair and Mrs Pearlman is distraught.

Discuss the following points with your colleagues:

- Who was at fault, Mrs Pearlman for not disclosing the fact she had previously bleached her hair or Joy for not testing the hair?
- What could happen as a result of this unfortunate situation?
- What could Joy offer Mrs Pearlman to try to improve the condition of the hair?
- How could this situation have been avoided?

Coping with perming and neutralising problems

Perming problems

The chart below identifies the problems that might occur with perms and what action you should take.

Problem	Reason	Action
Perm slow to take	Cold salon temperature; wrong selection of perm lotion; lotion evaporated; insufficient lotion applied	Use added heat – dryer/climazone; re-damp with stronger lotion; re-damp with same lotion
Perm processing too quickly	Hair too porous, allowing lotion to enter hair shaft too quickly; hair too dry when lotion applied; very hot salon	Remove any extra heat; remove cap if used; rinse hair
Hair breakage	Too much tension; lotion too strong for hair type; over processing	Use restructurant or deep penetrating conditioner
Rubber banding marks	Wound too tight	Use restructurant
Hairline and scalp irritation	Cuts, abrasions on scalp; cap and wool left around hairline; too much lotion applied	Rinse immediately using cool water
Fish hooks	Hair ends buckled or bent during winding	Remove by cutting
Frizziness	Over processing; lotion too strong; rods too small	Cut if possible; use restructurant or deep penetrating conditioner
Uneven curl formation	Lotion applied unevenly; rod tension uneven	Re-perm if hair is in good condition
Too tight curl	Over processed; rod size too small	Deep condition; assess hair condition for relaxing

Perming problems and how to deal with them

Neutralising problems

The chart below identifies the problems that may arise with neutralising and what action you should take.

Problem	Reason	Action
Frizziness	Over processing	Cut if possible
Uneven curl formation	Neutraliser applied unevenly	Use restructurant or deep penetrating conditioner; re-perm if hair in good condition

Neutralising problems and how to deal with them

Your questions answered

How long do I have to complete my perm on assessment?
When post-damping (applying the perm lotion after winding the rods), you have 45 minutes to complete the winding only. If pre-damping, your wind should be completed in 35 minutes to deem you commercially competent.

Will I be asked questions on what the chemicals do to the hair when I'm perming?
Yes, you need to fully understand what the perm lotion and neutraliser do to the hair when you are perming to be competent in this perming unit.

Will perm winding get easier?
Yes, it is like any new skill, it gets easier with a lot of hard practice. Remember, practice makes perfect!

How many perms do I have to do on assessment?
You have to successfully complete at least three full-head perms on assessment.

Test your knowledge

1   What personal protective equipment should you wear during the perming and neutralising processes?

2   What perming information should be recorded on your client's record card?

3   Why is it important to keep your work area tidy during the perming and neutralising processes?

4   Why is it important to minimise wastage of perming and neutralising products?

5   Name two perming tests that should be carried out before *perming*.

6   Name a perming test carried out during *the perming process.*

7   State five critical influencing factors for perming.

Perming and neutralising

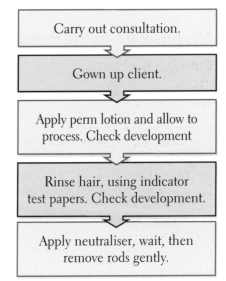

Carry out consultation.

Gown up client.

Apply perm lotion and allow to process. Check development

Rinse hair, using indicator test papers. Check development.

Apply neutraliser, wait, then remove rods gently.

8   State the three different types of perm lotion discussed in Element H12.2.

9   What two things are used to protect the client's hairline during perming?

10   Which three perm winds do you need to perfect for this qualification?

11   Why should you always check water temperature and flow during rinsing of perm lotion and neutraliser?

12   What types of heat can be used to help the perm process?

13   Name two perm lotion application techniques.

14   Why is accurate timing important during the perming and neutralising procedures?

15   How do you know how long the perm lotion should be processed for?

16   Why is it important to section accurately when winding a perm?

17   What result could perm rod rubbers positioned too tightly have?

18   State two reasons why you may achieve curls that are too tight.

19   How could you resolve the problem of a frizzy perm result?

20   How do perms work? Name the three stages of the perming process and explain what happens at each stage.

21   Which perm process involves applying and removing a curl re-arranger?

Perm, relax and neutralise hair (including African Caribbean hair) Unit H15/H16

This unit will give you all the information you need to carry out the processes that change the shape of the hair and give the client a completely new look. The information for the perming and neutralising processes is already covered in Unit H12 on pages 191-214. The following information concentrates on the relaxing and the neutralising part of units H15 and H16. Combined together, you will be able to achieve the underpinning knowledge and practical skills required to complete these creative services. Where necessary, you will be referred to the pages in Unit H12.

What you will learn
• Maintain effective and safe methods of working when perming, relaxing and neutralising hair H15.1 and H16.1
• Prepare for perming, relaxing and neutralising H15.2 and H16.2
• Relax hair H15.4 and H16.4

What are relaxing and neutralising?

Relaxing is the process of reducing or straightening the natural curl.

Neutralising is the chemical process that fixes the hair in a new position after it has been altered by either perming or relaxing.

However, these processes can be damaging to the hair if you do not understand what effect the chemicals have on the hair structure. It is very important to understand the hair structure, especially the cortex region where the chemical changes take place, in order to achieve a professional result. The correct use of after-care products such as restructurants is also extremely important. Before you begin this unit, look back at the section 'Facts about hair and skin' for a reminder of the hair's structure.

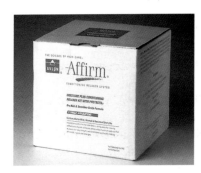

Relaxing product

Maintain effective and safe methods of working when perming, relaxing and neutralising hair H15.1/H16.1

Pages 191-214 cover everything you need to know in this unit about the perming and neutralising processes. Please read these thoroughly. For the relaxing process, you will also need to cover the following areas.

What you will learn
• How relaxers work
• Preparing your client
• Health and safety issues
• Organisation and stock control
• Commercial timing
• Maintaining a record card system

How relaxers work

Relaxing involves three stages:

The softening stage

The relaxer opens and swells the cuticle so that it can enter the cortex.

The bond breaking stage

The relaxer enters the cortex carrying water into the hair and breaking down some of the disulphide bonds. At this point the naturally curly hair is straightened using either your fingers or a comb. As the hair straightens, a new amino acid, Lanthionine, is formed. Lanthionine has only one sulphide bond which means that it can be removed from the hair by thorough rinsing as it combines with the water.

The fixing stage

Neutralising shampoo is used after the relaxer is rinsed from the hair. It restores the hair's natural pH balance, closes the cuticle and helps remove any remaining relaxer.

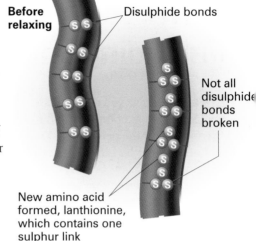

How relaxing works

Preparing your client

Gowning

The chemicals used in relaxers and neutralisers can cause a colour change in some fabrics. Therefore, it is important to ensure the client's clothes are fully protected with a towel, chemical gown (this is plastic coated and will stop any liquid penetrating through it), second towel for extra protection, and plastic cape.

Consultation

A thorough consultation is an essential start to a successful relaxing result. In addition to the normal areas to assess such as hair texture and porosity, you need to ask the client some specific questions relating to the relaxer:

- Do you have any relaxer or colour on your hair?
- How do you manage your hair at home – do you set, blow-dry, leave to dry naturally, use electric tongs?
- Is your skin sensitive to relaxing products?
- Are you on any long-term medication?
- How straight do you want your hair to be?
- Do you have any problem areas that do not relax very well?

Once you have the answers to these questions you can decide:

- if any hair tests are necessary
- which strength relaxer to use.

Health and safety issues

Relaxing and neutralising involves the use of chemicals and you have to know and understand your responsibilities when using these products. You must always read and follow the manufacturer's instructions for the particular product you are using.

It is vital that you follow all health and safety rules and regulations during the relaxing and neutralising process to ensure the highest level of client care possible.

Personal protective equipment (PPE)

When applying relaxers and neutralisers, it is important to protect yourself from the possible effects of the chemicals. You must wear an apron to protect yourself.

It is also very important to protect yourself from the occupational hazard of the skin complaint dermatitis, which has caused such severe skin problems for some hairdressers that they have had to change careers. If you always wear gloves when applying relaxer and neutraliser to avoid contact with these chemicals, you will minimise the risk of this happening to you.

Under the Personal Protective Equipment at Work Regulations, your employer has a responsibility to provide protective materials and gloves for you to use and you have a responsibility to wear them.

Control of Substances Hazardous to Health Regulations 2003

Under the Control of Substances Hazardous to Health Regulations (COSHH) 2003, you must read the data sheets provided by the manufacturer of the relaxer so that you know how to handle, store, and dispose of the chemicals used in the product.

Generally, relaxers should be stored in a cool, dry place away from bright sunlight. They should be used in a well-ventilated area and manufacturer's instructions must be followed. When disposing of any leftover relaxer or neutraliser, you should dilute the chemicals by flushing them down the sink with plenty of water.

Effective working methods

Refer to page 194 in Unit H12.

Working area

Your working area must be kept clean and tidy at all times to prevent hazards and potential accidents. Look back at Unit H12, page 194, and remind yourself of how you should maintain a clean environment at all times. What are the consequences of working unsafely in a muddle?

Organisation and stock control

It is important to build into your working day time to organise yourself for your client's service before they arrive.

When preparing your trolley for a relaxing service, include:

- large, wide-toothed comb
- sectioning clips
- barrier cream
- cotton wool
- towels
- gloves and apron
- water spray.

If you do not organise yourself in readiness for the relaxing, you will be wasting valuable time. Your employer will want you to use all of your time at work effectively and your clients will not want to be kept waiting.

Stock control

In order for the salon to function effectively, you are required to follow stock control procedures. Make sure you know what they are.

Check it out

What would you consider to be contraindications to relaxing? List five and keep in your portfolio.

Check it out

Make a note of your salon's stock control procedures, including:

- the person(s) responsible for re-ordering stock
- how *you* are required to report shortages of sundries and products
- the telephone number of your nearest hairdressing wholesaler or established representative
- how the salon keeps a check on the stock it has.

Place your findings in your portfolio.

Remember

The Data Protection Act states that all record card information should be accurate, up to date, kept for as long as the client is still attending the salon, must be accessible to the client, and is kept securely.

Commercial timing

It takes skill and accuracy to complete a relaxing process competently. As a Level 2 Hairdressing student, you have performance criteria for relaxing to meet before your assessor can be sure you are competent.

Relaxing (applying relaxer) = 20 minutes

The above timing is a target for you to work to and aim for. You should always follow manufacturer's instructions on timing.

Maintaining a record card system

It is especially important to keep your client's records up to date when relaxing. Record cards should contain all the relevant information such as date of the relaxing, products used, result of the relaxing, price of the relaxing and anything else you feel is relevant.

The record card needs to be filled in accurately so write down the information immediately after the client has left the salon. You will be amazed how quickly you forget things.

Health and safety

Gown client effectively to stop any chemicals staining clothes.

Carry out a thorough consultation and any hair tests necessary.

Always read the manufacturer's instructions for the relaxing products chosen.

Be organised and keep your area tidy as you work to avoid accidents happening.

Prepare for perming, relaxing and neutralising

H15.2/H16.2

In this element you will be provided with the information needed to prepare your client fully for relaxing and neutralising processes. You will have already covered preparing for perming on pages 198–204.

What you will learn

- Hair tests for relaxing and neutralising
- When not to relax
- Relaxing and neutralising products
- Preparing and protecting your client

Hair tests for relaxing and neutralising

You should always explain the importance of tests to your client so she is aware that you are checking to see whether the hair can withstand the chemical process you are going to carry out.

Elasticity test

This is to test the internal strength of the hair. Hair that has been damaged due to chemical treatments may have lost much of its natural strength. This type of hair may stretch to over two-thirds of its original length and may even break off. It is important to carry out this test. Hair that is in good condition will stretch and then return to its original length.

Take one strand of hair and hold each end firmly between the thumb and forefinger of each hand and gently pull. If the hair stretches more than two thirds of its original length then it is over elastic and may snap or break during relaxing.

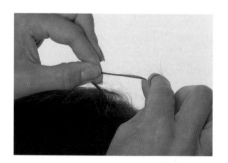

The elasticity test

Porosity test

This tests the condition of the outer layer of the hair shaft – the cuticle. If the cuticle is damaged, it becomes porous. Chemical products added to porous hair will be absorbed unevenly and may produce uneven results. Pre-relaxer treatments can be applied to porous hair prior to relaxing to help maintain an even absorption of chemicals.

Take a strand of hair and hold it by the point (where the hair has been cut) between the thumb and forefinger of one hand. Run the forefinger and thumb of your other hand from the root (where the hair grows from) down to the point. If the hair feels rough and bumpy, the cuticle scales are raised and open and this is an indication of porous hair. If the hair feels smooth, the cuticle is flat and closed and the hair's cuticle region is in good condition.

Incompatibility test for relaxing

Some chemicals do not work well together (they are incompatible) and may have a bad reaction if one is used over the top of another. Some colours, for example, contain metallic salts, which are incompatible with other chemicals. You should carry out an incompatibility test before relaxing if you are unsure of the products already on the hair or if the hair has a doubtful history.

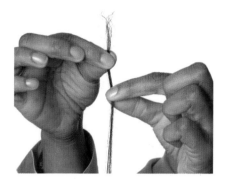

The porosity test

- Mix together (preferably in a glass bowl) 10 ml of hydrogen peroxide and 10 ml of relaxer.
- Place a small cutting of hair in the solution and wait. If heat is given off, the lotion fizzes and the hair breaks or dissolves or changes colour, then this is a positive reaction and the hair should NOT be relaxed with a product containing hydrogen peroxide. The hair contains metallic salts.

Pre-relaxer test

This tests for the reaction of relaxing products on the hair and should be carried out if you are unsure of the hair's history or condition, or if you are in any doubt about the suitability of the strength of the relaxer. The test will determine whether the relaxer is suitable and the speed at which the natural curl will be removed. It should be carried out where the hair is most resistant.

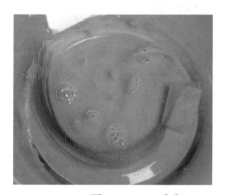

The incompatibility test

Take a small section of hair and pull through a slit in a piece of aluminium foil, placed as close to the scalp as possible. Apply the chosen strength of relaxer to the strand of hair and allow it to process on the hair for the amount of time given in the manufacturer's instructions (usually two to three minutes). Remove with a piece of dry cotton wool. If the test result is satisfactory, proceed with the full relaxing treatment. If the test is not satisfactory, repeat it, allowing the relaxer to process on the hair for a few more minutes. Keep a note of exactly how long the chemical has been on the hair until you get a satisfactory result. Always follow the manufacturer's instructions and never allow the relaxer to remain on the hair for any longer than is stated.

Once you have carried out the necessary tests and you are satisfied with the results, continue with the service. Remember not to apply relaxer to the hair used to do the test.

When not to relax

- When the scalp is damaged or the skin broken/damaged.
- When the hair is in poor condition.
- When the overall porosity of the hair is too high – over bleached.
- In the presence of metallic salts, for example, Grecian 2000.
- When the hair has poor elasticity.
- Only relax the re-growth on coloured or bleached hair to avoid hair breakage.

Reality check!

Always test the hair to check that it is safe to carry out the relaxing process.

Relaxing and neutralising products

Being able to choose and use the correct products suitable for both European and African Caribbean hair types is a particular feature of this unit.

Relaxing products

These have a very high alkaline pH, between 10 and 14, and, if used incorrectly, can be very damaging to the hair and skin. They contain sodium hydroxide, which is known as lye in the USA. Products containing lye are stronger and more likely to cause irritation to the skin and scalp. Many relaxing products imported into the UK have higher levels of chemical ingredients than are permitted in this country and some state that they have 'no lye'. This hides the fact that the relaxing product almost certainly contains other highly caustic chemicals such as potassium or lithium. Do not be misled into thinking these products will be kinder to the hair and skin. Relaxing products bought for use at home will be weaker than professional relaxers as they will contain less sodium hydroxide.

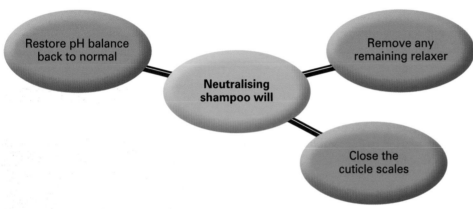

- Restore pH balance back to normal
- Neutralising shampoo will
- Remove any remaining relaxer
- Close the cuticle scales

Neutralising shampoo

This is used after the relaxing product has been rinsed out of the hair.

Neutralisers

Neutralisers come in many different forms. Some are ready to use out of the bottle, some need to be mixed with warm water, some need to be foamed up in a bowl and applied with a sponge, and some neutralisers are instant. The chemical ingredient in neutralisers may be either hydrogen peroxide or sodium bromate, both of which can lighten or fade hair colour. Most neutralisers used in African Caribbean perms usually contain sodium bromate, as this has a much gentler action on the hair than hydrogen peroxide. This is why the neutralising process differs with African Caribbean hair, as the rods are left in the hair throughout the neutralising process because the gentler action takes longer to process. Sodium bromate also has less hair lightening properties than hydrogen peroxide.

Preparing and protecting your client

The good practice outlined on page 193 of Unit H12 applies here.

You must always consider the effects of the chemicals you are using and their potential for harming your client. This will help you evaluate any risks and avoid accidents happening.

Preparing the hair for relaxing

Begin by correctly gowning your client (see Element H15.1).

Remember
Always read and follow the manufacturer's instructions before using a relaxing product.

Preparing for relaxing and neutralising

During consultation, analyse the hair and scalp, then question your client about any contraindications to relaxing and neutralising and record her responses.

⇩

Carry out any hair tests you feel are necessary from your consultation.

⇩

Choose your relaxer strength from the results of your consultation.

⇩

Prepare your client thoroughly and make sure you prepare the hair ready for relaxing.

⇩

Apply a pre-relaxer treatment if necessary from the results of your consultation.

⇩

Apply barrier cream around the scalp hairline before applying relaxer to stop scalp/hairline irritation.

⇩

Apply an anti-oxidant moisturising conditioner after neutralising to stop the chemicals working further (always read the manufacturer's instructions to check if this is recommended).

Barrier cream/protective base

This is a thick protective cream, which should be applied all the way around the client's hairline before applying relaxers (including nape area) to avoid irritation of the skin. Care must be taken to avoid putting the cream onto the hair as this will cause a barrier between the relaxer and the hair and will result in unsuccessful areas. Clients with sensitive skin will be more likely to have a skin reaction from the relaxer so always take the utmost care to avoid this happening. Some relaxing product manufacturers recommend you base all over the scalp with barrier cream before any chemicals are applied. This involves applying barrier cream very carefully using a cotton wool bud to the scalp only (if applied to the hair a barrier will stop the relaxer taking).

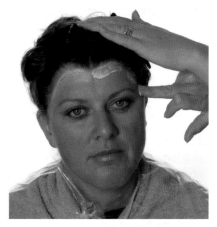

Applying barrier cream

Pre-relaxer treatment

These are used on porous hair in the same way as pre-perm treatments. They are used to:

- even out the porosity along the hair shaft to help the relaxer absorb at an even rate – results in an even result along the hair
- form a protective barrier along the cuticle region and help buffer/close any cuticle scales that are raised
- make the hair more pliable and easier to control.

Relax hair   H15.4/H16.4

Chemically relaxing hair is a permanent process that reduces the amount of curl. All relaxers contain hydroxide, which opens the cuticle scales, penetrates the cortex and breaks the disulphide bonds. The chemical ingredient in relaxers is usually sodium hydroxide (lye) but some relaxers may contain calcium hydroxide, potassium hydroxide, guanidine hydroxide and lithium hydroxide (all no-lye). Since these chemicals have a very high alkaline pH of 10 to 14, they can have a drying and damaging effect on the hair. Sodium hydroxide-based products are the strongest, fastest and have the highest pH value, very close to the pH of hair-removing creams (depilatories), so extreme caution must be taken when using these products.

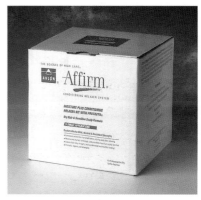

Relaxing product

Since relaxing is stronger than perming, it is advisable to explain to the client that once she has had relaxing products on her hair, it will be too fragile to withstand a perm.

What you will learn

- Analysing natural curl, critical influencing factors, and confirming amount of relaxing required
- Preparing the hair for relaxing
- Applying relaxing products to the hair
- Monitoring development of the relaxer and performing a strand test
- Rinsing relaxer from the hair
- Coping with relaxing treatment problems
- Treating re-growth

Analysing natural curl, critical influencing factors, and confirming amount of relaxing required

Carry out a hair and scalp consultation, taking into account critical influencing factors such as:

- any chemical treatments already on the hair
- elasticity
- porosity
- texture
- hairline
- scalp condition, cuts and abrasions
- hair growth patterns
- hair length
- the strength of natural curl, which may differ across the head.

The amount of curl and the condition of the hair will determine the strength of relaxer you choose.

Test timing

It is sometimes a good idea to ask your client to come in for a consultation prior to the appointment to enable you to carry out hair tests. This will allow you to determine whether you can carry out the procedure on the client before the appointment itself. Arrange this consultation when the client makes the booking – ask if it is possible for her to come in 24–48 hours prior to the appointment to allow you to carry out relevant tests. Explain what the tests are and why you have to do them.

It is important to discuss with the client the amount of curl to be removed. Not every client will want you to remove all their natural curl as this can make the hair hard to manage. A thorough discussion will determine the amount of curl the client hopes to remove, but you will also need to advise her regarding the strength of relaxer you feel it is appropriate to use.

Using your professional knowledge

If your client has colour-treated hair, for example, bleached, or sensitive hair, you would normally choose a mild strength relaxer. However, the client may also have very tight curly hair and want a very straight result from the relaxer. You would need to explain the reason why you wanted to use this particular product. As the hair is already sensitised with colour, a strong relaxer could cause breakage. For this reason, it is appropriate to use a mild formula that does not have the power to fully remove all the natural curl but will certainly soften the curl and leave the hair in a manageable condition.

Relaxer	Hair type
Mild	Coloured, bleached or sensitive hair
Regular	Normal hair (calcium or hydroxide based)
Super	Resistant, coarse or virgin hair (sodium hydroxide based)

Suitability of relaxers for different hair types

The pH factor for relaxers is 10–14 depending on their strength. The strongest relaxers contain the most sodium hydroxide and the result will be quicker to process, but there is a greater danger of chemical damage. If in doubt, it is always advisable to use a milder relaxer and have the option to leave it on the hair longer.

Preparing the hair for relaxing

DO NOT shampoo the hair before using a chemical relaxer. It is necessary to have the protection of the natural oils (sebum) on the scalp prior to the application of

Reality check!

Never relax hair that has been recently plaited as the hair will already be in a fragile state, especially at the roots. Wait at least two to four weeks before carrying out a relaxing treatment or you may find the hair snaps under the pressure used in relaxing. Recommend to the client a deep penetrating conditioner or restructuring treatment.

chemicals. For extra protection of the scalp, hairline and ears, always apply a protective base of barrier cream over the whole scalp using a cotton bud – make sure you work in a methodical and careful manner so that no barrier is applied to the hair that would prevent the relaxer from working (see pages 220–1).

Applying relaxing products to the hair

Always wear a protective apron and gloves before applying any relaxing product. The chemicals contained within a relaxer are caustic and will burn your skin and discolour your uniform.

Section the hair into four and secure with sectioning clips. With the desired amount of relaxer decanted into a bowl, start applying the relaxer to the most resistant/tightest curled area using a tint brush. Take small, methodical, neat sections and apply sufficient relaxing product until all the hair to be relaxed is covered. Take care not to apply to the scalp or ears. Apply to the front sections but leave the front hairline until last. Repeat the application throughout all the sections to ensure all the necessary hair is covered.

If applying to re-growth, only apply up to the line of the previous relaxer – DO NOT re-apply to already relaxed hair as this could cause the hair to break.

When working on porous hair, apply only to the healthiest part initially, as porous hair processes at a faster rate and therefore needs less development time.

Reality check!

Never use heat to aid processing time during relaxing treatments, as this will cause hair breakage.

Monitoring development of the relaxer and performing a strand test

Always follow the manufacturer's instructions for the development of relaxers. Most companies recommend you grip the hair, which has relaxer applied to it, between your index and middle finger and then using a scissor-like action, smooth the hair to reduce the curl. This procedure should be repeated until the desired straightness is achieved and the development time is complete.

To check that the desired straightness has been achieved, take a development test by removing some of the relaxer using a piece of cotton wool. Check the wave pattern, which should look smooth and shiny if processing is complete. NEVER EXCEED THE RECOMMENDED DEVELOPMENT TIME.

Rinsing relaxer from the hair

Use a backwash basin to avoid any chemicals entering the client's eyes. Using cool water, thoroughly rinse the relaxer from the hair. Do not massage the hair or scalp at this stage. Pay particular attention to the hairline and nape areas and make sure you have removed all traces of the relaxer from the hair. The hair is now ready to be neutralised.

Neutralising when relaxing

When the hair has been rinsed sufficiently and all the relaxer removed, you are ready to apply the neutralising shampoo. This does not rejoin the sulphur bonds as with neutralising after perming. The function of the neutralising shampoo is to return the hair to an acidic pH by neutralising the alkalinity of the hair caused by the harsh relaxing chemicals. Use the neutralising shampoo twice then shampoo with an after-treatment shampoo and apply a conditioner to smooth and moisturise the hair.

It is a good idea to use a timer that rings so that you know exactly how long you have rinsed for.

Reality check!

If any relaxer is left in the hair, it will continue working and over process, causing limp, damaged and often broken hair.

Step-by-step relaxing

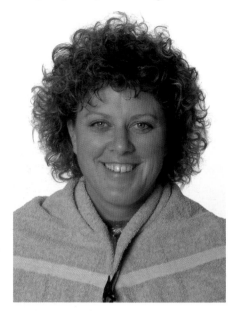

Carry out consultation and gown client.

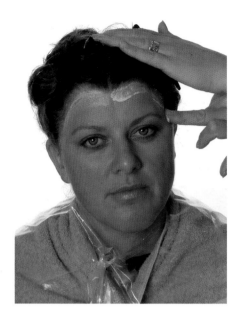

Apply the barrier cream to the scalp according to manufacturer's instructions to prevent irritation.

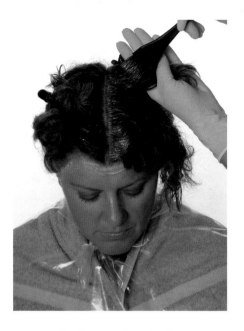

Section the hair and apply the product. Divide the hair – centre forehead to centre nape, ear to ear across the crown. Take small sub-sections. Start application from nape. Do not apply closer than 12 mm to the scalp.

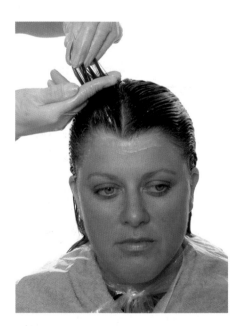

Smooth with fingers or comb and monitor development. Use a comb with wide-spaced teeth. Treat hair very gently. Leave on relaxer until the hair is as straight as required, but do not exceed the manufacturer's development time.

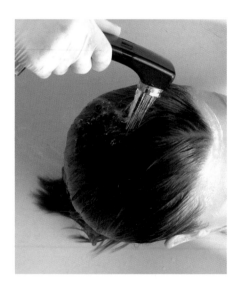

Rinse off relaxer at a backwash basin. Do not massage, but allow the force of the water to remove the product. Continue until all the water runs clear. Apply neutralising shampoo. Rinse and condition with moisturisers.

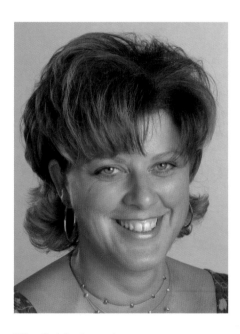

The finished result.

5   Name two tests that should be carried out before perming,

6   Name a perming test carried out during the perming process.

7   State five critical influencing factors for perming.

8   State the three different types of perm lotion discussed in Element H12.2.

9   What two things are used to protect the client's hairline during perming?

10 Which three perm winds do you need to perfect for this qualification?

11 Why should you always check water temperature and flow during rinsing of perm lotion and neutraliser?

12 Name two perm lotion application techniques.

13 Why is accurate timing important during perming, relaxing and neutralising procedures?

14 How do you know how long the perm lotion or relaxer should be processed for?

15 Why is it important to section accurately when winding a perm?

16 How could you resolve the problem of a frizzy perm result?

17 Which chemical ingredient is found in the strongest relaxing products available?

18 Should you use heat to help process a relaxing treatment?

19 What should you apply to the scalp prior to relaxing the hair?

20 Which bonds are broken during relaxing treatments?

21 What pH range do chemical relaxers have?

22 Why is it important to check the hair and scalp before relaxing?

23 Why should you ask the client about when she last shampooed her hair?

24 Why is it important to ask the client whether she has had her hair braided or had extensions added recently?

Change hair colour using basic techniques

Unit H13

Colouring can be one of the most challenging processes in hairdressing but also one of the most rewarding and exciting. Colour aids the appearance of texture, depth and movement of the hair. There are many different levels and techniques involved in colouring, from temporary colours, which will only stain the hair, to permanent colours that can be applied with foils, mesh, or even combed through the hair. This unit describes the procedures and introduces the basic principles of colouring.

What you will learn

- Maintain effective and safe working methods when colouring hair H13.1
- Prepare for colouring H13.2
- Add colour to hair H13.3
- Permanently change hair colour H13.4

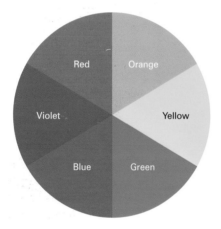

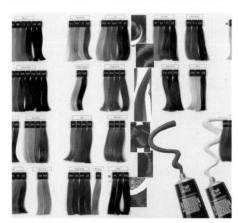

Maintain effective and safe working methods when colouring hair

H13.1

It is important to make sure that you work in a safe manner and environment when working with colour, as you are working with chemicals. You need to make sure you follow manufacturer's instructions and use the correct PPE for both yourself and your client. You need to be aware of COSHH and risk assessment policies to ensure your working practices adhere to health and safety regulations.

What you will learn

- Preparing the client for temporary, semi, quasi and permanent colouring treatments
- Ensuring health and safety
- Equipment you will be using
- Using your time effectively
- Carrying out a consultation
- Choosing suitable products and equipment
- Reporting low levels of stock
- General allocation of time for colour application
- Keeping accurate and up-to-date client records

Preparing the client for temporary, semi, quasi and permanent colouring treatments

Gowning

You should always make sure that the client is protected for any hairdressing service, but it is especially important when carrying out a colouring process. If the client is not correctly gowned, colour could fall onto her clothing and you could be held responsible for the damaged item. This is the correct gowning procedure.

- Use a chemical gown (if one is available).
- Place a plastic disposable cape around the client.
- Place a colouring towel over the top of the cape and secure.

Using barrier cream

Barrier cream is used to prevent any tint sitting on the client's face – dark tints will stain the skin. Some clients have very sensitive skin, which can become inflamed if a barrier cream is not used.

Apply the barrier cream, either with your finger or using a cotton wool bud. Make sure that the cream is evenly and thickly applied as close to the hairline as you can get without depositing any on the hair itself.

Remove the barrier cream *after* you have shampooed the tint from the hair and before you begin the cut or blow-dry. Make sure all traces are removed, as the cream can be very greasy.

Protecting yourself

You also have a duty to ensure your own health and safety within the salon. When preparing to carry out a colouring service, your PPE should consist of:

- an apron – to protect your clothes
- gloves – to protect your hands from chemicals and staining
- sensible shoes – flat, non-slip shoes to prevent any injuries to legs and ankles.

It is important that you wear the correct PPE when colouring hair, not only to protect your clothes but also to portray a professional image to the client.

Positioning

Ensure that the client is sitting in an upright position, enabling you to work freely around the head.

You may need to adjust the position of your client while working so that you can reach the more difficult areas of the head when colouring, for example, the top of the head. Do not be afraid to ask your client to tilt her head backwards or forwards so that you can apply the colour easily. Place your tools and equipment within easy reach.

You also need to consider your own posture and position when you are working at your unit. Read back through Unit G1 to remind you of this.

Ensuring health and safety

Protecting the client

Imagine the following situations:

- A client comes into the salon for a re-growth colour. You get out her record card only to discover that the last time she had a colour treatment in the salon was over a year ago. Your first responsibility is to ensure the health and safety of the

Remember
If you are not sure whether your client is allergic to barrier cream, use Vaseline (petroleum jelly).

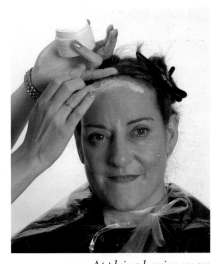

Applying barrier cream

Check it out
Discuss with your colleagues the correct and incorrect ways of positioning yourself and your client so that you reduce the risk of possible injury and fatigue while you are working.

client, so for her own wellbeing, you have to refuse the treatment until you have completed a current skin test.

- A second client comes into the salon, also for a re-growth colour. She is going straight to a dinner and dance from the hairdressers and has spent a long time on her make-up. She states that she does not want any barrier cream applied because it will ruin her make-up. Once again, this is a health and safety issue. You need to explain that the barrier cream is to protect her skin from staining and from becoming sensitive and that you are unable to carry out the procedure unless barrier cream is applied.

Applying the products

You will always need to take great care when using colouring products. Some are quite runny while others are thicker, but all need great care. Make sure you are aware of all health and safety rules that your salon and the manufacturers put in place when you apply these products.

Work area checks

- Put away or dispose of unwanted equipment before you receive your next client following the COSHH regulations if you need to.
- Check and, if necessary, mop up spillages of water or products on the floor.
- Sweep up any hair cuttings from the floor.
- Have ready the client's record card together with the appropriate equipment.
- Ensure your working area is clean and tidy to receive the next client.

Mixing colours

This should not be done by guesswork. Always prepare the colour as set out in the manufacturer's instructions. Quantities must be measured accurately. The wrong quantities may produce unwanted colour effects. It is essential to read the manufacturer's instructions to ensure that you use the product correctly. There are a variety of procedures and each is particular to the product. You will need to prepare the tint immediately before use. Do not allow it to stand for any length of time or it will lose its effectiveness.

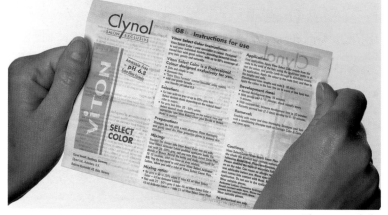

Always read the manufacturer's instructions

If you are using more than one colour, mix tints together in a bowl before adding hydrogen peroxide. Tint tubes have measurements marked on them to ensure that the correct amount of tint can be added. When you measure out hydrogen peroxide, read the amount at eye level to be sure of an accurate measurement.

When you are working with colouring products, you may find that it is better to mix up less colour than you think you will need. You can always mix up more colour later. For example, if you are working on long hair, perhaps putting two

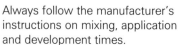

Quantities should be measured accurately

colours through using a foil technique, the service may take you slightly longer. While your product is in the bowl it is losing its strength and you may find this could produce a different colour result. In this instance, it is better to mix up a small amount of product then mix up more as it is required.

Reality check!

Always follow the manufacturer's instructions on mixing, application and development times.

Your salon will have legal requirements in place for the disposal of waste materials. Most salons will require you to dilute the product down the sink with water that is not used for any domestic services.

By law, all salons need to have risk assessment sheets on all products that are used within the salon. On these you will find all the relevant information on how to handle, store and dispose of products safely. Most salons will have these sheets located in a folder all together in an accessible location for everyone to access.

Minimise the risk of cross-infection

As with all hairdressing services, you need to be aware of the possibilities of cross-infection and infestation when you are working. To prevent the risk of either of these you will need to complete a thorough consultation to make sure that you are able to continue with the service. Refer to pages 92–94, for more information on cross-infections and infestations.

All tools and equipment should be cleaned and sterilised regularly. Washing in warm soapy water to remove old products can clean most of the equipment used for colouring. If you discover that your client has an infection or infestation when you are halfway through the application, you will be required to complete the service. In this instance, you will need to sterilise your equipment to prevent the risk of cross-infection.

Minimising harm or injury to yourself or others

When carrying out a colouring process, you may need to use extra equipment; it is your responsibility to make sure that the equipment is in good working order.

Safety considerations

- Check that plugs and cables are in good condition.
- Do not use electrical equipment with wet hands.
- Check temperature controls before you turn on equipment.
- Check the client is comfortable while you are using the equipment.
- Always allow equipment to cool before storing.

Products

When working with chemicals, follow all of the health and safety guidelines set down by the manufacturers and your salon or training institution.

Here are some guidelines.

- Complete a skin test on the client before carrying out any colouring process (apart from temporary colours).
- Mix only the amount of product that you think you are going to need – mixing too much is wasteful and uneconomic.
- Mix the product immediately before use – tint starts to oxidise (develop) as soon as it makes contact with the atmosphere.
- Place lids back on products as soon as you have measured out the amount that you require.
- Use the correct PPE.
- Store chemicals correctly when they are not being used – refer to manufacturers' COSSH sheets for information on handling, storage and disposal of products, the harm they could cause and how to treat in case of an accident (see Unit H5).

Check it out

In your salon, find out how you are expected to dispose of any waste materials left over from a colouring process.

Check it out

- Where does your salon keep its risk assessment folder?
- What colour is the folder?
- What does it contain?

Check it out

Thinking back to the sterilisation charts in other units, discuss and research in groups what you think would be the best methods of sterilising the equipment opposite.

Personal hygiene

As well as looking after your tools and equipment, you must also make sure that you take your own personal hygiene into account to minimise the risk of cross-infection and infestation.

- Long hair needs to be worn up to cut down on the risk of cross-infection.
- Minimum amount of jewellery to be worn.
- Flat shoes with tights may need to be worn for health and safety and hygiene purposes.
- You will be required to sterilise all tools and equipment after each client.
- Make sure your personal presentation and hygiene are of a very high standard.
- Make sure you use a breath freshening spray if you smoke or have had strong-flavoured food (e.g. curry, garlic or chilli) the night before!
- Wear cotton tops in the summer and use a good deodorant.
- Always wash your hands after a trip to the bathroom.
- Always keep cuts and open wounds covered with a plaster.

Most of these points are common sense and things that you will do on a daily basis without realising it.

Equipment you will be using

- Tint bowl
- Tint brush
- Sectioning clips
- Combs
- Towels
- Gloves
- Barrier cream
- Gowns.

Using your time effectively

Each salon allows a set amount of time for the different services that it offers.

Time allocation allowed for colouring services differs depending on the method of application and the products used. For example, applying a semi-permanent colour does not take as long as applying a full head bleach.

Carrying out a consultation

By completing a colouring consultation form, you will be able to answer all the following questions, allowing you to make the right choices and decisions for the colouring process.

- Identify and discuss your client's wishes.
- Is the process possible? Are there any critical influencing factors that may prevent the process, for example, previous chemical treatments, the condition of the hair?
- Can you achieve the target colour the client wants? Is the client's natural base shade too light or dark to achieve the target colour? How much grey is present in the hair?
- Decide on the products you will be using. How long does the client want the colour to last?
- What will your method of application be? Is it a re-growth colour or full head colour?

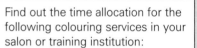

Check it out

Find out the time allocation for the following colouring services in your salon or training institution:

- temporary colour
- semi-permanent colour
- quasi-permanent colour
- permanent re-touch colour
- permanent full head colour
- highlights with cap
- highlights with mesh or foils.

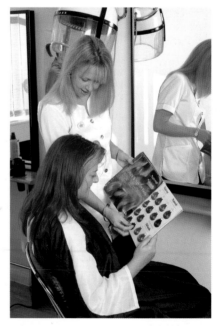

Can you achieve the colour the client wants?

Colouring consultation form

Client's name: _____ Address: _____

Contact tel. no: _____ _____

Date: _____ Date of last skin test: _____

Colouring

Natural base shade: _____

Natural tones: _____

Amount of white hair present

0–10% ☐   10–25% ☐   25–50% ☐   50–75% ☐   75–100% ☐

Colourant type

Temporary ☐   Semi-permanent ☐   Quasi-permanent ☐   Permanent ☐

Bleach ☐   Lightening ☐   Darkening ☐   Changing tone ☐

Product chosen

Name: _____

Shade no(s): _____

With/without heat: _____

Processing time: _____

Peroxide strength

10 vol (3%) ☐   20 vol (6%) ☐   30 vol (9%) ☐   40 vol (12%) ☐

Method of application

Full head ☐   Re-growth ☐   High/lowlights ☐

Foils ☐   Mesh ☐   Other ☐

Colour result and evaluation _____

After-care advice _____

Candidate evaluation _____

Assessor comments _____

Units assessed _____

Client evaluation

Were you satisfied with the treatment you received? Yes ☐   No ☐

Did the candidate consult with you about your requirements? Yes ☐   No ☐

Are you pleased with the finished result? Yes ☐   No ☐

Candidate's signature: _____

Client's signature: _____

Assessor signature and number: _____

Competent ☐

Not yet competent ☐

Style books and colour shade chart

During the consultation, you will find it helpful to use visual aids. A selection of style books will enable you to show the client different colouring techniques.

A colour shade chart plays a major role in your consultation. It will help your client to decide what depth or tone of colour she would like and it will enable you to match up to the client's natural colour. The chart will also help you to explain what can and cannot be achieved.

Most colour shade charts contain information and instructions on how to determine your colour choice, mix, application and development of the colour.

Choosing suitable products and equipment

When you begin a colouring service you need to take into account the type of product you will be using, as this affects how you prepare the hair for the application of the colour.

Check it out

From the information given in the chart below, what type of colour would you recommend to a client if she:

- had never had colour before and was worried about the maintenance of having a colour?
- had been on holiday and the ends of her hair were faded to a different colour from the roots?
- wanted to go two shades lighter than her natural colour?

Colouring treatments

Product type	Suitability	Effect
Coloured mousse Coloured setting lotions Hair mascara	Most hair types – not bleached or very porous hair	Lasts until the next shampoo. Does not lift hair, only deposits colour
Semi-permanent	Covers up to 30% white hair. Often used as a colour refresher for faded ends on fragile hair	Lasts 4–8 shampoos. Does not lift hair, only deposits colour
Quasi-permanent	Most hair types. Covers a high percentage of grey hair. Can produce a re-growth (a band of natural hair colour when the hair grows through)	Lasts 8–12 shampoos. Generally does not lift hair, only deposits colour
Permanent colours (para dyes)	Not suitable for over processed, dry, damaged hair. Will cover 100% white hair and lift up to three shades (lighten the hair by a maximum of three shades)	Grows out. Lightens hair. Adds depth and tone
Bleach	Not suitable for over processed, dry or damaged hair. Can be used to achieve seven shades of lift. Suitable for dark bases when a high lift tint will not achieve the required result	Lifts and lightens the hair, grows out
High lift tint	Suitable for base 6 (dark blonde) and above. Not recommended on very dry, damaged hair	Lifts and lightens the hair, will add tone. Grows out. Kinder than bleach

Mixing and measuring

Not all colours are mixed in the same way. Different manufacturers have different mixing and measuring procedures that apply to their own specific products. Just because one permanent colour that you have used is mixed in a certain way, do not assume that all colours are the same.

Remember

It is important to explain the lasting effects of colour to the client so that she can make the right choice for herself and the lifestyle she leads.

- Mousses and semi-permanent colours do not require mixing. They are used straight from the can or tube.

- Quasi-permanent colours are mixed with their own activators or developers. These usually contain only a very weak amount of hydrogen peroxide, but the same care must be used when applying as you would use for permanent colours.

- Permanent colours are mixed with 20, 30 or 40 volume peroxide (6%, 9%, 12%), depending on the target colour you wish to achieve.

When measuring out hydrogen peroxide and tint, make sure that you are accurate – do not guess. Read the amount in the measuring flask at eye level for accurate measurement.

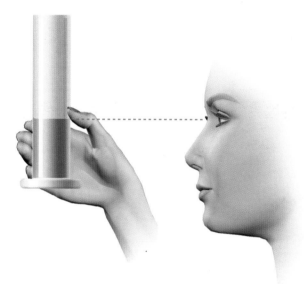

Read the amount in the measuring flask at eye level

When mixing a quarter or half a tube of tint, note where the marks are on the side of the tube and only squeeze out the tint to these guidelines.

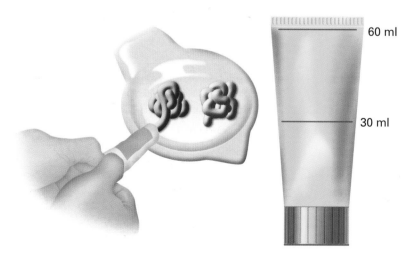

60 ml

30 ml

Tint tubes have guide marks to help you measure accurately

If you are using more than one colour, first mix the two tints together in a bowl *before* adding the hydrogen peroxide. This will ensure thorough mixing of the tints.

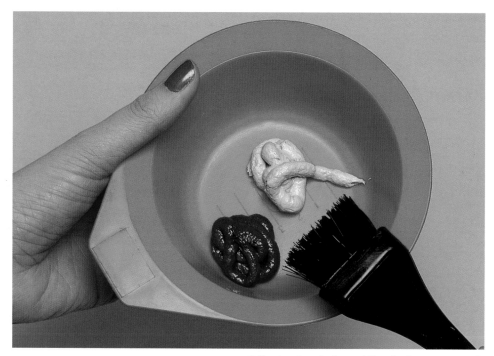

Mix the tints before adding hydrogen peroxide

Prepare the tint immediately before use. Do not allow the tint to stand for any length of time or it will lose its effectiveness.

Tools and equipment

The type of colouring effect that you want will determine the equipment that you use.

Equipment for colouring treatments

Type	Suitability	Effect
Highlighting/ lowlighting cap	Short to medium length hair (if hair is too short, it will produce a spotty effect). Used for the application of one colour	Strands of hair highlighted or darkened evenly over the head
Mesh or foil	All hair lengths except very short hair (less than 5 cm). Used for the application of two or more colours	Two or more colours woven or sliced through the hair
Block colouring	All hair lengths. Care must be taken; mask off the hair so that the colours do not run into each other	Hair is divided into two or more – a solid colour is applied to one half of the head and another colour to the other half and so on
Wide-tooth comb	All hair lengths, but especially short hair where other techniques cannot be used	Produces quite 'chunky' strands of coloured hair depending on the amount of tint applied to the comb

Using equipment that is safe for the purpose

During the colouring process you may need to use other electrical equipment to aid the development of your colour. By using this equipment you will be adding heat to the hair. You will need to make safety checks on the equipment.

You should carry out the following checks on equipment before you use it:

- check there are no frayed cables
- check the water levels if using a steamer
- check the sticker on the equipment is in date and authorised by a qualified electrical tester
- check the temperature at regular intervals.

As well as making checks on your electrical equipment, you will need to make checks on all other tools. Check that you do not have broken teeth on any combs as this may tear the hair and cause discomfort to the client. After a certain amount of time your tinting brushes may loose their bristles and this will hinder the distribution of your tint and may affect the colour result.

Reporting low levels of stock

The maintainence of adequate stock levels may not be your direct responsibility, but as part of a team, it is your responsibility to report any low or missing stock items and to make sure you are prepared for the services you are giving.

> ### In the salon
>
> Mrs Olinda is coming in for her Friday afternoon re-growth colour. She has been your client for months now and you have just found the colour that best suits her hair. Unfortunately, it has been a busy day and when you start to prepare for her you realise that the products you usually use are not in stock.
>
> Discuss with your group:
>
> - what actions you should take immediately.
> - what alternative product choice you could make.
> - how you would explain the situation to Mrs Olinda.
> - how you would ensure this does not happen again.

In most salons and colleges/training institutions you would report low stock levels to the person directly in charge of you. This could be your salon manager or tutor. If that person is not available, the best course of action is to leave a memo in whatever communication system you use. You would then have recorded that you identified that stock was low and notified the relevant person.

General allocation of time for colour application

As a trainee, the time allocations listed below are those you should be working towards and not what you are expected to achieve when you first begin.

- Temporary – these are applied as normal mousses or setting lotions, developed following manufacturer's instructions and rinsed.
- Semi-permanent – 15–30 minutes for consultation, preparation and application. Development time depends on the product you are using. Always read the manufacturer's instructions.
- Quasi-permanent – 15–30 minutes (as above).
- Permanent re-growth – 30 minutes for consultation, preparation and application.
- Permanent full head – 45 minutes for the first application, then a further 20 minutes to complete the application.
- Cap highlights – 30 minutes for consultation, pulling through the highlights and applying the product. Development time depends on the required end result and the product you are using.

Remember

A qualified electrician should check all electrical equipment every six months to comply with the Electricity at Work Regulations.

Check it out

In your groups, discuss the regular checks required to make sure tools and equipment are fit and safe for the purpose they are used.

Remember

Teamwork and supporting each other makes for a happy atmosphere in the salon.

- Mesh highlights – usually a maximum of one hour. Fresh tint may have to be mixed half way through as the product loses its strength after 30 minutes.

Keeping accurate and up-to-date client records

It is important to record all of the services that you carry out on a client for future reference. You should include:

- the client's name, address and a contact telephone number
- date of the client's last skin test
- date of last service
- products used and method of application
- cost of the service
- any retail products that were bought and their cost
- after-care advice given to the client
- comments by yourself or the client on the end result.

This information will enable you to:

Health and safety during colouring

Carry out your consultation.

⇩

Gown your client correctly to ensure she is protected from chemicals.

⇩

Ensure you are wearing the correct PPE.

⇩

Make sure that you follow the manufacturer's instructions.

⇩

Check on your client comfort at regular intervals.

⇩

Record card showing a client's colouring details

					TINTING	
Date of Skin Test: 4/8/01, 8/10/01				**Natural Colour:** Base 7		
Date	Brand used	Shades	Hydrogen Peroxide Vol.	Development Time	Remarks/Obvservations	Assistant
6.2.01	Majirel	1/4 tube 900's	40vol	40mins	Woven T-Zone with foil Hair contains natural warmth, ash tone may be needed next time	Tina
20.4.01	Majirel	1/4 tube 4.45	20vol	35mins	Chunky dark woven foils through T-Zone to break up re-growth	Tina
4.5.01	Goldwell clust	Free Bleach	2 flat scoops + 50cc 40vol		4.45 too dark added blonde	Michelle
10.9.01	Majirel + Bleach	4.45	20vol 40vol	35mins	Whole head woven foils, more blonde than dark. £55.00 Retailed serum, Inme shamp + Conditioner Retail £19.75	Pete
8.10.01	Skin test carried out					Jenna

Prepare for colouring

- make any changes necessary if required
- follow up any retail sales
- ensure the client receives excellent service every time.

What you will learn	
• Carrying out and recording all hair and skin tests • Choosing products, tools and equipment, taking into account critical influencing factors • Preparing the client and products prior to colouring	

In this element you will be looking at the hair and skin tests that you need to carry out before you begin the process. You will also be looking at how critical influencing factors will have an effect on the colouring process and the correct preparation of your products.

Carrying out and recording all hair and skin tests

Before carrying out any colouring process that will come into contact with the scalp (with the exception of temporary colours) you must carry out a skin test – sometimes called a patch test or hypersensitivity test. This is to check whether the client is allergic to the para dye (artificial colour pigment) that is contained in tints. The test is a safety precaution and must be carried out 24–48 hours prior to a colouring process.

Method

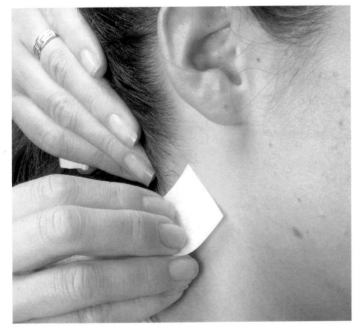

Clean a small area of skin with a medi-wipe just behind the ear. Mix together a small amount of dark tint with a few drops of 20 volume hydrogen peroxide (a dark tint is used because it contains more para dye).

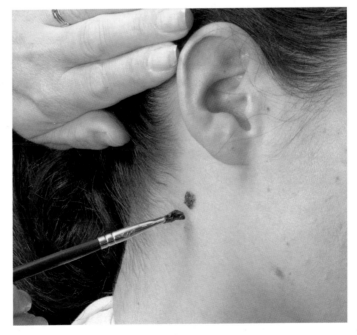

Using a brush or cotton wool bud, apply a small amount of tint behind the client's ear and allow to dry.

Positive reaction

Advise the client to leave the test for 24–48 hours unless there is any irritation. A positive reaction (the client is allergic to the product) would result in the following symptoms:

- redness
- soreness
- itching
- inflammation.

If your client experiences any of the above reactions, do not proceed with the colouring treatment.

Alternative methods of colouring may be offered where the tint does not come into contact with the scalp such as using a cap, mesh or foil. Great care must be taken anyway to ensure that tint does not come into contact with the skin.

Incompatibility test

The purpose of this test is to see whether the client has any metallic salts present on her hair. You would carry out this test only if you thought the client had been colouring her hair at home with a product that may contain metallic salts. Metallic salts are contained in hair colour restorers such as Grecian 2000.

Method

- Take a small cutting of the client's hair and secure the hair together with tape.
- In a glass bowl or container, mix together a small amount of hydrogen peroxide and alkaline perm lotion.
- Place the hair in the bowl so that the hair is covered with the mixture.
- Observe the mixture.

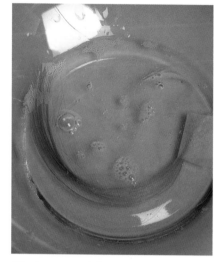

The incompatibility test

Positive reaction

This will normally occur within 30 minutes of the hair being placed into the mixture. You would expect to see any of the following:

- the lotion bubbles or fizzes
- the hair may change colour
- the hair may dissolve
- the solution may give off heat.

If any of these reactions occur, you should not proceed with any hairdressing process that involves using hydrogen peroxide.

Elasticity test

An elasticity test determines the condition of the hair. If the elasticity is poor, the internal links and bonds in the cortex have been damaged and the hair may not be able to withstand a chemical treatment.

Method

- Select a few strands of hair.
- Hold firmly between your thumb and index finger.
- Gently pull the hair.

If the hair stretches more than half of its length then it is over elastic and may break off. You may need to consult with the client to decide on your next step. You may be able to offer an alternative colouring service that will not cause further damage to the hair.

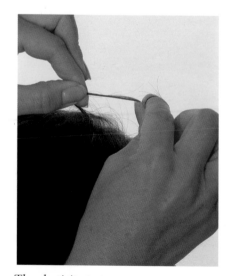

The elasticity test

Porosity test

This test also determines the condition of the hair. If the hair is very porous or unevenly porous, colour will be absorbed differently across the surface of the hair. The test will help you to work out what strength of hydrogen peroxide to use. If the hair is in good condition, you can colour the hair with a stronger peroxide strength. If the hair is over porous, you may need to rethink your colour choice and use a weaker strength of peroxide.

Method

- Select a few strands of hair.
- Hold them firmly in one hand near the points.
- With your other hand, slide your fingers down towards the roots.

If the hair feels smooth, the hair is in good condition; if the hair feels roughened, the cuticle scales are damaged.

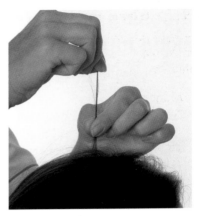

The porosity test

Strand test

The purpose of a strand test is to determine how well the colour is developing during the process.

Method

- Dampen a piece of cotton wool.
- Select a few strands of hair.
- Using some cotton wool, wipe off some of the tint from the hair.
- Hold the hair flat on your hand to see the colour result.

If the colour is not fully developed, leave for the further development time. If the colour is ready, rinse to remove the colour.

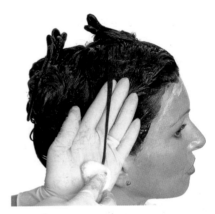

Strand test

Recording the result

After every hair or skin test has been completed, it is important that you complete the client's record card in full. Do not leave this until later – you could easily forget a piece of information that will be important for the client's next colouring service (look back at the record card on page 118).

Identifying critical influencing factors

When consulting with the client prior to a colouring service, you need to look at several other factors, not just hair condition, including:

- the age of the client
- the client's lifestyle
- cost.

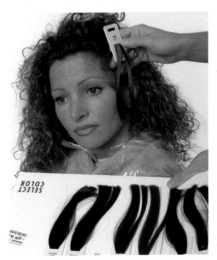

> ### Remember
>
> After completion of the hair or skin test, always fill in the client's record card. Include:
>
> - date
> - hair or skin test carried out
> - development time
> - results
> - advice or recommendations given.

Using a colour shade chart during a consultation

Choosing products, tools and equipment, taking into account critical influencing factors

When considering your choice of colour, you have to think about any existing colour that is already on the hair, as this will affect your end result.

- If the client has colour on her hair that has faded and just wants the colour 'freshened up', you will need to match up the existing colour with the shade chart and apply the colour following the manufacturer's instructions.
- If the client wants to tone down an unwanted red or ash tone in the hair, you will need to consult the colour wheel to find the neutralising colour and apply accordingly. You can only do this with a colour that is of the same depth or darker than the colour already on the hair. For example, if the client is a base 6 and her hair is looking slightly green and does not wish to go any darker, you will have to apply a colour that is also a base 6 with some warm tones in it.

Remember

Whenever possible, choose colours under natural light.

Virgin hair is hair that has not had any chemical treatment on it. You can use any colour on the shade chart although you must remember that you cannot lighten the hair when using temporary, semi- or quasi-permanent colours. You will be able to darken the hair or keep it on the same base and just change the tone.

The percentage of white hair that is present will also have an effect on your colour choice. When referring to the percentage of grey present in the hair, we are talking about the head of hair as a whole:

- if a client is completely grey, the hair is referred to as being 100% grey
- if three-quarters of the hair is grey, it is described as 75% grey
- if half of the hair is grey, it is 50% grey
- if only a quarter of the hair is grey, it is 25% grey.

Viton S grey scale

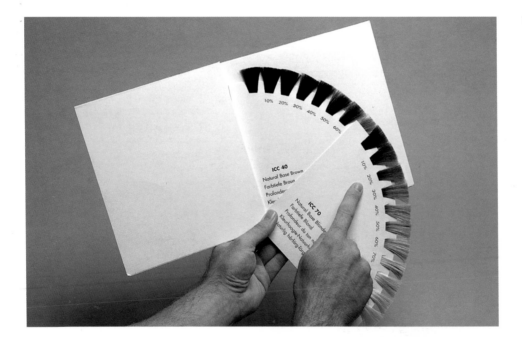

If a client had 75% grey present in her hair and you put a bright red fashion colour on the hair, what do you think would happen? It would probably turn pink! Since all colours can be intermixed, you would still be able to colour this client's hair but you would need to introduce some base colour into the fashion colour.

Permanent base colours (ICC 1–10) will cover 100% grey hair. Fashion colours, which are all the colours that have the primary and secondary tones in them, will only cover a certain percentage of grey hair if used on their own.

All the scenarios below are based on using a whole tube of tint.

If the client chooses 7.44 as the target colour that she would like to be and has 50% grey hair, you would need to use equal quantities of base 7 with the target colour (7.44). The base colour acts as the undercoat for the hair and the fashion colour as the topcoat, which is the colour that we see. If you did not apply the undercoat (base 7), you would be putting a very rich red copper on to white hair and it will produce a pink hue!

> **Remember**
>
> It is always important to read the manufacturer's instructions.

- 25% grey requires $\frac{1}{4}$ tube base colour $+ \frac{3}{4}$ tube fashion shade.

- 50% grey requires $\frac{1}{2}$ tube base colour $+ \frac{1}{2}$ tube fashion colour.

- 75% grey requires $\frac{3}{4}$ tube base colour $+ \frac{1}{4}$ tube fashion colour.

Colour and porous hair

The porosity of the hair will influence the way in which you apply the colour. If the hair is porous, it may mean that the cuticle scales are damaged due to previous chemical treatments. The hair will absorb the colour unevenly and the colour result could end up uneven and patchy. Extra care needs to be taken when applying colour to porous hair.

When choosing the target colour, you will also need to take into account the following critical influencing factors:

- temperature
- existing colour of hair
- percentage of white hair
- test results
- hydrogen peroxide percentage by volume
- porosity of hair.

> **Reality check!**
>
> When using added heat, always check the manufacturer's instructions for development times and also check for hot or cold spots that could lead to patchy results.

Temperature

You can assist the development of the colour by adding heat. You can use:

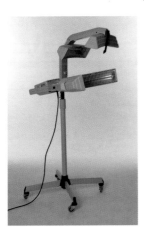

a climazone – dry heat speeds up the development of permanent colours

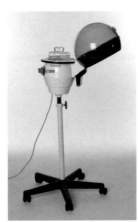

a steamer – moist heat is generally used for lightening products, for example, bleaches.

Existing colour of hair

If the client already has colour on her hair and wants to lift the colour, you need to be aware that permanent colour (tint) cannot lift permanent colour (tint).

Percentage of white hair

The amount of white hair present will determine how much base colour is used (remember the undercoat!), the percentage of hydrogen peroxide you use, and where you begin the application. When adding colour to the hair (covering white hair), start at the most resistant area (where the white hair is most obvious).

Preparing the client and products prior to colouring

Test results

Before permanent colouring you will need to carry out:

- a skin test to determine whether the process can be carried out
- an incompatibility test (if you suspect metallic salts are present on the hair).

Other preparation activities that you need to carry out before you begin the colouring service include:

- making sure you are organised to receive the client – client record card and colour shade chart
- the correct gowning procedure for the client – to protect the client's clothing
- ensure you have the correct personal protective equipment (PPE) for yourself
- applying barrier cream to the client's skin.

Applying colour to wet hair

Always read the manufacturer's instructions, as these will tell you whether you should apply the colour to wet or dry hair. They will also give all the information that you require on how to mix your products, what peroxide strength to use, and any other information that you require.

- Shampoo the hair with a soapless shampoo. A soapless shampoo will not affect the pH balance of the hair as this product has a neutral pH and does not leave a residue on the hair. DO NOT use a conditioner, which would act as a barrier on the hair preventing the colour from taking.
- Towel-dry the hair to remove excess moisture.
- Section the hair (if required) into four (the hot-cross bun) to move the bulk of the hair out of the way so that you can work more easily.
- Apply the product following the manufacturer's instructions.

Colouring products applied to wet hair include:

- temporary colours, for example, coloured mousses or setting lotions
- semi-permanent colours, for example, Wella Colour Fresh
- some quasi colours.

Applying colour to dry hair

- Brush the hair through, removing all tangles.
- Section the hair into four (the hot-cross bun).
- Apply the colour following the manufacturer's instructions.

Colouring products applied to dry hair include:

- hair mascaras and coloured sprays
- all permanent colours, for example, high lift tints, bleaching products
- some quasi colours.

Reality check!

If adding colour, add where the hair is most white. If lightening, add where the hair is darkest.

Check it out

What other types of protective equipment must you use when using colour in the salon and why should you use them?

Preparing for the service

Carry out the appropriate tests.

Record the test results.

Seek advice if unsure about contraindications or results of hair tests.

Choose the correct products, tools and equipment for the service.

Make sure the client is protected for the service.

Add colour to hair

H13.3

Adding colour to the hair means adding or depositing colour on to the hair but not lifting the natural colour of the client's hair. You need to think about factors such as the amount of grey in the hair or any previous chemical treatments.

What you will learn
• Preparing the client for a colouring treatment • Principles of colouring • Choosing the product and application • Development and removal • The finished result

Preparing the client for a colouring treatment

It is a good idea to carry out the consultation *before* you gown the client so that you can take into account her personality; for example, the way your client dresses is a good indication of the type of lifestyle she may lead.

You should also complete a full colouring consultation form and carry out porosity and elasticity tests during the consultation (see pages 240–41).

Refer to a colour shade chart to enable the client to see the colour choices available to her. It will also enable you to match up to the client's existing colour and choose one to enhance and complement her skin tone.

When deciding whether to choose temporary or semi-permanent colours, you will need to take into account the following critical influencing factors:

- the client's existing hair colour
- the percentage of white hair
- the porosity of the hair.

The above factors will not only influence your colour choice but also the application of the colour.

Principles of colouring

To understand how these factors will influence your colour choice, you need to have an understanding of the principles of colouring.

What is colour?

White sunlight is made up of all colours. You can see those colours in the sky when a rainbow is formed. They are known as the colours of the spectrum.

In hairdressing, indigo is not used because it is too difficult to distinguish from blue and violet. The six colours that you will use are made up of primary and secondary colours.

The primary colours are:

- red
- yellow
- blue.

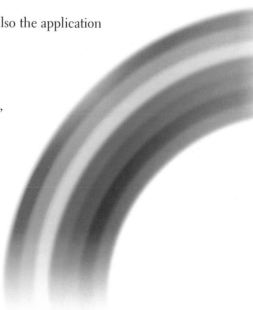

Red
Orange
Yellow
Green
Blue
Indigo
Violet

These colours cannot be made by mixing other colours together.

The secondary colours are:

- orange
- green
- violet.

Mixing two primary colours together makes a secondary colour, for example, red plus yellow makes blue. All other colours are made by mixing primary and secondary colours together, for example, red plus yellow plus blue makes brown.

The warm colours on the colour wheel are red, yellow and orange.

The cool colours on the colour wheel are blue, green and violet.

A principle of the colour wheel is that opposite colours on the spectrum neutralise one another. For example, use a cool, ash (green) tone to neutralise hair with too much warmth in it (too many red or gold tones). Hair that is looking green can be made to look warmer by using a warm tone.

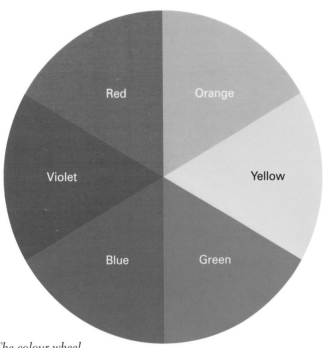

The colour wheel

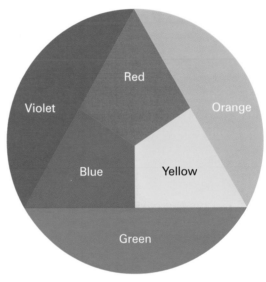

Mix primary colours to obtain secondary colours

Natural hair colour

The cortex contains all the colour pigments in the hair. These are called melanin. Melanin is broken down into two types of colour pigments:

- Black and brown are called eumelanin – they are the cool tones in the hair (ash or matt).
- Red and yellow are called pheomelanin – they are the warm tones in the hair (auburn or golden).

The amount of each of the four colour pigments in the hair determines the natural colour of the hair. For example, a person with a lot of eumelanin and a little pheomelanin will have medium to dark ash brown hair. A person with more pheomelanin than eumelanin would be a medium to light golden blonde.

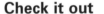

Choosing the product and application

International Colour Chart system

Colour chart by Wella

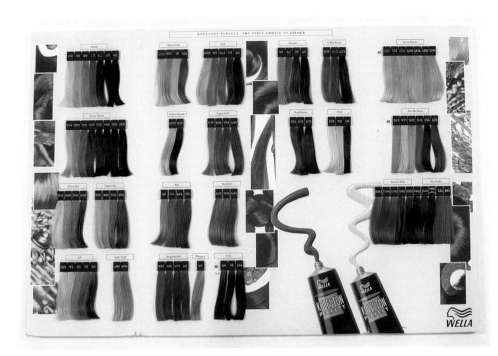

The International Colour Chart (ICC) system is a guide to colouring that is used all over the world. Although each manufacturer has a slightly different system, all use a similar numbering system. Basic hair colours are numbered 1–10, 1 being the darkest colour (black) and 10 being the lightest colour (very light blonde). As a stylist, learning what these numbers stand for will enable you to pick up any colour chart and know exactly what depth of colour you can hope to achieve.

The names that are given to colours, such as 'Sahara blonde' and 'Black tulip', are more for the benefit of the client, although they will help you to picture the colour in your mind when you first start colouring.

How to use the ICC system

For each colour, the first number on the chart describes its depth, for example:

- 6 = blonde
- 4 = light brown
- 2 = dark brown.

The depth of the colour is the same as referring to the base colour. It means the colour that you are starting from before you begin the colouring process, how light or dark the hair is.

The next number on the chart after the base number tells you the primary tone of the colour, for example, 6.3 or 6/3 = golden blonde. There are six tones:

- ash/green, blue base
- mauve
- gold
- copper
- mahogany
- red.

Check it out

Write down the numbers 1–10. Using a shade chart, note next to each number the colour that it refers to. Compare this to other shade charts, if available, and discuss any differences.

Sometimes there is a third number on the chart. This tells you the secondary tone, for example, 6.34 or 6/34 = copper gold blonde. Primary and secondary tones have nothing to do with primary and secondary colours. Sometimes colours may be 8.44 or 8/44. In these colours, the primary tone (the most intense tone) and the secondary tone (the least intense tone) are the same. This gives the colour an intense tone.

Hydrogen peroxide percentage by volume

The chemical formula for hydrogen peroxide is H_2O_2 (H = hydrogen; O = oxygen). The chemical formula for water is H_2O. It is the oxygen in hydrogen peroxide that is used in hairdressing.

The strength of hydrogen peroxide is measured in percentage strength or volume strength. Percentage strength equals the amount of oxygen given off by 100 ml of hydrogen peroxide solution. For example, 6% strength/volume = 6 ml of oxygen from a 100 ml solution.

The higher the percentage or volume, the more oxygen is released from the hydrogen peroxide.

Hydrogen peroxide is stabilised with a mild acid to stop it giving off oxygen in the bottle, but it is very important that you put the top back on after use or it will oxidise in the bottle and lose its strength. Never pour hydrogen peroxide back into the bottle – this will also allow the peroxide to oxidise in the bottle, losing its strength.

Hydrogen peroxide softens (swells) and opens the cuticle. It can be used prior to applying permanent colour to resistant hair.

Temporary colours

Temporary colours have large molecules that coat the cuticle. They do not dramatically alter the colour of the hair but will add stronger tones. Temporary rinses will add colour but will not lighten the hair.

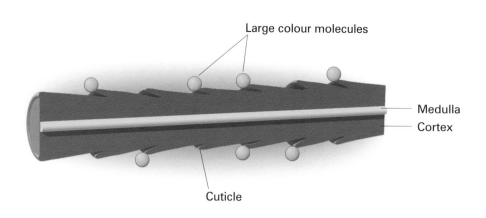

Large colour molecules

Medulla

Cortex

Cuticle

Temporary colour molecules coat the cuticle with a colour

To apply to porous hair:

- shampoo the hair and divide into four sections (hot-cross bun).
- pour the setting lotion into a bowl and using a tint brush, apply the lotion to the hair in sections approximately 1 cm deep. This will ensure that the lotion is applied evenly to all of the hair.

For non-porous hair, the setting lotion can be applied from the bottle and sprinkled onto the hair.

Temporary colours can be removed from the hair at the next shampoo, but if the hair is porous, there may be a build up of colour. Some sprays and paints will brush out.

Application of coloured mousses and hair mascaras

Because coloured mousses and hair mascaras stain the hair, they will also stain your hands – always wear gloves! Shampoo the hair and towel dry to remove excess moisture. Divide the hair (if appropriate) into four.

> **Reality check!**
>
> Make sure you do not get coloured mousse on the client's skin, as it stains. If this happens, remove with damp cotton wool.

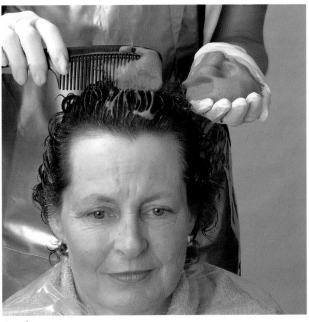

Applying mousse

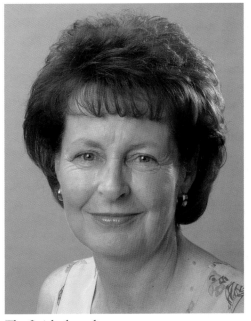

The finished result

Application of semi-permanent colours

Semi-permanent colours are available as:

- cream
- mousse
- liquid – synthetic organic dyes.

They have large and small colour molecules that stain the cuticle and partially penetrate into the cortex.

Semi-permanent colours are always applied to wet hair. They last from four to eight shampoos, but if the hair is porous, there may be a build up of colour. They cover up to 30% grey hair. Such products add colour to the hair but will not lighten it.

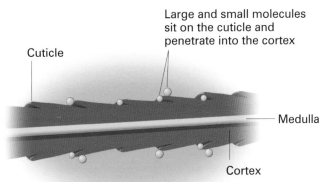

Large and small molecules sit on the cuticle and penetrate into the cortex

Cuticle

Medulla

Cortex

Semi-permanent colour molecules stain the cuticle and partially penetrate the cortex

Step-by-step application of semi-permanent colours

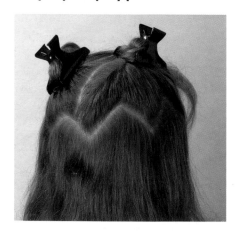

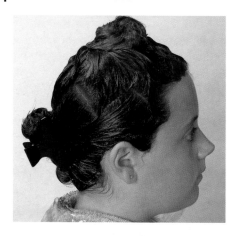

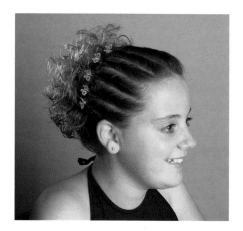

Section the hair and make sure that both you and the client are wearing the correct PPE. Begin to apply the colour onto previously shampooed hair.

When all the colour has been applied, the development time begins. Make sure you consult the manufacturer's instructions. When development is complete, rinse the colour and use an anti-oxy conditioner to seal the colour.

The end result. Check that there is no excess colour on the skin and style the hair using the correct styling and finishing products. Confirm the look with the client.

Very long hair may require two or more bottles. The hair should be sectioned off and the application begun at the nape area moving up towards the crown. Always inform the client if you are going to have to use more than one application, as this will incur extra costs.

Development and removal

When applying temporary colours, there is *no* development time. With semi-permanent colours, read the manufacturer's instructions to check the development time, then make a note of the time of the finished application and when the colour needs to be rinsed. In busy salons stylists often use a timer that rings when the development time is completed.

Reality Check!

When applying any colouring product to the client's hair, make sure:

- the client is fully protected with the correct gown, towels and barrier cream
- the hair is towel-dried so that the colour will not drip off wet hair
- the client's position is adjusted so that you can see where you are applying the tint
- any of the product is removed *immediately* from the skin with damp cotton wool so that it will not stain.

In the salon

Miguel was a junior in his salon, training to become a hairdresser. One of his main jobs was to shampoo, neutralise and rinse colours for the other stylists. He was rinsing a colour for one stylist when another one asked him to neutralise a perm for him. Miguel knew that it was important to neutralise the perm quickly when it was ready so stopped rinsing the colour even though he knew there was a bit of colour still on the scalp. When the stylist came to blow-dry the hair of the client who had had the colour, she found the hair would not dry. On closer inspection, she realised that this was because the client still had colour on her hair.

Miguel was asked to take the client back to the basin to remove the excess colour from the hair and the stylist was then running late for her next appointment as a result.

- What are other implications of not rinsing colour properly from hair?

While the colour is developing, you should make sure that the hair is not piled too tightly on the head. To help a colour develop properly, air needs to be able to circulate through the hair.

Rinsing

Once the colour has developed, take the client to the basin to remove it. Make sure that the client is still well protected – a towel and plastic cape should be covering the client's clothing. Ensure that she is seated comfortably at the basin. Check that you have all of her hair in the basin and that she is sitting far enough back so that you can reach to remove the tint.

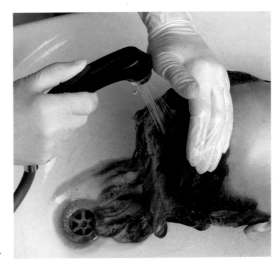

Rinsing off the colour

Step-by-step rinsing

1 Check the water temperature.
2 Dampen the hair.
3 Massage to emulsify the colour.
4 Rinse until the water runs clear.
5 Use an anti-oxy conditioner. (If you shampooed the hair prior to colouring, there is no need to shampoo again.)
6 Check that you have rinsed all of the tint from behind the ears and in the nape area.
7 Towel-dry and style the hair.

The finished result

Only once you have styled the client's hair will the actual colour be fully clear to you and the client – wet hair always looks darker! It is a good idea to take the client to a window so that she can see the colour in natural light. Let the client hold the hand mirror so that she can have a good look. Confirm with her that she is happy with the result.

Adding colour to hair

> Confirm the desired effect with the client.
>
> Prepare the client and the hair in the appropriate manner for the service.
>
> Use a suitable application/technique for the service and length of hair.
>
> Make sure the manufacturer's instructions are followed to develop and remove the colour.
>
> Identify any colouring problems that may occur.
>
> Seek advice if you are unable to resolve the colour problem.
>
> Confirm the end result with client.

Permanently change hair colour   H13.4

When changing hair colour permanently, the world is your oyster! There is a wide variety of products and techniques, from highlighting to bold and dramatic looks, such as putting slices of colour through the hair.

Colouring is only limited to your imagination.

There are additional factors to be considered when permanently colouring the hair because you will be chemically changing the colour molecules in the hair.

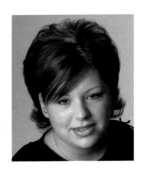

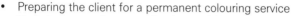

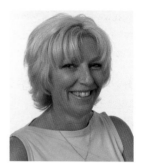

What you will learn

- Preparing the client for a permanent colouring service
- Techniques, products, application and development
- Product removal
- Coping with problems
- Confirming and recording the end result

Preparing the client for a permanent colouring service

The consultation

The consultation for a permanent colouring service should be slightly more in depth than for temporary and semi-permanent colours. This is because of the wider choice of products available and the effects you can achieve. For example, you can:

- lighten (permanently)
- darken (permanently)
- change tone (permanently).

First, you should check whether the client has an up-to-date skin test. This is to protect against any allergic reaction to the para dye that is contained in permanent colours. If she does (and there was no positive reaction), you are free to carry on the consultation.

Next, you should find out whether the client wants to:

- go lighter than her natural base colour
- go darker than her natural base colour
- stay at the same depth as her natural base colour, but add a warm or cool tone.

The target colour to be achieved will determine the strength of hydrogen peroxide that you will use.

During the consultation:

- use a colour shade chart
- match up the client's natural base shade to the shade chart
- decide whether you are lightening, darkening or adding tone
- decide on the technique that you will use
- agree with the client if it is a full head colour or re-growth colour
- check whether the client wishes to have more than one colour in her hair
- find out if the client will be able to maintain the colour
- double-check with the client that you have chosen the right colour.

Permanent tint is permanent! If the client does not like the result, she will have to grow the colour out.

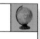

Reality Check!

Permanent colour enters the cortex. It contains pigment molecules which expand and become trapped in the cortex making colour change permanent.

Reality check!

All manufacturers recommend that a skin test is carried out 24–48 hours before a colouring service is carried out.

As well as the colour consultation, you will need to complete the standard client consultation form, which will give you information on the hair's porosity, texture, amount of grey present and previous chemical treatments.

Preparing the client for highlighting and lowlighting processes

As well as completing a colouring consultation form (see page 233), there are additional questions that you will need to ask the client in order to complete this specific colouring service:

- Does she want colour added or the hair lightened?
- How much colour would she like to see?
- How thick or fine and how many high/lowlights does she want to see?
- Has she had this procedure before? If not, you should explain the procedure to her.

You need to decide whether to use the highlighting cap or mesh or foils. Choose foils or mesh for hair that is very long and if more than one colour is required. A cap should be used if the hair is too short to weave and you are using only one colour. It is cheaper to use the cap method, as it is not so time consuming. If the client wants foils or mesh for short hair and only one colour, that is her choice, but you should make her aware of the extra costs involved.

You select the colour the same way as in other colouring services. You will need to:

- match up the client's natural base shade to determine what depth of colour she is
- choose the target colour – the colour the client wants as the end result
- determine from this if you are going darker than the client's natural base colour or if you are lifting the hair
- decide how many shades you are lifting or darkening – this will determine the strength of hydrogen peroxide that you will use
- work out what percentage of grey hair (if any) the client has – this will determine how much base colour (if any) you need to use.

Gowning and hair preparation

Once you have completed the consultation, gown the client with a chemical gown, towel and plastic cape. Prepare her hair for the service.

- Brush the hair through to make sure there are no tangles.
- Make sure your highlighting cap is covered with talc, otherwise the rubber will tug the hair.
- Place the highlighting cap on the client, making sure you have placed the hair in the parting the client wears her hair in.
- Only at this point should you mix the tint!

High/lowlighting procedures should be completed on dry hair. If you are pulling through the cap, brush the hair through beforehand to remove hairspray or tangles.

It is not recommended to use the highlighting cap on below-shoulder-length hair. The hair is likely to tangle causing discomfort to the client. Instead, you would recommend using foils or mesh. Also, it is not recommended to use the highlighting cap on hair that is very short. This could result in the hair looking spotty (leopard spots!).

Reality check!

Complete an in-depth consultation to confirm the service that you are going to carry out before you begin to mix up any product.

Products, techniques, application and development

Permanent colours

All permanent colours are applied to dry hair. There are two main types:

- creams and gels – synthetic, organic
- metallic dyes – inorganic.

Synthetic dyes are known as para dyes.

Para dye facts
- They must be mixed with hydrogen peroxide to work.
- They are alkaline and so open up the cuticle and penetrate into the cortex.
- They can lighten up to three shades above the base colour.
- They can cover any amount of grey hair.
- They will darken the hair or add tones to natural colour.
- They can cause a serious allergic reaction.

Para dyes have small molecules that allow them to enter the cortex. When they start to develop, they mix with the oxygen from the hydrogen peroxide and join together to form large molecules that are then trapped inside the cortex.

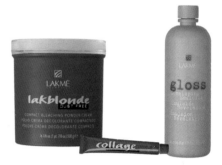

Colouring products

Inorganic dyes

Metallic dyes contain, as their name suggests, metal salts. They are commonly found in 'colour restorers' but are sometimes mixed with semi-permanent colour and with henna.

Metallic salts are not compatible with hydrogen peroxide. How bad the reaction is depends on the type of metal salt on the hair. Some turn the hair green; others will fizz and bubble producing enough heat to dissolve the hair. If you suspect that the client has used a colour at home that may contain metallic salts, you must carry out an incompatibility test on the hair (see page 240).

Reality check!

A skin test must be done 24–48 hours before applying a para dye.

Quasi-permanent colours

Quasi-permanent colour molecules are small enough to enter the cortex but do not change the natural hair colour permanently.

Quasi-permanent colours have a lasting quality that falls between semi-permanent and permanent colourants. If used once, they will usually last between eight and twelve shampoos, but if used regularly, they will build up on the hair and cause a re-growth.

Some stain the cuticle, while others can enter the cortex and may change the natural colour pigment.

Most quasi-colours require a skin test to be done before they are used. Also carry out an incompatibility test if you suspect metallic salts are present on the hair.

Most quasi-colours are mixed with a developer, which contains very weak hydrogen peroxide. It is important to read the manufacturer's instructions, as there are no general rules for these products. They can be mixed as colour baths.

High lift tint

Use a high lift tint when you require a higher lift than normal. A high lift tint can lighten the hair up to four shades depending on the base colour of the hair (the darker the base, the less lift you will be able to achieve). High lift tints are usually recommended for use on hair of a base 6 (dark blonde and above) and upwards.

These tints are usually mixed one part tint to two parts hydrogen peroxide, that is, 50 ml of tint to 100 ml of hydrogen peroxide. They usually require a longer development time (always check the manufacturer's instructions) and can benefit from the use of added heat.

Hydrogen peroxide percentage by volume

The amount of lift required determines the strength of hydrogen peroxide to be used:

- 20 volume or 6% = 1 shade of lift
- 30 volume or 9% = 2–3 shades of lift
- 40 volume or 12% = 3–4 shades of lift.

If you have a higher strength hydrogen peroxide than you require, you may dilute it to the correct volume by using distilled water (never tap water) – see the following chart to help you check the correct quantities of water to peroxide to dilute peroxide if you ever run out. Only dilute the amount you require and never store diluted mixture – it will be destabilised and give off oxygen, creating a potential fire hazard. It also loses its strength when stored. The chart gives the correct ratios of water to hydrogen peroxide to mix to give you the correct dilutions of hydrogen peroxide required.

Remember

Only use distilled water when diluting hydrogen peroxide – tap water contains impurities.

Hydrogen peroxide you have (by volume)	Peroxide		Water			Hydrogen peroxide strength you may require (by volume)
40 (12%)	3	+	1	=		30
40	1	+	1	=		20
40	1	+	3	=		10
40	1	+	7	=		5
30 (9%)	2	+	1	=		20
30	1	+	2	=		10
30	1	+	5	=		5
20 (6%)	1	+	1	=		10
20	1	+	3	=		5
20	1	+	7	=		2.5

Dilutions of hydrogen peroxide (H_2O_2)

Remember

Never store diluted hydrogen peroxide solution. It is a fire hazard.

Bleaches

Bleaches lighten the hair and will lift tint out of the hair. The bleaching process is one of oxidation. It is permanent. The hair must be in good condition and strong in order to withstand the bleaching process.

The two most commonly used bleaches are:

- powder – used for highlights/foils
- gel – used for full head bleaching (scalp application).

Both types are mixed with hydrogen peroxide to activate them. They are alkaline and so open up the cuticle and allow the oxygen they give off to penetrate into the cortex. Once inside, the oxygen combines with the hair's natural hair colour pigment, melanin. This forms a new colour pigment – oxymelanin – which is colourless. The oxygen combines first with the black pigment, then the brown, next the red and lastly the yellow.

When a full head bleach is done, the colour result is often too yellow. This is because the bleach lifts out the natural colour pigments in the hair, with yellow being the last one it lifts out.

Bleaches are applied to dry hair and will continue to lighten until completely removed from the hair.

Porosity, elasticity and possibly incompatibility tests need to be carried out prior to the process.

Bleach can also be used to pre-lighten the hair if you require a strong, vibrant fashion colour and the client's hair may be too dark to achieve this with a normal tint – see the chart below.

Fashion tone required	Pre-lightening tone required
Burgundy, plum	Dark orange
True red	Orange
Auburn, bright copper	Bright orange
Warm copper	Gold
Chestnut, warm gold	Dark yellow
Sandy, gold, beige	Yellow
Ash, pinky rose	Pale yellow
Pale silver, platinum, blue, violet	Palest yellow

Choosing the correct pre-lightening tone

Check it out

Discuss with your group why it is important not to lift the client's hair too light when pre-lightening.

Applying high/lowlights and colouring techniques

Highlighting cap

During the consultation you would have established how much colour the client wishes to see in her hair. If she requires only one colour, you can use the highlighting cap.

To determine how much colour the client wants, ask these types of questions:

- Do you want to see more natural colour than high/lowlights?
- Do you want to see equal amounts of coloured and natural hair?
- Would you like more colour to show than your natural hair colour?

The client's answers will give you a good indication of how many high/lowlights are required and how thick to pull each strand through the highlighting cap. The hooks you will be using vary in size – the numbers on the hooks indicate their size. Thicker highlights require a slightly bigger hook, and vice versa.

Once you have brushed the hair, confirm with the client where she wears her parting (if any) and position the hair accordingly. When you have placed the cap on her and have checked that she is comfortable (ears are not bent back!), you can begin to pull the high/lowlights through.

Reality check!

Before placing a highlighting cap on the client, sprinkle a little talcum powder on it. This will allow the cap to slide onto the hair easily.

Step-by-step highlighting

It is always best to begin at the nape area. This is because as you work up the head you will be able to see where you are going without having to hold any hair up out of the way.

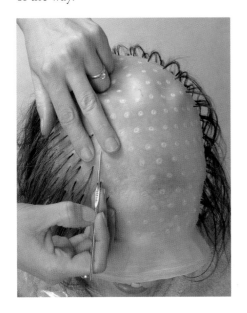

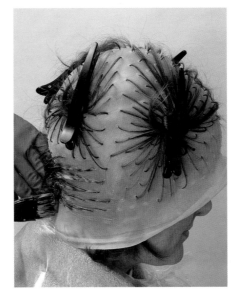

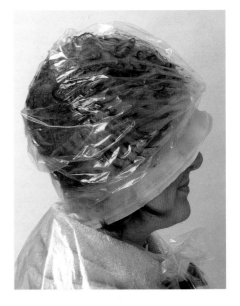

Pull the high/lowlights through the highlighting cap. Once you have finished pulling through all of the high/lowlights required, section the hair into four to allow for easy application of colour. Mix up the product you are going to be using.

Begin applying the colour at the nape area taking sections 1 cm deep. By doing this you will ensure even coverage of all of the hair.
When you have completed the application, loosen the hair slightly with the end of your tint brush to allow air to move through the hair. (This will allow the hair to develop evenly.)

Place a plastic hat over the top to help the body heat process the colour. Always read the manufacturer's instructions for development times.

Mesh and foils

If you are adding two or more colours to the hair, you will have to use foils or mesh.

You ask the same questions as for the highlighting cap and prepare the hair in the same way.

When you have established the thickness of the strands of hair to be coloured, section the hair into four (hot-cross bun). The amount of hair that you want to colour will determine how thickly or finely you weave out sections of the hair that are to be coloured.

As with any colouring process, gown the client correctly, then mix the colours required.

Beginning at the nape area, drop a fine mesh of hair about 2 cm deep. Pick up this section of hair and using the end of a pintail comb, select the strands you wish to apply colour to.

If using two or more colours, you will need to alternate the colours as you apply them.

If you require a lot of colour in the hair, you would weave every section. If the client did not want as much colour in her hair, you would leave a section in between each packet.

Remember

Lightening products expand as they process, so great care must be taken to ensure that the product does not seep onto the surrounding hair and create a patchy result.

Check it out

When using easi mesh, the blue band at the top of the packet is your guideline for where to apply the product to. It is slightly sticky and secures the packet when closed. If you apply the product over the top of the band, it will not be as secure in the hair. Some products expand on development and by using this band as your guideline, you will prevent seepage of the product going onto the rest of the hair (bleeding).

Step-by-step slicing using foils

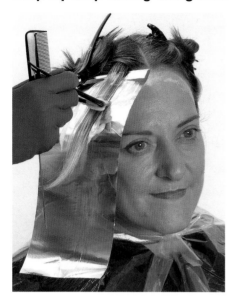

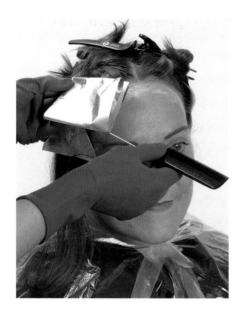

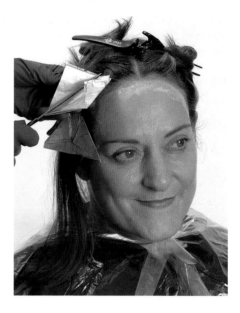

Cut the foil to the required length and place to the root, as close as possible. Place the colour on the section of the hair making sure you allow for the expansion of the colour so it does not seep out of the packet.

Fold the foil in half using the tail of your comb.

Fold in either side of your packet to seal in the colour, also securing the packet to the head.

Step-by-step weaving using mesh

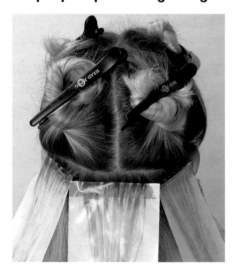

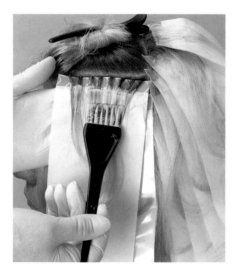

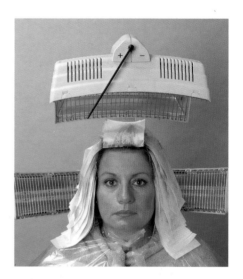

Section the bulk of the hair out of the way and begin to apply the mesh in the nape of the neck.

When you have worked up to the crown, move to the side sections and begin to place your mesh starting from the bottom and working your way up to the parting and repeat on the opposite side.

A climazone (added heat) may be required to help with the development of the colour.

Critical influencing factors

When deciding on the product and technique to use, you will need to take into account the following critical influencing factors:

- temperature
- existing colour of hair
- percentage of white hair
- hydrogen peroxide percentage by volume
- length of hair
- test results.

Temperature

When colouring the hair, there are 'hot spots' in the nape area and the top of the head that you need to be aware of. In the case of a full head of foils, where you begin at the nape area, this hair will start to process as soon as you apply the product to the hair. By the time you reach the front of the head, the first section of hair may be near to the end of its development time. If this is the case, you need to apply the product quite quickly and you may need to think about using added heat on the last packets applied.

A climazone offers an excellent way of adding heat only where you require the heat to be directed. Because you turn off the arms that you do not require on the climazone, you can process specific parts of the head, allowing the hair to 'catch up' with itself.

When completing a high/lowlighting service with a cap, by placing a plastic disposable hat over the top, the body heat of the client is trapped inside, which will assist the development of the colour.

If using a product, such as bleach, and the hair is not lifting as much as you would want, place the client under a steamer to help the bleach to develop.

Existing colour of hair

When deciding on the target colour for the client, you should know the following:

- tint will not lift tint
- you can only achieve three shades lift with a fashion colour
- high lift tint will give you four shades lift if on a base of 6 or above
- if going darker than the base colour, it is only advisable to go three shades darker so that the colour will still suit the client's skin tone.

Percentage of white hair

The amount of white hair present will determine the strength of peroxide you use and if a base colour needs to be added to the hair.

If the client wishes to go darker or stay at the same depth as her natural colour to cover white hair, you will be adding colour not lifting the hair. However, you will still need to use hydrogen peroxide to open the cuticle and allow the tint into the cortex.

Porosity

The porosity of the hair determines how well the colour takes. If hair is in good condition, the cuticle scales lie flat and the colour will coat the hair evenly, reflecting the light back to show healthy, shiny hair. If hair is in bad condition, the cuticle scales may be open, the colour will not take evenly and the light reflected back will bounce off in all directions making the hair look flat and dull.

Remember

A hood dryer can dry out bleach, so a steamer is the better option if one is available. When using added heat, always carry out health and safety checks.

Reality check!

Always check the manufacturer's instructions for the product you are using. These will tell you the strength of hydrogen peroxide required. For example, Majirel colours from L'Oreal:

- amount of white hair = 50%
- adding colour or darker colour = 20 volume or 6% hydrogen peroxide.

The instructions will also tell you the quantities of colour to mix together. For example, 50% or more white hair = $\frac{1}{4}$ to $\frac{1}{2}$ of the basic shade to be mixed with one tube of the target shade.

Hair in good condition

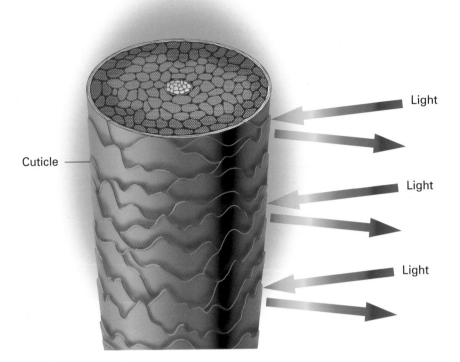

Cuticle

Light

Light

Light

Healthy cuticle scales reflect the light to show shiny, healthy hair. Scales in poor condition bounce the light back in all directions giving the hair a flat and dull appearance

Hair in bad condition

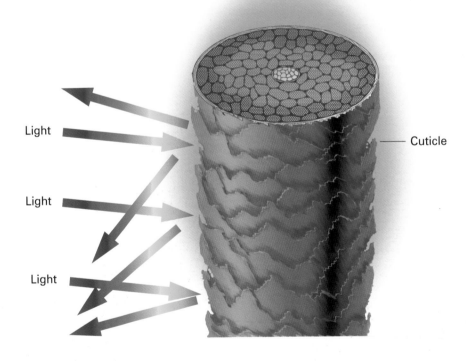

Light

Light

Light

Cuticle

Length of hair

As discussed in high/lowlighting techniques, the length of hair plays an important part when deciding which technique and the method of application to use. Also, the longer the hair is, the older it will be! The older the hair is, the more likely it is to be porous. This may not be from chemical treatments but day-to-day wear and tear.

Test results

- Porosity test – the hair's condition will affect the application and development of the colour and will determine whether you should use added heat. If the hair is in poor condition, the colour will penetrate the hair more quickly than in hair that is in good condition. It will be 'active' in the cortex for a longer period of time and could cause damage to the hair if left unchecked! Using added heat helps to lift the cuticle scales to allow the colour to penetrate but is not recommended on porous hair.
- Elasticity test – hair with poor elasticity will be further damaged by a high volume of hydrogen peroxide, so it is important to do this test to make sure that the hair can withstand the treatment you will be carrying out. For example, highlighting the hair involves lifting the natural colour. Generally, clients want to see a relatively high degree of lift, which requires a stronger volume of hydrogen peroxide. The elasticity test will help you determine whether it is safe to go ahead.
- Skin test – this should be carried out before any colouring process (except temporary colouring). However, if the colour is not going to be in direct contact with the skin, a skin test is not always required. *Note:* You do not need to complete a skin test for a bleaching treatment, but you must check that the client is not experiencing any discomfort during the process.
- Incompatibility test – this test should always be carried out if you suspect there are metallic salts present on the hair and you are going to be using a product that contains hydrogen peroxide.

Application of products
Basic techniques
There are many techniques that you can use when applying colouring to hair.

Step-by-step re-growth application

> **Check it out**
>
> Should you use added heat on porous hair?

> **Check it out**
>
> Which products contain metallic salts?

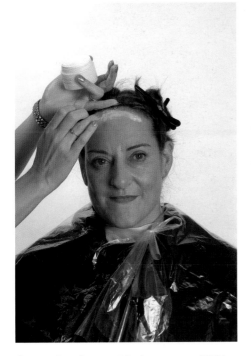

Gown the client with the correct PPE, section the hair into four and apply barrier cream all around the hairline.

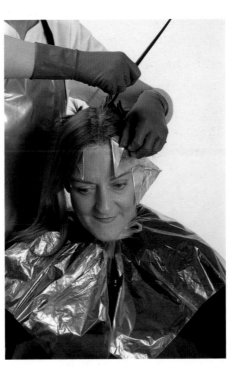

Begin to apply the tint through the partings of the four sections, making sure that you do not put colour onto previously coloured hair.

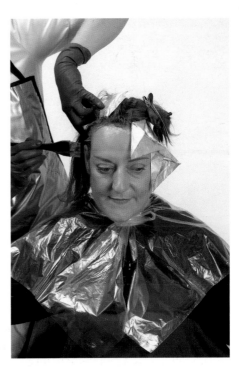

Continue to apply the tint to the outside hairline, making sure you do not get tint onto the skin where barrier cream has not been applied.

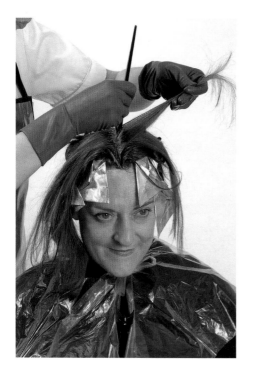

Beginning at the crown area, take a small section, work your way down the back of the head, applying the tint to the re-growth areas only, and continue through the side sections.

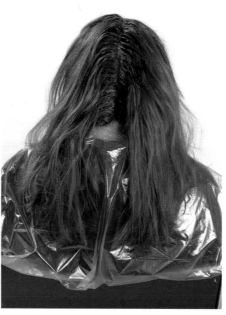

When all of the re-growth area has been covered, cross check your application by going back through your sections in the opposite way in which you applied the tint to ensure complete coverage.

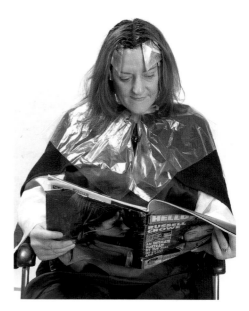

Leave your client to develop according to the manufacturer's instructions. To ensure client comfort, give her a magazine and a drink if she wants one.

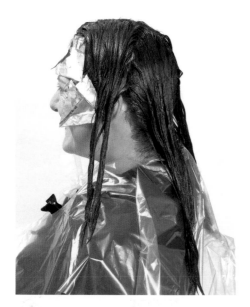

To refresh the colour through the mid-lengths and ends, mix up a weaker solution of the tint and work through the sections of hair and develop for the appropriate time.

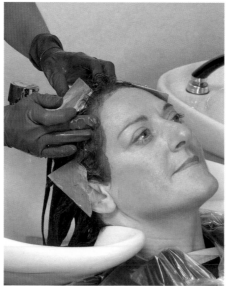

When the colour has fully developed, take the client to the basin and emulsify the tint around the hairline and through the rest of the hair. Shampoo with TLS shampoo and condition with an anti-oxy conditioner.

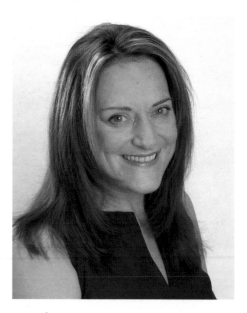

The finished result. Ensure all the product is removed and there is no tint on the skin, then style as desired.

Application of permanent tint or bleach to virgin hair

In order to get an even colour result, you need to take into account:

- the length of the hair
- the porosity of the hair
- body heat.

On hair that is over 2.5 cm long, the roots will develop more quickly than the ends of the hair. This is because heat that escapes from the scalp speeds up the development time. The hair that is furthest away from the scalp takes longer to develop because it does not have the benefit of body heat.

Hair that is more porous will develop more quickly than hair that is in good condition.

On long hair, the ends (because the hair is older) will be more porous than the mid-lengths and will process more quickly.

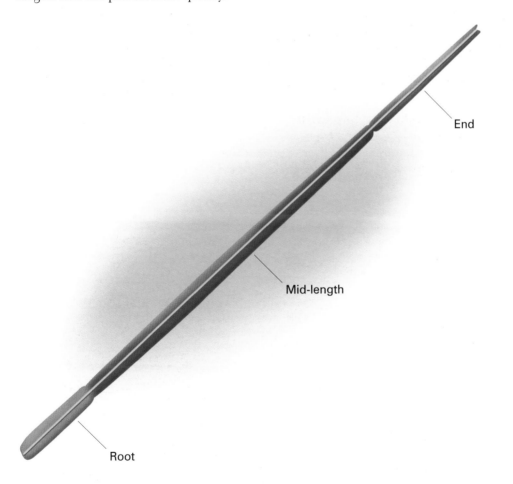

Hair may be divided into the root, mid-length and end

End

Mid-length

Root

Full head tint or bleach should be applied to the hair in the following order:

1 mid-lengths

2 ends

3 roots.

When using lightening products, do not allow one application to overlap the other. This can cause breakage to the hair as you are effectively double processing the hair.

> **Remember**
>
> Always read the manufacturer's instructions for development times.

Step-by-step application of bleach

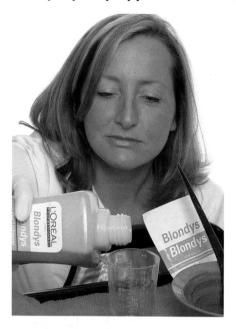

Wearing the correct PPE, mix the product, making sure you measure out the quantities to ensure the correct measurements.

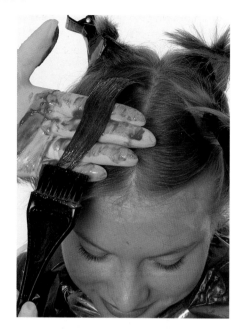

Section the hair into four and begin to apply the bleach mixture to the darkest area of the hair. Apply the colour up to an inch from the roots, to the mid-lengths and ends only.

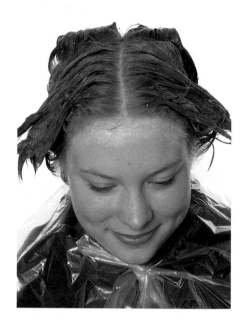

Continue to apply all of the bleach, making sure that the root area is left and develop the bleach following the manufacturer's instructions.

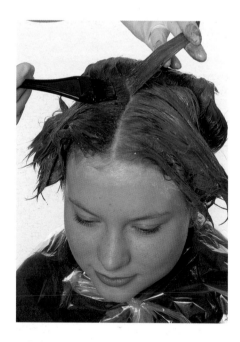

When the bleach has lifted on the mid-lengths and ends, mix up fresh bleach and begin to apply to the root area, again beginning at the darkest area.

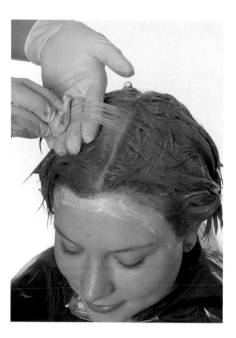

Check the development time of your colour by removing some of the product with damp cotton wool. Check the colour match from roots to ends and in several different places on the head.

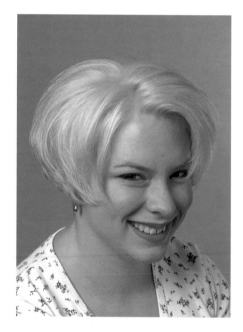

Remove the product with tepid water, not massaging too vigorously. Shampoo with TLS shampoo and use an anti-oxy conditioner. Style the hair in the appropriate manner using the correct styling and finishing products.

Changing tone

To change the tone of the hair and achieve a vibrant result, you should use a quasi-colour. Because quasi-colours have a small amount of hydrogen peroxide in the developer, they allow the colour molecule to enter into the cortex and deposit the tone.

Step-by-step changing tone

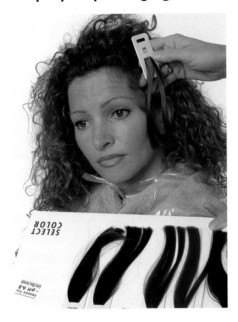

Consult with your client for the desired colour and use the colour swatches to hold against the skin for the colour choice.

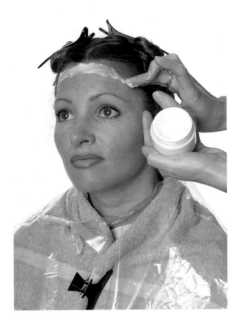

Gown yourself and the client. Section the hair into four and apply barrier cream to the hairline area.

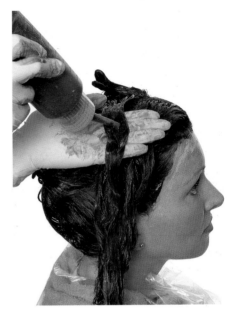

Apply the colour directly from the applicator flask to the hair, working from roots straight through to the ends of the hair.

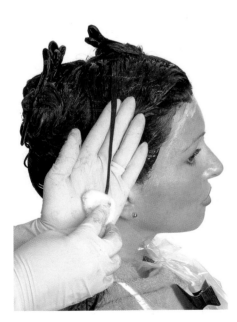

Check the development of the colour halfway through its development time by removing some of the product with damp cotton wool.

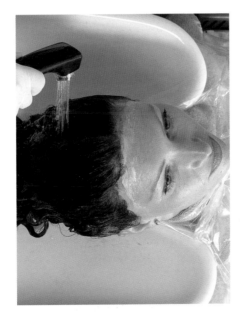

Rinse the colour from the hair, checking the water temperature. Rinse until the water runs clear.

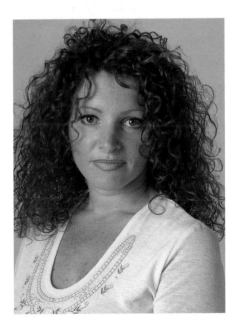

The finished result. Check the colour result with the client and style as desired.

Applying colour

When applying any colour to the client's hair, make sure that you use the correct protective equipment and take great care when applying the colour. Do not apply any tint beyond the barrier cream.

When mixing, make sure you use the correct quantities so that the mixture is of the right consistency and will not drip on the client's face or clothing.

When developing the colour, you should complete a strand test halfway through the development time. This will enable you to determine how well the colour is developing and if added heat is required.

When using added heat:

- check the temperature controls before you put the client under a heat source
- do not allow the product to dry out. This is especially important with bleaches and it is best to use a steamer for this reason
- use a timer
- monitor the development at regular intervals.

Reality check!

Do not operate electrical equipment with wet hands. Unplug equipment when you have finished and allow to cool before storing.

Product removal

When the colour is fully developed and you are happy with the result, remove the colour from the client's hair.

1. Take the client to the basin.

2. Moisten the tint with warm water and gently massage to loosen and emulsify the tint. Pay particular attention to the front hairline and nape area. Tint removes tint, so this is the best way of doing it.

3. Rinse the tint until the water runs clear.

4. Shampoo the hair twice using a TLS shampoo, again checking that you have removed all traces of tint from the nape area, behind the ears and the front hairline.

5. Condition with an anti-oxy conditioner to stop further oxidation and return the hair to its natural pH.

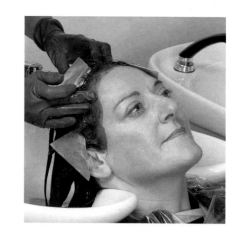

Development and removal for highlighting effects

Once you have finished applying the colour, check the following:

- Are the towel and cape protecting the client still in place and not covered in tint? If they are, change them.
- Is there any product spilt on the trolley you have been using? If so, clean it up.

If using a highlighting cap, lift up the front so the client can see again and secure with a pin curl clip (make sure that it is to the side of the head so that it does not mark the skin).

If using foils or mesh, you should secure any that are around the client's face with a pin curl clip.

Check the manufacturer's instructions for development times. You should monitor the development process all the way through. Take regular strand tests to check that the colour is developing evenly all over the head.

Step-by-step removal for highlighting effects

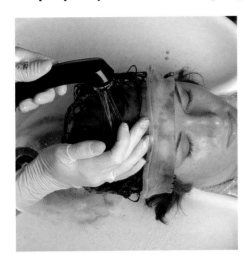

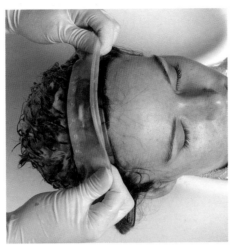

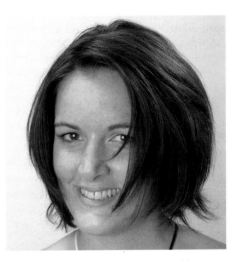

When the colour has processed, take the client to the basin and rinse the product from the cap. Make sure you ask the client to close her eyes or shield her face with your hand to protect from splashes.

To remove the cap, apply some anti-oxy conditioner to the hair and gently ease the cap from the client's head, checking that there is no discomfort. Use a shampoo for coloured hair and apply an anti-oxy conditioner.

The finished result. Style the client's hair and confirm the look.

Rinsing

At this point, you should also remove any capes or towels that are no longer necessary to the client. You will make the client more comfortable and ensure that colour from the towels is not transferred onto the client's clothing. Remove any excess barrier cream. If you do not, you will leave a greasy residue around the hairline that could have an effect on the hair when you are blow-drying. You can remove any skin staining with a medi wipe.

Coping with problems

Problem	Cause	Action
Uneven result	Porous hair; uneven application	Spot colour lighter areas
Scalp irritation	Allergy to product	Remove product with lukewarm water
Coverage not good, especially on white hair	Resistant hair; uneven application	Pre-soften with peroxide or pre-pigment with base shade; spot colour light areas
Hair breaking	Hair in poor condition; peroxide too strong; incorrect application of bleach; too much heat	Remove product and re-use restructurant
Too yellow	Wrong choice of bleach or peroxide; not developed for long enough	Re-apply bleach or use a violet toner
Seepage of product	Incorrect masking of area not to be coloured; incorrect mixing of product, incorrect use of foils or mesh	Spot re-colour on problem areas
Colour fade	Porous hair	Comb tint through; use quasi-colour

If you identify a colouring problem but are unable to correct it, you should refer to the person in charge, either the salon manager or your lecturer. Explain the problem and the course of action that you may have already taken. The manager/lecturer will then be able to help you to deal with the problem. If the problem is caused because of the client's hair and was unforeseen, you will need to make a note on the client's record card so that future stylists will be aware of potential problems. If the colouring problem was one caused by you, it will help you to see that all treatments must be followed in a logical order with great care and attention to detail, and it will be something that hopefully you will not repeat!

Coping with problems when highlighting

If some areas are processing slower than others, use added heat. When using foils or mesh, if you find that part of the hair has processed more quickly than another, remove the product from the part that has developed while leaving the rest to continue developing. It is important that you remove the foils and colour from the hair without disturbing the rest of the colouring process.

To do this, you will need:

- damp cotton wool – to remove the colour from the hair
- sectioning clips – to hold the packets out of the way as you work
- the correct personal protective equipment
- a bin close at hand – to dispose of cotton wool.

1 Section the hair away from where you will be working so that you can get to the packets that need to be removed.

2 Open up the packets. Making sure you have a towel across your hand, spray the packets with a water spray and gently slide them out.

3 Using damp cotton wool, wipe away the colour from the hair. Do not over wet the hair, as it will drip (think health and safety!).

4 Continue in this way until you have removed all of the packets that have developed. Leave the rest of the hair to carry on processing, checking at regular intervals.

Confirming and recording the end result

You should be able to tell from your client's reaction whether she is pleased or not with the result, but you also need to ask such questions as:

- 'That's a really good result, what do you think?'
- 'Shall I book you in for a root re-growth colour in five weeks?'

As soon as possible, fill in the client's record card. For the service, you will need to make a note of the following:

- if bleach was used, how long the bleach took to develop fully
- the number of colours used and in what order for full head foils
- any extra costs incurred for using more than one colour
- any problems encountered during the service.

> **Check it out**
>
> From the table, can you identify the colouring problems that you could deal with, within the limits of your own authority? Which of the problems in the chart would have to be referred to a senior member of staff or lecturer?

The colouring service

> Carry out any necessary hair and skin tests prior to the service.

> Use the appropriate colour application techniques to achieve the desired result.

> Take strand tests at appropriate intervals during the development.

> Ensure that the product is fully removed from the client's scalp.

> Confirm the desired effect with the client.

Your questions answered

What do I do if my colour looks brassy after using a high lift tint?
You will need to refer to your colour wheel and look at the opposite colour on the wheel, as this will be the neutralising colour to counteract the gold in the hair. This can be in the form of a toner to tone down unwanted golden tones in the hair.

What do I do if my client comes in and has not had a skin test?
You will need to explain to the client that you are unable to carry out the service and explain in detail why. You could offer a temporary colour and carry out a skin test so that you can re-book another appointment.

What can I do if my client's hair is in very poor condition but she insists on having a colouring treatment that is going to cause more damage to her hair?
You can only advise your client of the consequences of what will happen to her hair and advise on how she might achieve the same result using another less harmful product.

How will I know what colour to use on a client if she has not had a colour before and leaves it up to me?
This is when your consultation skills come into their own. If you ask all the right questions and use a shade chart as reference for the client, you will find that between you, you will find all of the answers!

What do I do if I have not got the right peroxide strength for a client?
You will need to refer to the table on page 255 and dilute down a higher strength of peroxide to achieve the one you want.

What can I do if my client has a very dark base and wants to achieve a very vibrant red?
Manufacturers are bringing out new products all of the time, but if you cannot find one that will achieve your target colour because of the client's natural base colour, you will have to pre-lighten the hair, then apply your target colour over the top.

I'm really scared of using a colour and it going wrong!
This is all down to having good product knowledge. If you read the manufacturer's instructions and follow them, you will find that it is difficult for the colour to turn out incorrectly. Do not be afraid, with colour there is always something that can be done, for example, the use of temporary, semi or quasi products to help you to achieve your target colour.

I always find it hard to remember the opposites on the colour wheel, what can I do to help me remember?
Think of this saying, one that you might remember from school:

Richard Of York Gave Battle In Vain.

The first letter of each of the words is the letter of the colour for the colour wheel: red, orange, yellow, green, blue, indigo and violet. We do not use indigo because it is too similar to violet and blue. Draw a circle and divide it into six equal portions, write the colours in the correct order into the six segments and there you have your colour wheel!

I always get confused by the terms 'target colour', 'depth of colour' and 'base colour'.

If you think of a bull's-eye on a target, that is what you are aiming for, the colour that you want to achieve. Depth and base are both referring to the same thing, i.e. how light or dark the natural hair colour is. Another term that you need to be aware of is the 'tone' of the colour. This refers to the natural golds or ashes that are present in the hair which are equally as important to identify, as they will influence your final colour result.

Test your knowledge

1   What is a colour wheel and why would you use one?

2   What is an incompatibility test?

3   What are the two names given to the hair's natural colour pigments?

4   Why are hair and skin tests important?

5   Why is it important to record the service given to your client?

6   How do the different hydrogen peroxide strengths affect colouring and lightening effects?

7   Why is it important to use products economically?

8   Why is it important to section the hair prior to a colouring service?

9   Why is it important to mix and measure products following the manufacturer's instructions?

10   How and when should you use added heat during a colouring process?

11   What PPE should be used during a colouring process?

12   Why is it important to identify critical influencing factors prior to a colouring service?

13   What are your responsibilities under COSHH Regulations?

14   Why is it important to position yourself correctly while carrying out a colouring service?

15   What are the responsibilities under the current Electricity at Work Regulations?

Dry hair to shape to create finished looks for men

Unit H14

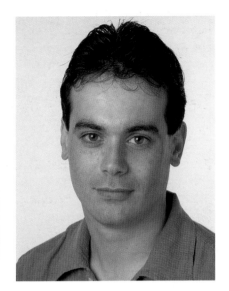

In many unisex salons you will be required to carry out blow-drying services on men's hair. These services are offered to produce an end result from a cutting service and should complement the style in which the hair is cut.

In this unit you will be looking at using different styling techniques to create a wide range of finished looks, taking into account any critical influencing factors and working with a range of styling and finishing products. Many of the products, tools and techniques that you will use are very similar to those in ladies' hairdressing (see Unit H5).

What you will learn

- Maintain effective and safe methods of working when drying hair H14.1
- Dry and finish hair H14.2

Maintain effective and safe methods of working when drying hair

H14.1

What you will learn

- Variations for men's services

The essential underpinning knowledge and skills you will need are covered in Unit H10, pages 131–165. They are:

- Preparing your client, page 131
- Your position while working, page 132
- Personal hygiene, page 137
- Safe working area, page 132
- Safe use of tools, page 140
- Organisation of working area, page 136
- Consultation, page 137

Variations for men's services

However, there are one or two variations for men's services that you need to be aware of.

Products

There are fewer products that you will need, as drying and finishing hair is a more limited service for men. As a stylist, you need to know the effects of different products on different hair types to help you ensure the treatments you carry out are successful. There is a wide range of products available, from those that make the hair more pliable to those that protect the hair from added heat and the effects of atmospheric moisture.

Reality check!

Always follow the manufacturer's instructions. These give you all the information you need to use the product correctly.

Product	Application	Suitability	Comments
Gel (wet or dry look)	Apply to wet hair at the roots and spread thoroughly	Firm hold – good for short spiky styles	Suitable for all hair types
Mousse	Apply to wet hair and comb through evenly	Medium to firm hold – gives body and bounce to hair	Ideal for all hair types except very thick hair
Glaze	Apply evenly to towel-dried hair	Firm hold – dries hard and adds body to hair	Ideal for slicking back unruly hair
Dressing cream	Apply small amount evenly with hands	Light hold – large amounts will produce a slicked back look	Leaves hair sticky to touch
Blow-drying lotion	Apply before blow-drying	Gives hair a softer look and feel	Some products contain chemicals that protect hair from heat
Hairspray	Apply sparingly onto styled hair from a distance of 20 cm	Holds finished style in place	Brushes out; will have drying effect on hair
Hair gloss	Apply small amounts on wet hair to mid-length and ends of hair	Reduces frizz and increases shine	Ideal for African Caribbean hair; too much will leave hair greasy
Moisturiser	Apply to hair before styling	Makes hair soft and shiny; loosens tangles	Useful for conditioning African Caribbean hair
Activators	Apply to wet or dry hair	Used to maintain curl or replace moisture in permed or naturally curly hair	Defines curl; adds moisture and shine to hair

Styling and finishing products

Tools

Choosing the right tools

As well as understanding how styling products affect the way hair behaves, you also need to know the effects different types of equipment can help you to achieve.

When blow-drying, the length of hair dictates the size of the brush that you would choose. This is why most stylists have a wide and varied range of brushes. To start with, you will only need a basic range of brushes. As you gain experience and master different techniques, you should add to your equipment.

Timing

Organising your time effectively

Organising yourself and your time at work is an important part of your role as a stylist. Every salon allows a set amount of time for every process that is carried out, from shampooing to colouring.

A good trolley layout with all the necessary equipment will allow you to spend more time with the client on the service.

Most salons allocate the following timings to each service:

- Shampoo and conditioning = 5 minutes
- Blow-drying = 20–30 minutes.

Preparing your client

Ensure you have correctly gowned your client for the service.

Complete a consultation, identifying the correct styling and finishing tools and products for the service.

Ensure your personal standards follow the health and safety rules and regulations.

Work within a commercially viable time.

Tool		Effect	Suitability
Denman brush		Use for a smooth finish	Hair only requiring a slight curve or straight finish; curl cannot be achieved
Vent brush		Produces a soft, casual, 'broken-up' effect	Good for quick casual result; not very suitable for curling
Circular brush		Good for producing a curled effect. The smaller the brush, the tighter the curl	Large, round brushes are ideal for long hair, small brushes for shorter hair. Any round brush can tangle in the hair
Dressing-out combs		Use for backcombing and teasing the hair into style	Used for all dressing-out techniques
African Caribbean and wide-toothed combs		Used to de-tangle hair	Suitable for straight and curly hair

Styling tools and techniques

In the salon

One of your clients with longer than shoulder length hair has come in for a wash and blow-dry. During the consultation he mentioned that he did not want a lot of body or volume, just a very soft casual look. You left home late this morning and cannot seem to find what you need. Nothing seems suitable for this client. Other stylists around you are very busy and the client needs to be out of the salon as soon as possible. You decide to try to work with the equipment that you have to hand and see if you can get away with it. You use a brush that ends up giving you lots of height and volume.

In your group, discuss the following:

* What would have been the correct tool to use?
* How would you handle the situation if it happened to you?

Remember

Always have your equipment with you or readily available. You must be prepared for all eventualities.

Dry and finish hair

H14.2

In this element you will learn how to carry out a consultation, use equipment safely and effectively, apply the correct styling and finishing products and take into account critical influencing factors.

What you will learn

* Consultation
* Blow drying
* Styling and finishing products
* Critical influencing factors
* Communicating with the client throughout the blow-dry

Consultation

The consultation is the first communication that you have with the client. It is important to spend time questioning him on his requirements and expectations of the service. It is also the time when you need to complete a blow-drying analysis. It may be useful to prepare a checklist to help you.

During the consultation, check:

- for anything that may not let you carry out the service such as infections and infestations
- the type of hair you are working on – look at the texture and density of hair as this will influence the choice of styling product
- any critical influencing factors that may influence the blow-dry such as head and face shape
- how the client is currently wearing his hair – if he wants the same style, you have an advantage by seeing the hair before it is shampooed
- how much natural movement there is in the hair – this will affect your product choice and the choice of brush size
- whether there are any natural partings – it is always better to allow the hair to fall into its natural partings as the style will last longer and look more natural.

Types of questions to ask during the consultation

- Would you like a styling product on your hair?
- How would you like your hair blow-dried? (Use style books to help.)
- Do you get any problems with particular parts of the hair? (Let the client identify what they consider to be awkward areas.)

Blow drying

For tools, see page 273.

You need to be able to control the hair as you blow-dry it. The way in which you manage the hair is very important, as this will affect the finished result. Here are some tips to help you.

- Rough-dry excess moisture from the hair before you begin to style it.
- Take small sections to allow the heat of the hairdryer to dry/penetrate the mesh of hair.
- The airflow from the hairdryer should flow over the cuticle in the direction of the hairstyle, not against it, otherwise this will roughen the cuticle scales making the hair look fluffy and dull.
- Try not to direct the heat from the hairdryer directly onto the scalp, as this will cause great discomfort to the client.
- Do not over dry the hair. When a mesh of hair is dry, you will not be able to alter its shape.
- Adjust the height that the client is sitting at to enable you to work around him effectively.
- Always warn the client if you are going to adjust the position of the seat.

Remember

Men do not always have such elaborate blow-dries as women. You will need to be more aware of where double crowns and natural partings sit so that you are working with the hair and the style is manageable for the client.

- When blow-drying the nape of the hair, position the client's head downwards so that you can work freely in that area.
- Remember to change hands (with the dryer and brush) so that you can work effectively around the head.

Step-by-step blow-dry

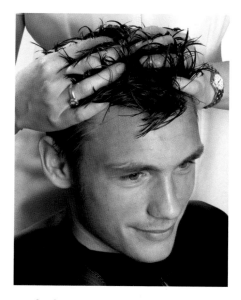

Apply the desired amount of product and distribute evenly through the hair.

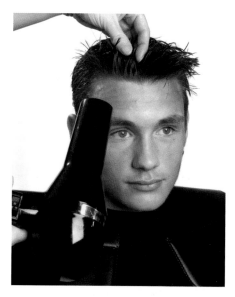

Dry the hair into the desired style making sure that the hairdryer is at the correct angle so that the airflow produces the correct amount of root lift.

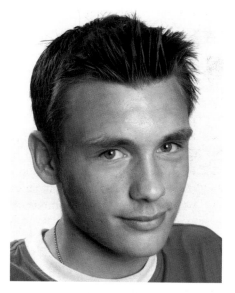

Confirm the finished result with the client.

Styling and finishing products

It is important that you understand the drying techniques, products and equipment available to help you to achieve a wide variety of styles (see pages 132–3).

Check it out

Gather together some styling products that you have in your salon or college/training institution. Draw up a chart using the headings below, then fill it in deciding which products are suitable for the hair types listed

Hair type/style	Product(s)	Application	Benefits to the hair
Short and spiky			
Curly/permed			
Fine flat hair			
African Caribbean hair			
Dry porous hair			

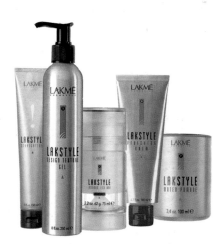

Styling and finishing products

Styling aids

Since the hair has the ability to absorb water (allowing you to shampoo it), it can also absorb atmospheric moisture. Atmospheric moisture is humidity (water) in the air (atmosphere) from rain, the shower and the bath. Styling products will put a barrier on the hair, preventing the effects of atmospheric moisture returning the hair to its natural state.

Sets and blow-dries may not last long, because as soon as the hair comes into contact with

atmospheric moisture

it will start to

drop.

The use of setting or styling products will help to produce a longer-lasting set or blow dry. There are several types of products but all modern products work in the same way.

They coat the outside of the hair shaft in a

plastic film.

This prevents

atmospheric moisture

penetrating the cuticle layer.

Modern products are made of plasticisers, e.g. Polyvinyl Pyrolidone, a clear film which dissolves in hot water and shampoo. It is therefore easily removed from the hair. They soften the hair shaft allowing shapes to be formed readily, preventing the hair from becoming 'fly away' which makes it more

manageable

when it is dressed out.

They also

protect

the hair from

added heat.

Critical influencing factors

When choosing products, equipment and blow-drying techniques, you should take into account the following factors:

- hair texture – very fine hair will need a product that stops it becoming fly-away.
- haircut – the length of the layers and style will determine what brush size to use.

- head and face shape – this will influence your drying technique and how you style the hair.
- hair growth patterns – a firm-hold product may be needed to help you disguise a double crown or a fringe with a cowlick.
- hair length.

Communicating with the client throughout the blow-dry

Throughout the blow-dry service you should check the following:

- Are you working towards the style desired by the client? Is his parting in the right place?
- Are you achieving the amount of texture and spikiness that the client requires?
- Is the heat of the hairdryer comfortable for the client?
- Would the client like any finishing products?
- Is the client happy with the finished result?

Your questions answered

When blow-drying, I put too much lift and body into the hair. How can I prevent this?
Check that the styling equipment and products you choose are suitable. You may be able to tame the hair by using a finishing product such as wax – this will help to calm down the hair and add texture to it.

What should I do if I get a client wet when I shampoo?
Remove all wet garments from the client, that is, towel, cape and gown. Then use a hairdryer very carefully to dry the collar of his shirt. Hold the collar away from his neck with your hand so that you are protecting his neck from the heat. Make sure you keep the airflow moving so that you don't burn his skin or clothing. Place a dry towel and gown around the client. Do not forget to apologise. To make sure this does not happen again, you will need to change the position and technique you are using.

What should I do if a client does not want to talk to me?
You will need to learn to read people's body language and decide whether the client is in the mood for a chat or would prefer to relax and have his hair done in peace and quiet. If a client is not in the mood to talk, you should respect his wishes.

What happens if I run over the time allocation?
You will be behind for the next client and may have to ask for some assistance from a colleague. You should make a note on the client's record card that his service takes slightly longer. When booking the next appointment take this into account and allow yourself some extra time. However, it may be that you need to adjust your working methods – look carefully at the reasons why you overran.

What would happen if I put wax on wet hair?
You would end up with an oil slick! The wax would sit on the hair preventing the hairdryer from drying the hair so you would have a sticky wet look. Should this happen, to remove the wax, add neat shampoo to the hair to break down the wax and then shampoo as normal.

Remember
Always show the client the back and profile of the finished result using a back mirror.

Dry and finish hair

Consult with your client before and during the service.

⇩

Apply suitable styling and finishing products following the manufacturer's instructions.

⇩

Effectively control the hair taking into account critical influencing factors.

⇩

Confirm the finished look with the client.

⇩

Give the appropriate after-care advice.

Test your knowledge

1   Why is it important to carry out a thorough client consultation?

2   What effect do you achieve when blow-drying with a vent brush?

3   Why is good organisation important?

4   How long should you take to carry out a blow-dry in the salon?

5   What is a critical influencing factor?

6   How can you ensure client comfort throughout the service?

7   What safety considerations need to be taken into account when drying hair?

8   Why is it important to sterilise tools and equipment?

9   What are your responsibilities under the Control of Substances Hazardous to Health Regulations?

10   What checks should you make on electrical equipment before using it?

11   What are the effects of humidity on the hair?

12   How can products help to protect the hair from the effects of humidity?

Cut hair using basic barbering techniques

Unit H7

Many hairdressing salons are unisex and require stylists to have cutting skills in both ladies' and men's hairdressing. Many of the skills that you have can be adapted to suit both types of hairdressing.

This unit will help you to develop your cutting skills using clippers with attachments, clipper-over-comb techniques and scissor-over-comb techniques. It covers critical influencing factors, such as male pattern baldness, and considers the health and safety laws and regulations that you will need to follow when cutting men's hair.

What you will learn
• Maintain effective and safe methods of working when cutting hair using barbering techniques H7.1
• Cut hair to achieve a variety of looks H7.2

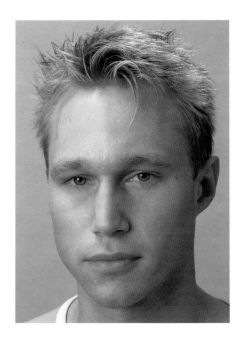 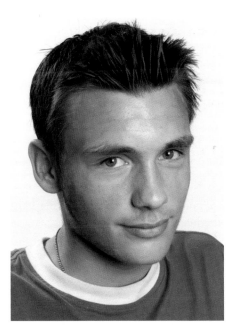 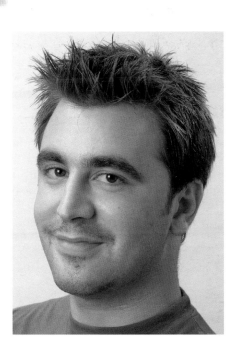

Maintain effective and safe methods of working when cutting hair using barbering techniques

H7.1

It is essential to take health and safety into account when cutting men's hair. You should know which sterilisation methods to use to avoid cross-infection or infestation and how to dispose of used sharps (blades). This element also looks at the tools and equipment suitable for men's barbering and how to maintain and care for your equipment.

What you will learn

- Preparing the client for a cutting service
- Health and safety issues
- Safe working methods
- Good organisation and time management
- Protecting yourself
- Identifying factors that may influence the service prior to cutting
- Critical influencing factors

Preparing the client for a cutting service

With any hairdressing service, you need to prepare the client for the service. Whether you are carrying out a haircut on dry or wet hair, you will need to protect the client and his clothing from hair cuttings.

For a dry cut:

- place a cutting square around the client's neck – this is usually secured with a Velcro strip (make sure that all the client's clothing is covered).
- over the top of the cutting square place a cutting collar – this is to prevent hair cuttings falling down the client's neck.

For a wet cut:

- use a cutting square, then place a towel over the top and secure with a jaws clip.
- after shampooing, towel-dry the client's hair and then remove the towel, replacing it with a cutting collar. (See Unit H9 for shampooing procedure and product choice.)

You also need to be aware of the hair cuttings that fall onto the client's face which need to be removed throughout the service. You will require a neck brush so that you can gently brush away the loose hair cuttings as they fall. You should check that the gown is secure at all times, especially if you have moved the client from one seat to another. This again is to prevent any hair cuttings from falling down his back.

If hair cuttings are sticking to the client, a small amount of talc can be used to help you remove them. Dip your neck brush into the talc making sure you do not overload the neck brush and engulf him in talcum powder! The talc will absorb the moisture that is making the hair stick to the skin and will allow you to remove the hair cuttings.

Positioning

The way in which your client is positioned in the chair is very important when carrying out a cutting service. You should make sure that he is:

- comfortable
- seated with the base of his back against the back of the chair
- seated with both feet flat on the ground or footrest.

By ensuring that your client is sitting correctly, you will be able to work comfortably for the duration of the haircut.

There are times when you will require the client to put his head forward or slightly to the side. You will need to ask him to do this and gently direct his head into the position you require. Never move or push his head forward without saying what you are doing.

You also need to consider your own posture and position when you are working at your unit.

Some salons may have their workstations situated close together. You then have a trolley alongside you, which will take up space. If you work on a client without bending your knees, you may find that you will be bumping into your colleague and it will also put a strain on your back. This may result in spinal problems and fatigue.

Remember, it is important to bend from the knees to portray a professional appearance and reduce the risk of injury or unnecessary fatigue.

Health and safety issues

As part of your professional image and in order to maintain a good service to your clients, you need to keep your work area clean and tidy at all times. First impressions count, so when you take your client to your workstation, he will want to see a clean and tidy workstation. You will need to find the time between each client to tidy up your equipment, remove hair cuttings from your work area, and generally present yourself in a professional manner.

It is important to remove hair cuttings from the floor as these pose a health and safety issue. If not removed, your client could slip resulting in a nasty injury and potential court case for the salon.

Potential hazards in the salon

- Hair cuttings not swept up from previous client.
- Trailing leads from electrical equipment.
- Client incorrectly gowned for a service.
- Rucksacks or coats left on the floor.
- Spillages from previous treatments, for example, a water spray used during a cut might have left the floor wet.

Safe working methods

Tools and equipment

You will require a variety of tools and equipment to help you complete a haircut successfully. You need to understand their uses and how to care for your equipment so that you will minimise the risk of damage to your tools, yourself, or others.

Scissors

The most important piece of equipment for a hairdresser is scissors.

Scissors vary in design, size and price. The best way to find out if a pair of scissors suits you is to pick them up and see if they are comfortable to hold. Hands and fingers vary in size so holding them is the only way to tell if they suit you.

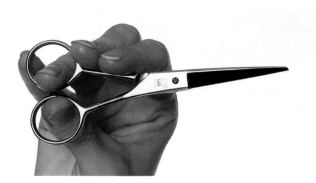

Standard haircutting scissors

281

Thinning scissors

The purpose of thinning scissors is to remove bulk from the hair. There are two main types: those that have two notched (serrated) blades and those that have one ordinary blade and one notched blade. The spaces between the notches vary in size and determine the amount of hair that is removed.

Scissors with two notched blades will take off more hair than thinning scissors with one notched blade and one ordinary blade. Notched scissors with wide spaces between them will remove more hair than thinning scissors with smaller spaces between them.

Thinning scissors are also called:

- texturising scissors
- serrated scissors
- notched scissors.

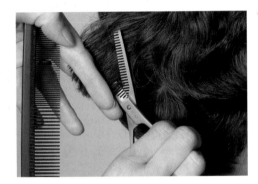

Thinning scissors

Razors

The most commonly used razors are open or cut-throat razors, shapers and safety razors. You should only use a razor on wet hair.

The more modern razor has a disposable blade and a guard over it so only a small amount of the hair is cut. This also gives added protection and prevents cuts.

The disposable razor is easy to use. Once the blade becomes blunt it can be replaced quickly and easily, ensuring you do not tear the client's hair.

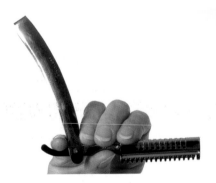

The correct way to hold a razor

Reality check!

Razors must be kept sharp at all times – if the blade becomes blunt it will tear the hair and cause discomfort to the client.

Reality check!

Never keep scissors or razors in your pockets (think health and safety!).

Electric and rechargeable clippers

Clippers are generally used for short, graduated styles. They are used on dry hair only. They can give the effect of a scissor-over-comb cut and are used in both men's and ladies' hairdressing.

Clippers work by the bottom blade remaining fixed while the top blade moves at a very high speed. You can add clipper attachments to vary/alter the length of the cut, depending on the size of the grade that you attach – the higher the number is on the grade, the longer the hair will be left; the lower the number on the grade, the shorter the hair will be cut.

Rechargeable clippers are generally smaller than electric clippers and give a closer haircut. They can be used to trim behind the backs of the ears and other hard-to-reach areas. Different heads are available for these clippers for use in hair sculpting. After use they should be replaced on their stand for recharging.

You should oil both types of clippers after every use to maintain them and to make sure that they run smoothly. This will help to prolong their life.

Clipper attachments

Clipper attachments, also know as grades, are added to your clippers to allow you to cut the hair at different lengths. They are available in different sizes ranging from a grade 0.5 (the smallest) up to a grade 8 (the largest).

You attach them to the clipper head making sure that they are sitting firmly and correctly to the clippers and then you are ready to begin the haircut. Clipper attachments should not be used if they have missing or broken teeth as this will result in an uneven haircut.

You should confirm with the client the size of the clipper grade as you attach it to your clippers to double check that you heard correctly and are using the correct grade.

You can sterilise the clipper attachments by brushing off the hair cuttings, then either using a sterilising spray or removing them from the clippers and immersing them in barbicide solution for the recommended time.

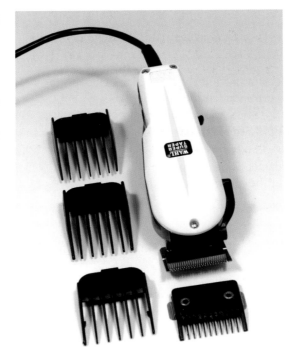

Electric clippers and attachments

Reality check!

- Check your clippers regularly to make sure that they have not been knocked out of alignment. (If the moveable top blade is above the bottom still blade, this will cut the client.)
- If your clippers are out of line, check the manufacturer's instructions to re-set them.
- Do not use clippers with broken teeth as they can pull, tear or cut the scalp.

Tools – their uses and how to care for them

Tool	Uses	Care
Scissors	Most cutting techniques – club cutting, freehand texturising, etc.	Remove hair cuttings, oil frequently
Thinning scissors	Removes bulk not length from hair	Remove hair cuttings, oil frequently
Razor	Removes length and bulk from hair	Remove hair cuttings, oil frequently
Clippers	For short graduated styles	Remove hair cuttings, oil after use

Neck brush and water spray

A neck brush removes cuttings from the client and is necessary for the duration of the haircut.

Use a water spray to damp down hair that dries too quickly. If the hair is allowed to dry out halfway through, you will not achieve even tension.

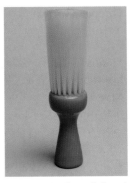

A neck brush

Using equipment safely to minimise damage to tools

- Do not use electrical equipment with wet hands.
- Check plugs and wires are not loose/damaged before use.
- Use the correct piece of equipment for the job you want to do.
- Replace equipment carefully after use, ensuring it is clean and in good working order.
- Switch off electrical items when not in use and unplug to avoid trailing wires.
- When putting away electrical equipment, avoid folding flexes too tightly as this will cause them to short circuit if they get damaged.

In accordance with the Electricity at Work Regulations 1989, all electrical equipment should be checked every six months by a qualified electrician, who should then place a sticker on the equipment to show that it is safe to use. A record of the visit should be kept by the salon for future reference.

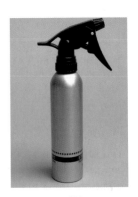

Water spray

Sterilisation and cleaning of tools and equipment

You have looked at how to prevent cross-infection of blood by covering any open cuts when working. You also need to be aware that tools must be sterilised to ensure that you minimise any risk of infection or infestation that can be passed on by your equipment. The table below shows the best methods for sterilising tools.

Methods of sterilising and cleaning tools and equipment

Tool/equipment		Method of cleaning/sterilisation
Neck brush		Wash bristles in soapy water and immerse bristles in barbicide solution for specified time (20 minutes) and allow to dry
Water spray		Wash out bottle with barbicide solution. Rinse well before use
Sectioning clips		Wash regularly in soapy water and immerse in barbicide solution for specified time (20 minutes)
Cutting comb		Wash in hot, soapy water to remove dirt and grease. Ultra-violet cabinet; barbicide solution
Scissors		Ultra-violet cabinet; autoclave; alcohol/sterile wipes or sprays
Thinning scissors		Ultra-violet cabinet; autoclave; alcohol/sterile wipes or sprays
Razor		Ultra-violet cabinet; autoclave; alcohol/sterile wipes or sprays
Clippers (and attachments)		Remove loose hair cuttings then spray blades with sterilising clipper spray

Disposal of used sharps

'Sharps' is the term used in hairdressing to describe the blades used in safety razors.

Salons should supply a yellow sharps bin for the disposal of blades. It is a hard plastic bin that cannot be pierced, which is collected by the local health authority and incinerated. If you put a disposable blade from your razor/hair shaper in an ordinary black bin liner, the person emptying the bin may cut themselves and be at risk of cross-infection.

Good organisation and time management

You need to be prepared for every client, which means you must have the right tools available to cover every aspect of the men's cutting services that your salon offers.

Good organisation means:

- all equipment is clean and sterilised
- record cards are at hand
- a tidy working area which is free of excess waste (cut hair) and has no slippery surfaces or potential hazards.

Using your time effectively

You should always be organised and ready for the client's arrival. Each salon has its own time allocation for services offered, for example, most experienced stylists will allow only 20 minutes for a dry cut and a maximum of 45 minutes for a cut and blow-dry. As a trainee, you should be aware of the time it takes you to cut a client's hair. If you took two hours for a basic cut, your salon would soon be out of business!

However, it is expected that you will take longer than an experienced stylist for your first cuts.

These are the usual timings allowed for the following services:

- wet cut = 30 minutes
- cut and blow-dry = 45 minutes
- dry trim = 20–30 minutes.

Protecting yourself

For your own health and safety you need to be aware of potential hazards to yourself, for example, the possibility of cross-infection from blood-borne diseases such as Hepatitis and HIV.

Prevention is better than cure. You can have a vaccination for Hepatitis A and B if you are in a high-risk group, of which hairdressing could be considered one. You are at risk because of the potential of cuts from scissors and sharps – this increases the risk of exposure to blood.

If you have an open cut, make sure that it is covered with a dressing so that if you accidentally cut a client you will not be at risk from cross-infection of blood.

Check it out

Investigate the sharps bin in your salon or training institution.

- Where is it kept?
- What colour is it?
- What should you put into it?
- How often is it collected?

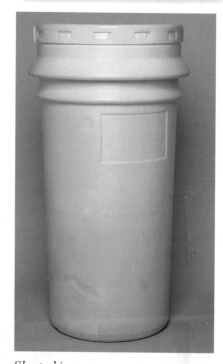

Sharps bin

Remember

A basic cut should take no more than 30–40 minutes.

Check it out

Find out how long your salon allows for the following services:

- wet cut
- cut and blow-dry
- dry trim.

Check it out

What would you do if you accidentally cut a client? Discuss this together before you read on.

In the salon

Tara was cutting a client's hair when the client jerked his head sharply and she nipped the top of his ear with her scissors. Although there was a lot of blood, she tried not to panic, but took the following actions:

- put on protective gloves
- applied a small amount of pressure to stem the blood flow with a clean towel she had to hand
- called for Estelle, next to her, whom she knew was a first aider.

In your group, discuss why these three actions would have been necessary. After the incident, what further action should Tara have taken and why?

Your personal health and hygiene needs to be of a high professional standard at all times. You need to make sure that all equipment that you use is clean and sterile for each client to minimise the risk of cross-infection or infestation between clients. You will need to make sure you have good personal hygiene standards, that is, the use of deodorants and breath fresheners, and ensure your appearance reflects your profession.

Identifying factors that may influence the service prior to cutting

When you carry out a consultation on your client, you need to be aware that there may be factors that may not let you carry out the service. You should be checking the hair and scalp for any infections or infestations and looking for any strong hair growth patterns or problem areas that could be classed as a critical influencing factor.

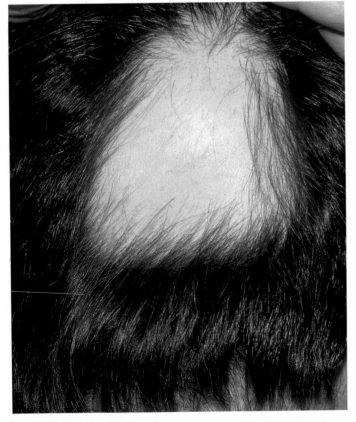

Alopecia

Condition	Description	Cause	Treatment
Pityriasis capitis (dandruff)	Small, itchy, dry scales (white or grey)	Overactive production and shedding of epidermal cells – stress related	Dandruff shampoo, e.g. selenium sulphide or zinc pyrithone; oil conditioners or conditioning creams applied to the scalp
Seborrhoea (greasiness)	Excessive oil on the scalp or skin	Overactive sebaceous gland – stress related	Shampoos for greasy hair; spirit lotions
Psoriasis	Thick, raised, dry, silvery scales; often found behind the ears	Overactive production and shedding of the epidermal cells – possibly passed on in families, recurring in times of stress	Medical treatment; coal tar shampoo
Male pattern baldness	Receding hairline, thinning hair, baldness	Hereditary, i.e. passed on in families	Medical treatment is being developed
Sebaceous cyst	A lump either on top or just underneath the scalp	Blockage of the sebaceous glands	Medical treatment may be advised; treat gently during salon services
Fragilitis crinium (split ends)	Split, dry, roughened hair ends	Harsh physical or chemical treatments	Cutting and reconditioning treatments
Damaged cuticle	Cuticle scales toughened and damaged, dull hair	Harsh physical treatments	Reconditioning treatments; restructurant
Alopecia areata	Bald patches	Shock or stress	Medical treatment; high frequency treatment
Trichorrhexis nodosa	Hair roughened and swollen along the hair shaft, sometimes broken off	Harsh use of chemicals; physical damage,	Restructurant; reconditioning the cut hair whenever possible
Monilethrix	Beaded hair – a very rare condition	Uneven production of keratin in the follicle – hereditary	Treat very gently within the salon
Tinea capitis (ringworm)	Pink patches on scalp, develops onto a round, grey, scaly area with broken hairs – most common in children	Fungus (not a worm) – spread by direct contact (touching) or indirectly through brushes, combs or towels	Highly contagious; medical treatment required
Impetigo	Blisters on the skin, which weep and dry to form a yellow crust	Bacteria entering through broken skin	Highly contagious; medical treatment required
Pediculosis capitis (head lice)	White or light brown specks attached to the hair shaft close to the scalp; often at nape of neck and behind ears; itchiness – very common in children	Small parasites (with 6 legs, 2 mm long), which bite the scalp and suck blood from the host. The females lay eggs (nits), which stick to the hair close to the scalp (they need warmth to survive). Cannot jump but are spread by direct contact (head to head) or indirect contact (from brushes, combs, etc.). Can live for 2 days off the scalp. Once infected, lice multiply rapidly	Highly contagious; refer to pharmacist

Condition	Description	Cause	Treatment
Folliculitis	Small yellow pustules with hair in centre	Bacterial infection from scratching or contact with infected person	Medical treatment required
Warts	Small, flesh-coloured raised lumps of skin	Virus spread by direct contact or touch	Only contagious when damaged; treat with care in salon
Scabies	Red irritating spots and lines on the skin	Animal parasites (itch mites) burrowing in the skin	Highly contagious; medical treatment required
Barber's itch (sycosis)	Small yellow spots around the follicle; general irritation and inflammation; possible burning sensation	Bacterial infection of the hair follicle; generally found in beard area	Medical treatment required

Conditions, infections and infestations of the hair and scalp

Critical influencing factors

A critical influencing factor is anything that you may have to take into account that will have an effect on the end result that you hope to achieve. For example, if a client had extremely fine hair, you would not carry out thinning techniques on this type of hair. If the client had a crown that wanted to stand up on end, you would not want to cut the hair too short as it would enhance this!

These are all classed as critical influencing factors because they will have an influence on how you will carry out the service and what techniques and methods you will use.

Hair density

When you talk about the hair's density, you are referring to the amount of hair that an individual client has per square inch on his head. On some heads of hair you can see the scalp through the hair. This means that the client does not have very dense hair. On other heads there may be a lot of hair per square inch meaning the client has very dense hair.

It is sometimes easy to get density and thickness of the hair confused. You will need to remember that density refers to the amount of hair on a head and thickness refers to the texture of an individual hair not the amount of hair the client has.

Hair texture

You should examine the hair's texture very carefully during your consultation with the client because this may affect the cutting technique that you choose to use. If you decide on a particular cutting technique because of the hair's texture, you will have identified a 'critical influencing factor'. For example, if the client has very fine hair, you may choose the club cutting method to increase bulk in the hair (a critical influencing factor). On the other hand, you would not want to increase bulk in thick hair (also a critical influencing factor), so you might choose a thinning technique for this hair texture.

You can determine the texture of the hair by separating a few strands of hair and placing them across the palm of your hand. The texture of the hair usually falls into three categories: fine, medium, and thick. You will need to look at the hair closely and decide which one of these categories it falls into.

Elasticity

You need to test the elasticity of the hair to see how good the internal strength of the hair is (remember, porosity testing determines the condition of the outside of the hair shaft). Refer to Unit G7 for hair tests. If the hair is in bad condition, you may choose not to use razoring techniques on it. This is because if the hair is very fragile it may not be able to withstand this method of cutting which can put extra stress on the hair.

Head and face shapes

When consulting with the client before deciding on the length of the cut, you should take into consideration the client's head and face shape because these can become 'critical influencing factors' in your choice of length for the cut. For example, if a client wanted a crew cut, you would need to take into account the client's head shape – a bumpy head becomes more obvious with a crew cut.

The four most common face shapes are: square, round, oblong and oval. You will need to decide which face shape your client has to determine which style will best suit him. For example, to balance out a square face you will need to style the hair to make the 'squareness' of the face less obvious.

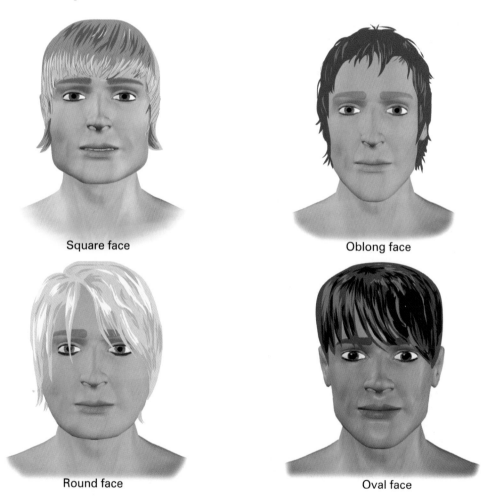

Square face

Oblong face

Round face

Oval face

Styles for the four most common face shapes

Hair growth patterns

On some heads the hair growth patterns are very apparent. For example, if the client has a cowlick in the middle of his fringe and the fringe has jumped or parted as a result, this will be obvious to you. The client may also have blow-dried his hair so well that he has disguised a double crown or strong hairline movement.

You need to look very closely at potential problem areas when the hair is dry and take a second look as a safeguard if you wet the hair. By deciding to leave length because of the client's hair growth patterns, you will be identifying a 'critical influencing factor'.

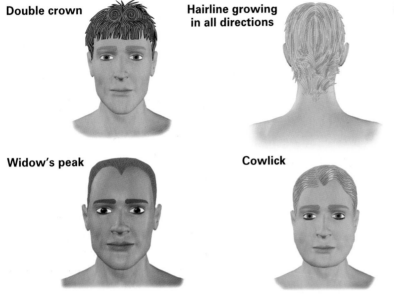

Double crown

Hairline growing in all directions

Widow's peak

Cowlick

Hair growth patterns

Check it out

Working in pairs, look at each other's hair growth patterns and try to identify any critical influencing factors.

Potential factors to consider when cutting hair with strong growth patterns are:

- the nape hairline may grow unevenly meaning that the hair would need to be tapered into the neck.
- There may be a cowlick in the fringe area so the fringe needs to be made heavier to keep weight to help the hair stay down.
- There may be a double crown so the parting may have to be changed to distribute the hair more evenly either side of the head to disguise the double crown.

Presence of male pattern baldness

Where a client's hair recedes at the temples or may be slightly thinning at the crown area, you will need to take this into account as a critical influencing factor. The client may ask you to style his hair in such a way that you would be emphasising the male pattern baldness.

Male pattern baldness is the term used to describe a hereditary factor that can affect male clients at a very young age. Most men can look at their fathers or grandfathers to see how their hair will thin or recede (or not). Some clients may be sensitive to this so you should:

- be tactful
- suggest a variation on the style suggested by the client if you think his idea would emphasise the baldness
- leave the hair slightly longer to compensate for these areas.

Not every client who has male pattern baldness will be concerned about it and you may find that they wish to have a very short haircut, such as a crew cut.

A crew cut

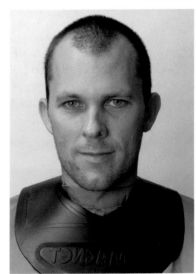

In the salon

A trainee had a client in for a dry trim. She carried out a consultation and discovered that the client was thinning on his crown area (think of monks!). To overcome the problem she did not remove too much length from this area and suggested that he might want to grow his hair into a graduated wedge style. The client was very pleased that the trainee had suggested another style and gave her a very good tip. Immediately he booked another appointment four weeks later with the same stylist.

• What can you learn from this?

Remember

Always remember to carry out a thorough consultation.
• You need to be able to identify male pattern baldness.
• Be tactful at all times.
• Do not be afraid to offer advice and suggest new styles.

Working within a commercially viable time

You will have researched how long your salon or training establishment allows for the services that it offers and this will be the time frame that you will be trying to work within.

By breaking the service down into fragments it should show you how much time you will have to spend on each stage and give you a timescale to work towards.

What you do not want to do is constantly watch the clock. This will not only get you flustered but will also make the client feel uncomfortable. All you need to do is be aware if you are on track and not running over on one part of the service, which will have a knock-on effect on the rest of the day's services.

Health and safety of cutting

Ensure the client is correctly gowned.

⇩

Position yourself and your client to minimise fatigue while working.

⇩

Keep your work area clean and tidy throughout the duration of the service.

⇩

Use the correct tools for the service.

⇩

Complete the service within a commercially viable time.

Cut hair to achieve a variety of looks   H7.2

This element covers the barbering techniques you will need to carry out to complete the unit. It looks at cutting techniques used specifically for men's barbering. You will need to take into account the presence of male pattern baldness and different hair growth patterns that will determine the neckline shape of the haircut. This element also looks at a wide range of cutting techniques and effects on different types of hair.

What you will learn

• Preparing the client for a cutting service
• Cutting techniques
• Cuttiing effects
• Meeting client expectations and ensuring comfort

Preparing the client for a cutting service

Consultation

Before you can begin any service you need to complete a consultation with your client. This is to establish:

- the client's wishes
- the technique/method of cutting that you will be using
- the tools and equipment suitable for the job.

A suggested consultation checklist is given on page 175.

During the consultation check for any infections or infestations that may not allow you to carry out the service.

Hair preparation

You need to be aware of the advantages and disadvantages of both wet and dry methods of cutting – see the table below.

Advantages and disadvantages of cutting wet and dry hair

Wet hair		Dry hair	
Advantages	**Disadvantages**	**Advantages**	**Disadvantages**
More precise lines	Client may be uncomfortable if salon temperature is too cool	Hair will be same length when finished	Hair flies everywhere
Hair is easier to manage and control	Unable to see bulk/weight lines in hair (especially permed/ naturally curly hair	Easier to see what needs to be removed from hair	Cut can be uneven
Hair can be manipulated into style during cutting			Hair can be hard to control and keep even tension
			Client may have greasy/dirty hair

Accurately establishing and following cutting guidelines

When you are ready to begin your cut on the client, you need to make sure that you work in a methodical manner. You will need to section the hair so that you can see your guidelines clearly, making sure that they are neat and level. Hair that you are not working on will need to be secured out of the way. The sections (meshes) of hair you are working on need to be combed through so that even, clean tension is maintained throughout each section. The sections of hair should be no more than half an inch deep, this will help you use each section as a guideline for the next section of hair you are going to cut.

By following these guidelines you will be able to work around the head, using your time to the maximum benefit and ensuring you achieve the required result.

Cutting techniques

Club cutting

This method leaves the ends of the hair blunt and level. It is sometimes called the blunt cut. The technique is most commonly used for removing length from the hair and is ideal for fine hair as it gives the appearance of increasing bulk. It can also help to reduce the tendency of the hair to curl.

Check it out

- Why is club cutting a good technique to use on fine hair?
- Can this technique be used on either wet or dry hair?
- Does this method of cutting help to encourage curl into the hair?
- What effect does this technique have on the ends of the hair?

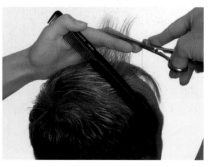

Club cutting

Club cutting can be used on wet or dry hair. It is very suitable for curly hair because the sections are combed through and held with tension, ensuring that the ends of the hair are blunt and level. This technique can be used on any hairstyle that is cut with scissors.

Freehand cutting

This technique is mainly used on straight hair. This is because curly hair will not sit in one place; the curl in the hair means it will lift and not remain in a way in which it can be cut free hand.

As the name of the technique suggests, you do not hold the hair with tension – the hair is combed into place and cut free hand. The freehand technique gives you a truer indication of where the hair will sit when dried because you will not have used tension by pulling the hair down. This is an ideal method to use on fringes as they have a tendency to 'jump up' when dried and is also better suited to one-length looks that are cut above the collar. Cutting hair above collar length requires a very blunt even line – by combing the hair down flat on to the neck and cutting free hand, you will be able to achieve this precise line.

Freehand cutting can be used on wet or dry hair.

Scissor-over-comb

This technique is used to cut hair very short following the natural contours of the head. It is most frequently used in the nape area or around the ears and is often used in men's hairdressing to taper the hair into the hairline.

The technique can be used on wet or dry hair, although you will achieve a better result on dry hair, as the cutting line is clearer.

Step-by-step scissor-over-comb technique

Reality check!

When club cutting, sections taken must be combed through so that the hair is smooth and held with even tension to ensure an even result.

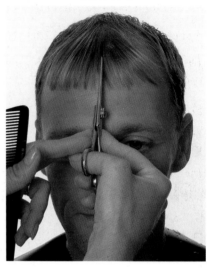

Freehand cut

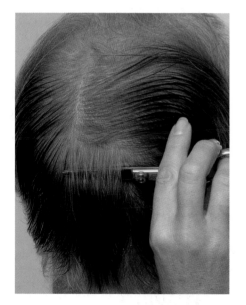

Comb all of the hair into style and place your scissors into the hair to pick up a mesh of hair for cutting.

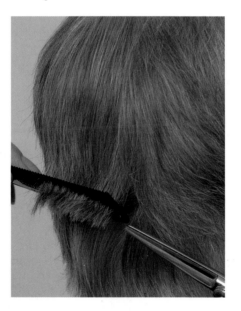

Replace the scissors with your comb to support the section of hair you are going to cut, holding the hair out at 90° to the head.

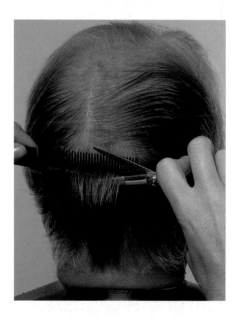

Remove the desired amount of hair keeping your comb in position.

Clipper-over-comb

With the clipper-over-comb technique, clippers are used instead of scissors to give a similar effect to scissor-over-comb. Both techniques allow you to cut the hair shorter than if you were holding the hair between your fingers.

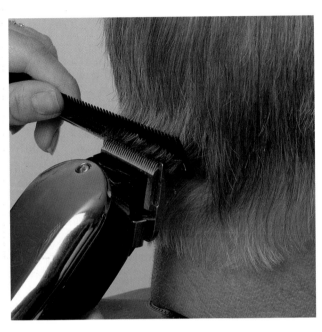

Comb is used to support the hair and then the clippers are used to remove the desired length of hair

Remember

Always remember health and safety when using electrical equipment such as clippers.

Reality check!

- You should sterilise and oil your clippers after every client.
- Only use clippers on dry hair.

Thinning

There are various cutting techniques that can be used to thin the hair as well as using thinning scissors and razoring techniques (for information on tools, see pages 281–3).

Some of the thinning techniques that you will be using are also referred to as texturising techniques. The thinning method of cutting removes bulk from the hair without removing the overall length. Thinning is normally carried out on dry hair because it is more obvious where the bulk/weight is in a haircut (the only exception is when using a razor).

Avoid using thinning techniques on front hairlines, natural partings or the crown area as they will produce unwanted spiky effects.

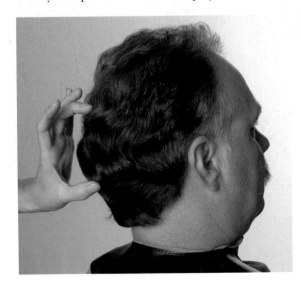

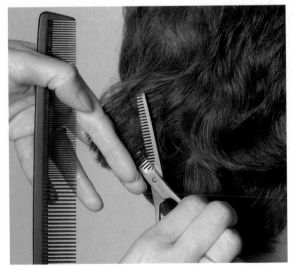

Thinning scissors remove bulk from the hair

Technique	Suitability	Benefits
Weave cutting	Not for the whole head because of size of the meshes of hair. Can be used on wet or dry, long, short, straight or curly	Shorter pieces of hair will stand up supporting the remaining hair
Pointing/chipping	Ideal for straight hair	Breaks up hard lines in the hair
Castle cutting	Can be used on wet or dry hair	Breaks up hard lines in the hair
Razoring	Only to be used on wet hair. Not recommended for very fine hair. Ideal for thinning large areas of hair, curly or straight	Will encourage the hair to curl. Removes a lot of bulk, leaving the ends soft and feathered
Thinning scissors	Not recommended for very short or very fine hair. Ideal for medium to long hair and for large areas of thinning. Suitable for straight or curly hair	Removes bulk without removing length. Overuse will result in the ends becoming wispy

Thinning techniques

Tapering technique (slither cutting)

This method of cutting is a sliding movement that goes backwards and forwards along the hair. Hair is tapered by holding the section of hair in the crutch of the scissors (where the bottom of the blades meet). Begin the sliding movement a third of the way down the length of the hair from the points, opening and closing the blades slightly as you slide the scissors.

Cutting effects

Uniform layer cut

This cut produces layers of hair the same length all over the head.

Step-by-step uniform layer cut

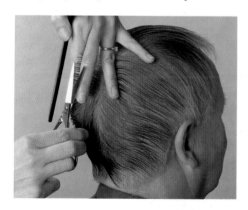

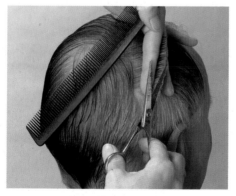

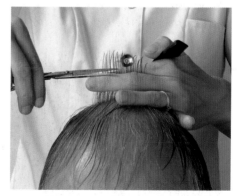

Begin by taking a section of hair just below the crown in the centre of the head and hold out at 90° to the head. Remove the required amount of hair by cutting above the fingers while keeping the hair at this angle.

Working around the head in orange segments, continue to use a piece of the old guideline with your new hair and remove length from the new sections. Work in this manner through either side of the central back sections.

Going back to the top crown section, take a mesh of hair and hold it up at 90° to the head and remove the unwanted length. Use this section to follow down through the sides to blend the top section with the sides.

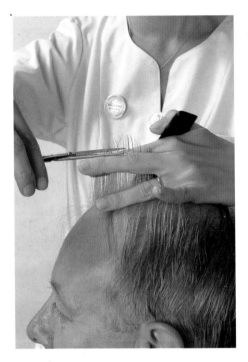

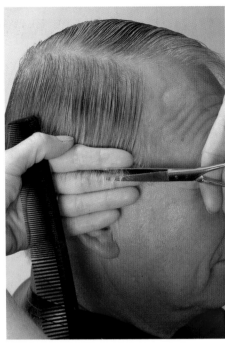

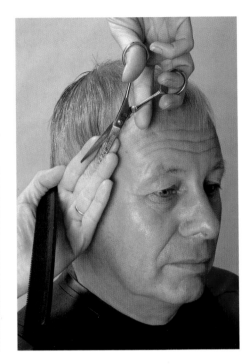

To blend the top in with the front of the hair, take a section in the opposite direction and continue the cut by holding the hair at the same angle, blending in the two sections of hair.

The perimeter length needs to be held flat to the head and unwanted hair removed following client requirements, to give a clean outline.

The hair is pulled forward at the sides to remove any strands of hair that may fall forward onto the face.

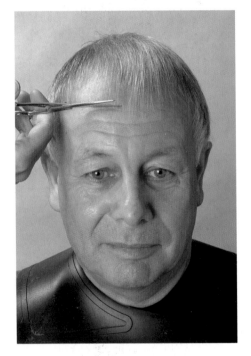

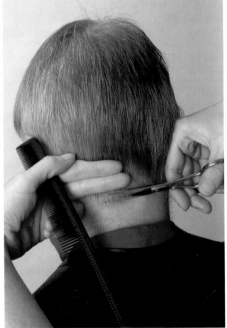

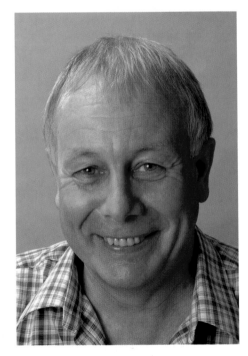

The fringe area can be cut free hand, again to remove unwanted stray pieces of hair, checking the desired length with your client.

The nape line will also need to be cut to blend with the rest of the haircut and produce a clean and tidy hairline. Comb the hair flat onto the neck and remove the unwanted hair outside the desired neckline shape.

Confirm the finished result with the client.

Graduated layer cut

This cut produces a tapered look in the nape and at the sides, keeping more length and weight in the hair at the top of the head.

Step-by-step graduated layer cut on straight, dry hair

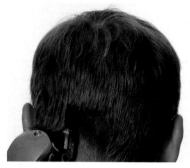

Determine the amount of hair that needs to be removed. Using clippers with grade or the scissor-over-comb technique, begin at the centre back section of the head.

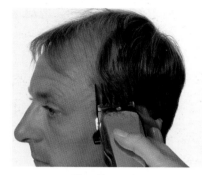

Move round to the side sections of the head and continue to cut the hair making sure you do not go too high, blending with the back sections. Repeat on the opposite side.

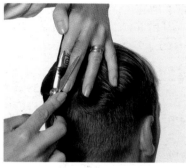

To blend the top of the haircut, you will need to hold the hair at a 45° angle, with the shortest point blending into the already cut hair.

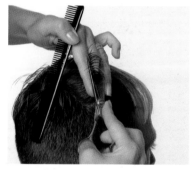

Continue to blend the hair, taking orange segment slices, working your way around the head, cutting the hair at the 45° angle.

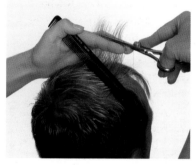

Move through to the top sections beginning at the crown area holding the hair up at a 90° angle and remove the required amount of hair. Follow this section down to blend in the sides of the hair.

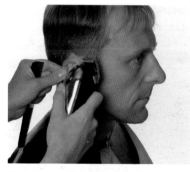

To tidy the hair around the ears and neckline, you can use the edge of the clippers, moving the ears to help you get in close to the head.

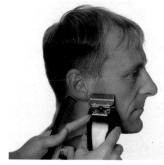

Sideburns need to be balanced on either side of the head by using the edge of the clippers flat to the head and creating a clean sharp line.

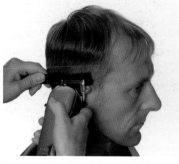

If you want the hair to be tapered in closer to the head, use the clipper-over-comb technique to achieve this.

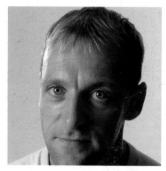

Confirm the finished result with the client and apply appropriate finishing products to complete the look.

Adapting your cutting techniques to take into account critical influencing factors

You have looked at cutting methods/techniques and critical influencing factors – now you need to put the two together.

When you are going to carry out a hair cutting service on a client, you need to establish during your consultation what critical influencing factors (if any) that you have to consider.

It is important to check through the client's hair before and after you shampoo the hair. This is because some critical influencing factors may be apparent only on wet hair and others only on dry hair. If a client has straightened his hair and you have carried out your consultation on straight hair, you may discover, when you take him to the basin and wash his hair, that he has a very strong natural wave which means you may need to use different cutting methods or techniques to the ones you had discussed.

Alternatively, if you do not carry out your consultation until the client's hair has been shampooed, you may not see potential problem areas that disappear when the hair is wet. It is important to carry out your consultation on dry hair and then re-check the hair when it is shampooed to make sure you have identified all the potential critical influencing factors.

Adjusting your position and crosschecking the cut

As you are progressing through the cut, you will need to adjust the position in which you are working in relation to the head. Although heads come in different shapes and sizes, they are all round. If you stand 'square' on to a head of hair and try to cut the hair in this position, you will not achieve a balanced shape. You need to move around the head as you work so that you are covering all angles of the haircut. This will help you to achieve an accurate cut, ensuring that you have even distribution of weight and balance throughout the style.

Crosschecking the haircut as you work will also help you to achieve even distribution and weight throughout the style.

To crosscheck a haircut you will need to take sections/meshes of hair in the opposite direction to the way in which you have carried out your haircut. You still hold them at the same angle as you did for the original haircut and continue to work in small methodical sections so that you are covering the whole of the haircut.

Your mirror is another good tool to use to check the shape, weight and balance of the haircut. If you stand directly behind your client and lift sections of hair, you will be able to use the mirror to confirm that they are of the same length, that you have used the same angle on both sides and that you have achieved a balanced result. When you are more experienced, you will be able to carry out this process without using your mirror and check your sections through by feel, looking to see if the hair is 'sitting' in the style you have cut. You will be able to see if the weight left in the hair is working, giving you the effect both you and the client wanted to achieve.

By crosschecking and using your mirror to check the weight and angles of your cut, you are giving yourself and your client the opportunity to make any changes to the haircut before you get to the drying stage. It is important to check with your client that he is happy with what you have done and is ready for you to dry his hair into the finished result.

Check it out

In pairs, discuss any potential problems that you may come across, such as double crowns, very fine hair, strong nape growth patterns and thick naturally curly hair. For each of the problems that you identify, make a list of the cutting methods and techniques that you would use to minimise the effects of the problems identified.

Check it out

In your groups, discuss the types of questions that you can use to confirm with the client that he is happy with the desired look.

Remember to think about using open questions rather than closed questions, which will help you to gain more of a response from your client.

Neckline shapes

Cutting an accurate neckline shape in men's barbering is very important. Everyone's hairline grows differently and you will need to take this into account. It is always best to follow the natural growth pattern of the hairline. Any hair that is outside of the neckline shape will need to be removed by using clippers to give a clean, accurate finished result.

If the client doesn't have a preference, you could suggest one of the following neckline shapes. Clipper-over-comb/scissor-over-comb techniques can be used to achieve these effects.

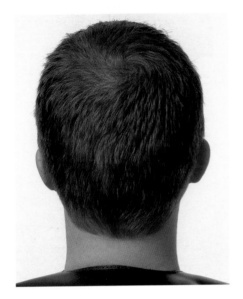

Rounded neckline

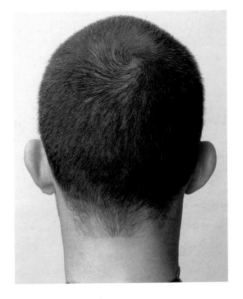

Tapered neckline

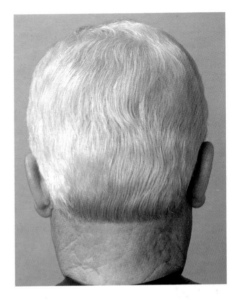

Square neckline

Step-by-step rounded neckline

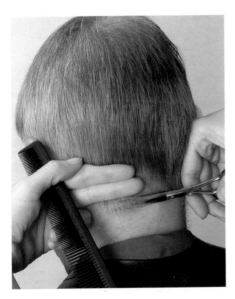

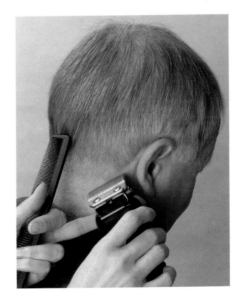

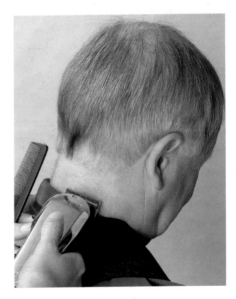

The hair is combed flat to the head and the extra length removed following the natural shape of the hair-growth pattern.

Clippers are turned over so that a sharp edge can be given to the previously cut neckline shape.

Clippers are used to remove unwanted hair from outside the previously cut neckline shape.

Sideburns

When cutting men's hair, you will be required to shape and balance the client's sideburns. You can use:

- scissor-over-comb techniques
- clipper-over-comb techniques
- freehand techniques
- club cutting techniques.

Scissor- and clipper-over-comb techniques will reduce the bulk from the sideburns, while club cutting and freehand cutting will remove length.

It is not always a good idea to judge the length of the hair by looking at where the hair sits in relation to the client's ears, as they can be uneven. It is best to look at your client straight on in the mirror with a finger at the bottom of each sideburn to determine the correct balance and length.

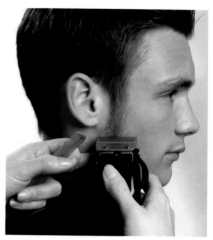

Shaping sideburns

Meeting client expectations and ensuring comfort

Client comfort is important throughout the treatment. If the client is not seated correctly, he is wet from the shampoo, or is covered in hair cuttings, he will not be comfortable.

Throughout the treatment you should confirm with the client that he is happy with the way the service is progressing. These are the type of questions you could ask:

- Are you comfortable?
- Have I removed enough length? (Only cut one section of hair before asking this question!)
- Where would you like your fringe to sit? (Use eyebrows as a guideline.)
- How does the whole cut feel? (Let the client run his fingers through his hair.)

It is also important to use the back mirror to show the client the profile and back of his hair, again reaffirming that he is happy with the cut that you have completed.

When using the back mirror:

- hold it at the height of the client's head
- spend time letting the client see all angles of the haircut
- do not stand too far back.

After-care advice

Giving after-care advice is an important part of the whole service. You would not expect to go to a hi-fi shop, purchase a stereo system and not receive information or instructions on how to use the equipment that you have bought. The same goes for giving information to your client following any service given in the salon.

The information on aftercare that you should give includes:

1 How often he should come back into the salon for a trim to maintain the look.

2 Which products are best suited to his hair type and will help him to re-create the look you have achieved.

3 What the best tools (for example, correct size of brushes) and equipment are for achieving the look.

Remember

A cutting collar will prevent hair going down the client's back and a neck brush will allow you to remove stray hair cuttings throughout the cut. If the client is comfortable, you will be more able to achieve an accurate cut.

Check it out

Think back to your last visit to the hairdressers. How did the stylist check that you were happy and comfortable during your treatment? Did this make you feel more reassured during your visit? If the stylist did not ask you any questions, how did this make you feel?

Basically, you are trying to give information that will aid the client to maintain his hair and achieve the desired effect.

You can talk to him about the use of products and drying techniques during the service and give him information on how much the average head of hair grows each month so that he will have a better understanding of why it is important to come into the salon for regular trims.

Your questions answered

What do I do if a client wants a haircut that is not appropriate for his type of hair?
Tactfully you would try to steer the client towards a style that you feel would enhance his features and be suitable for his hair type.

How can I tell whether the client has a double crown or whether he has slept on his hair awkwardly?
When you shampoo the client's hair, a double crown would still be apparent. If it was where the client had slept on his hair, it would disappear when you wet the hair.

I do not understand what is meant by the term 'cross checking the hair'.
Cross checking the hair means that you are going back through the haircut, taking sections in the opposite direction to the way in which you originally cut the hair, to make sure that all aspects of the haircut have been covered.

Test your knowledge

1 *Why is it important to seat your client squarely in the chair when cutting?*

2 *List three advantages and three disadvantages of cutting wet hair and dry hair.*

3 *What are the three other names given to thinning scissors?*

4 *Do thinning scissors remove length or bulk from the hair?*

5 *Do you use clippers on wet or dry hair?*

6 *Where do you dispose of used blades from your safety razor?*

7 *Why is it important to keep your work area clean and tidy?*

8 *Why is it important to fill in an accident report form?*

9 *What do the Electricity at Work Regulations cover?*

10 *What different sterilisation methods are available to you?*

11 *How many different neckline shapes can you achieve?*

Remember

On average, the hair grows half an inch each month. Some clients' hair will grow quickly and some not so quickly, so knowing this will aid you when you are consulting with your client and assessing how much hair to remove since his last trim.

The cutting service

Suitably prepare your client.

Work in a methodical manner following guidelines.

Adapt your cutting techniques to take into account any critical influencing factors.

Check the weight, balance and shape of the haircut.

Create a neckline shape suitable to the natural hairline.

Confirm the cut and give suitable after-care advice.

Cut facial hair to shape using basic techniques

Unit H8

In this unit you will learn how to cut beards and moustaches. Many unisex salons and barbers offer these services as part of a complete package to their clients. The cutting techniques you will be using are the same as those for cutting hair, but there are other factors that you will have to consider such as strong hair growth patterns, face shapes and the client's features. Your cutting techniques will need to be adapted to take these into account.

What you will learn
• Maintain effective and safe methods of working when cutting facial hair H8.1
• Cut beards and moustaches to maintain their shape H8.2

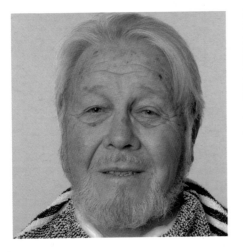
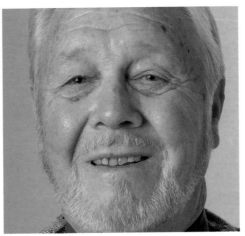

Maintain effective and safe methods of working when cutting facial hair

H8.1

When carrying out any hairdressing service, it is your responsibility to ensure the health and safety of your client and yourself while working. This element addresses all of the health and safety issues that you will need to consider when carrying out barbering services. You will look at the risk of cross-infection and infestations that can be passed from one client to another. This element also covers the preventative actions you should take to avoid cross-infection.

What you will learn
• Preparing the client for a beard or moustache trim
• Health, safety and hygiene
• Organising your working time
• Protecting yourself and the client
• Tools and equipment
• Identifying factors that may influence the service prior to cutting
• Safe disposal of used sharps

Preparing the client for a beard or moustache trim

Gowning

You should ensure that you correctly gown the client for this service to prevent any hair from entering the client's clothing or falling down his neck and causing irritation.

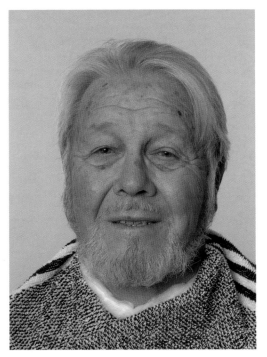 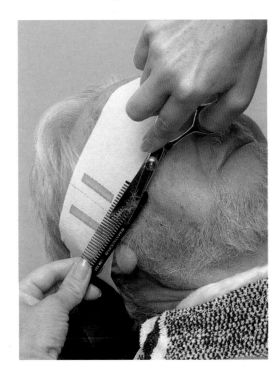

Correct gowning for a beard and moustache trim

When gowning for a beard or moustache trim:

- place a cutting square around the client and secure with the Velcro strip or use a jaws clip
- place a towel across the front of the client, tucking it slightly into the gown (but not too tightly)
- over the top of the towel use either a strip of cotton wool or neck tissue to prevent cuttings from falling beyond the gown onto the client's skin
- cover the client's eyes with a protective strip to prevent cuttings falling into them.

It is also important to ensure that you remove any hair cuttings from your client as you work, so make sure you have a neck brush.

Positioning

To enable you to work comfortably on the client during a beard or moustache trim, it is important that he is positioned correctly in the chair. Ensure that the client is sitting squarely with both feet flat on the floor. This will prevent him from leaning to one side, making it awkward for you to work.

If your salon or training institution has a men's barbering chair, you need to recline the chair into the position that you require, then ask the client to sit down. *Note*: If you sit the client in the chair first and then recline the chair, the weight of the client may make the chair tip too far back causing an injury to yourself or the client. Once he is seated, you need to make adjustments to the chair. Ask him to sit forward before you recline the chair any further.

You also need to consider your own posture and position when you are working at your unit.

Some salons may have their workstations situated close together. You then have a trolley alongside you, which will take up space. If you work on a client without bending your knees, you may find that you will be bumping into your colleague. It will also put a strain on your back if you are not standing in the correct position which could cause spinal problems and fatigue.

Health, safety and hygiene

Health, safety and hygiene are the most important factors to be considered in the salon. You need to demonstrate good hygiene practice whenever you are working. Every client must be treated with care and attention from the beginning to the end of his treatment and good health and safety practices must apply to all clients.

Potential hazards in the salon

- Hair cuttings not swept up from previous client.
- Trailing leads from electrical equipment.
- Client incorrectly gowned for a service.
- Bags or coats left on the floor.
- Spillages from previous treatments, for example, a water spray used during a cut might have left the floor wet.

Using equipment safely to minimise damage to tools

- Do not use electrical equipment with wet hands.
- Check plugs and wires are not loose/damaged before use.
- Use the correct piece of equipment for the job you want to do.
- Replace equipment carefully after use, ensuring it is clean and in good working order.
- Switch off electrical items when not in use and unplug to avoid trailing wires.
- When putting away electrical equipment, avoid folding flexes too tightly as this will cause them to short circuit if they get damaged.

In accordance with the Electricity at Work Regulations 1989, all electrical equipment should be checked every six months by a qualified electrician, who should then place a sticker on the equipment to show that it is safe to use. A record of the visit should be kept by the salon for future reference.

Cleaning and sterilisation of cutting tools

After each client, tools and equipment should be cleaned and sterilised to prevent cross-infection.

- Remove all hair cuttings.
- Wipe scissors and razors with spirit, alcohol wipe, or with sterilising spray.
- Dry metal tools thoroughly before putting them away.
- Change disposable blades after use and dispose of in the sharps bin.
- Spray clipper blades with sterilising spray after use.
- Wash all brushes and combs after use then sterilise them.
- Never use dirty or broken tools.

Check it out

In your groups, discuss the potential injuries that you could develop by positioning yourself incorrectly while you are working. How can you overcome these situations and what is the best method of working to maintain a posture that will help to prevent any injuries or cause you fatigue?

Remember

If an accident or a sudden illness occurs, it should be entered on an accident report form in case there is a claim for personal injury at a later date.

Check it out

Look around your immediate work area and list any potential health and safety hazards that might lead to harm or injury to your client.

Remember

It is essential to keep your work area clean, tidy and free of waste.

Tool/equipment		Method of sterilisation
Sectioning clips		Wash regularly in soapy water and immerse in barbicide solution
Cutting comb		Wash in hot, soapy water to remove dirt and grease. Ultra-violet cabinet; barbicide solution
Scissors		Ultra-violet cabinet; autoclave, alcohol/sterile wipes or sprays
Clippers (and attachments)		Remove loose hair cuttings then spray blades with sterilising clipper spray

Methods of sterilising tools and equipment

Organising your working time

At the start of each day, you need to organise yourself so that you are ready to receive your first client. You should:

- check the appointment book to see who your first client is
- get out the client's record card (if appropriate)
- ensure you have all the correct tools and equipment for the service.

By making sure you are organised you will save time in the salon.

Using your time effectively

You should always be organised and ready for the client's arrival. Each salon has its own time allocation for services offered. As a trainee, you should be aware of the time it takes you to carry out a beard or moustache trim. If you took two hours for a basic trim, your salon would soon be out of business! However, it is expected that you will take longer than an experienced stylist for your first trims.

To make full use of your working time, you should always be prepared to receive your client. Tools and equipment should be clean and sterilised and within easy reach. If you are not prepared correctly, this will 'eat' into the appointment time that you have with your client and could result in you running late for your later appointments.

Protecting yourself and the client

You need to have a high standard of personal cleanliness. Nails should be well trimmed and jewellery should be minimal. Clean overalls, uniforms or clothes, should be worn with short sleeves, the forearms being bare. Hands should be washed between each client. Any wounds or open sores on your hands should be covered with a suitable dressing, otherwise they may be a source of infection to the client or the client may infect you.

For your own health and safety, you need to be aware of potential hazards to yourself, for example, the possibility of cross-infection from blood-borne diseases such as Hepatitis and HIV. Prevention is better than cure. You can have a vaccination for Hepatitis A and B if you are in a high-risk group, of which hairdressing could be considered one. You are at risk because of the potential for cuts from scissors and sharps which increase the risk of exposure to blood.

Before carrying out a beard or moustache trim, always cover the client's eyes – facial hair is coarser than normal hair and can fly up into the client's eyes! If you wish, as an extra safeguard, ask the client to close his eyes.

During the trim, you should be aware of the client's and your own position while you are working. Make sure that you stand in such a way that you don't strain your back. Remember to bend from your knees and not your back. Ensure that you have positioned the client correctly so that he is comfortable and you can work around him without difficulty.

Your personal standards of health and hygiene minimise the risk of cross-infection, infestation and offence to clients and colleagues.

You may be required to wear a uniform in many establishments. This may be so that you follow the college or salon's health and safety policies.

Some hygiene requirements that should be expected:

- Long hair to be worn up to cut down the risk of cross-infection.
- Minimum amount of jewellery to be worn so that water and hair cuttings will not become trapped underneath causing bacteria to grow.
- Flat shoes with tights may need to be worn for health and safety and hygiene purposes.
- You will be required to sterilise all tools and equipment after each client.
- Make sure your personal presentation and hygiene are of a very high standard.
- Make sure you use a breath freshening spray if you smoke or have had strong-flavoured food, such as curry, the night before!
- Wear cotton tops in the summer and use a good deodorant.
- Always wash your hands after a trip to the bathroom.
- Always keep cuts and open wounds covered with a plaster.

Most of these points are common sense and things that you will do on a daily basis without realising it. It is important to continue to follow good health and hygiene practices to maintain a professional appearance to clients and colleagues.

Tools and equipment

Electric and rechargeable clippers

Clippers work by the bottom blade remaining fixed whilst the top blade moves at a very high speed. You can add clipper attachments to vary/alter the length of the cut, depending on the size of the grade that you attach – the higher the number is on the grade, the longer the hair will be left; the lower the number on the grade, the shorter the hair will be cut.

Rechargeable clippers are generally smaller than electric clippers and give a closer haircut. They can be used to trim behind the backs of the ears and other hard-to-reach areas.

You should oil both types of clippers after every use to maintain them and to make sure that they run smoothly. This will help to prolong their life.

Check it out

Make a list of what you think are the important safety issues in terms of your equipment that you would need to check on a daily basis.

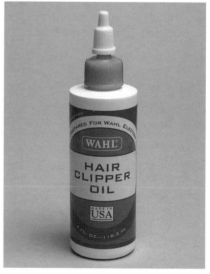

Use clipper oil after each use of the clippers

Clipper attachments

Clipper attachments also known as grades are added to your clippers to allow you to cut the hair to different lengths. They are available in different sizes ranging from a grade 0.5 (the smallest) up to a grade 8 (the largest).

You attach them to the clipper head making sure that they fit firmly and correctly to the clippers. You are ready to begin the beard trim. Clipper attachments should not be used if they have missing or broken teeth as this will result in an uneven haircut.

You should confirm with the client the size of the clipper grade as you attach it to your clippers to double check that you heard correctly and are using the correct grade.

You can sterilise the clipper attachments by brushing off the hair cuttings, then either using a sterilising spray or by removing them from the clippers and immersing them in barbicide solution for the recommended time.

Identifying factors that may influence the service prior to cutting

Before beginning the consultation, you must always check the client for any skin conditions that may not let you carry out the service (see page 313).

Your client's features will determine the size and shape of the beard or moustache.

- Check the natural growth of the hair – this may determine the shape of the moustache or how to finish off the neckline shape of a beard trim.
- Check the density of hair – this may influence the cutting technique that you use. For example, if the beard is not very thick, you may want to use a scissor-over-comb technique so that you can leave the beard or moustache longer in places where the hair may be more sparse. However, if the beard is very dense, you may want to use clippers to give an even finish all over.

Safe disposal of used sharps

'Sharps' is the term used in hairdressing to describe the blades used in safety razors.

Salons should supply a yellow sharps bin for the disposal of blades. It is a hard plastic bin that cannot be pierced, which is collected by the local health authority and incinerated. If you put a disposable blade from your razor/hair shaper in an ordinary black bin liner, the person emptying the bin may cut themselves and be at risk from cross-infection.

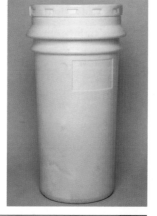

Sharps bin

Reality check!

- Check your clippers regularly to make sure that they have not been knocked out of alignment. (If the moveable top blade is above the bottom still blade, this will cut the client.)
- If your clippers are out of line, check the manufacturer's instructions to re-set them.
- Special sterilising sprays should be used on your clippers after every use.
- Do not use clippers with broken teeth as they can pull, tear or cut the scalp.

Remember

Only use clippers on dry hair.

Cutting checklist

Ensure your client's clothing and eyes are protected.

⇩

Correctly position your client.

⇩

Use the correct tools that are fit and safe for the purpose.

⇩

Identify factors that are likely to affect the service before cutting.

⇩

Work within a commercially viable time.

In the salon

Ushma had just completed a moustache and beard trim on a client. She was new to the salon and did not know where the sharps bin was kept. She was in a hurry to get ready for her next client so to save time, Ushma threw the used sharps into the nearest bin.

- What should Ushma have done?
- What might be the consequences of her actions?

Check it out

Find out how long your salon allows for the following services:

- beard trim with clippers
- beard trim using scissor-over-comb technique
- moustache trim
- full beard and moustache trim.

Cut beards and moustaches to maintain their shape

H8.2

This element looks at the cutting techniques required to complete a beard and moustache trim. As with other barbering services, you will need to take into account critical influencing factors.

What you will learn
• Preparing the client • Cutting techniques • Critical influencing factors • Adjusting your position to ensure an even, accurate, balanced cut • Meeting client expectations and ensuring comfort

Preparing the client

It is important that you follow the natural growth patterns of the hair.

- Comb the client's beard or moustache in the direction that it grows – this will also detangle the hair ready for cutting.
- Always complete a beard and moustache trim on dry hair.
- Check that the client is comfortable and that he is in a position that you can work around comfortably.
- Check that the client is correctly gowned and protected for the service.

Check that your clippers are safe to use – make sure that the top moveable blade is not protruding above the bottom blade.

Consultation

During your consultation with the client you are not only determining how much hair he wants removed or the shape of the beard or moustache he would like, you are also looking for any adverse skin conditions that may not allow you to carry out the service. If you suspect that the client has an infection or infestation, notify your salon manager or tutor. You will need to explain to the client as tactfully as possible why you are unable to carry out the service and recommend that he goes to see his GP.

Carrying out your consultation

Here are some guidelines to get you started.

- Refer to the client by name.
- Make eye contact, either face to face or through the mirror.
- Ask simple questions – do not use technical words that the client may not understand.
- Listen carefully to the answers to your questions and show an interest.

The consultation will involve finding out exactly what the client requires from the beard or moustache trim. You should ask the following questions:

- How short do you wish your beard or moustache to be? This will determine the clipper grade you will use to remove length.
- What neck shape would you like to see? Tapered, round or square?
- When did you last have a beard or moustache trim? This will give you an indication of how often the client likes to have a beard or moustache trim and how quickly his facial hair may grow.

Reality check!
Never use electrical equipment on wet hair. (Always think health and safety!)

During your consultation with the client you should have established the length and shape of the beard or moustache that you will be trimming.

Choosing your equipment and techniques

If the client had a very long, thick beard and wanted it cut very short, you would need to choose your equipment very carefully. You could use clippers with an attachment to shorten the beard, but you need to be aware that you might tug or pull the hair on a beard that is very long and thick. In this instance, you would be better off removing some of the length using a scissor-over-comb technique and then using the clippers for a closer finish.

In another instance, if the client had a very fine, soft beard that was not very long and was thin in places, you would choose to cut the beard using the scissor-over-comb technique. By using this technique you are able to leave the beard slightly longer in places to compensate for the thinner areas where the beard may not grow so thickly.

Normally scissors are used for moustaches because it is only a small area, which is not suitable for clipper work, that you are trimming. You would also use scissors to cut and blend any sideburns into the beard area.

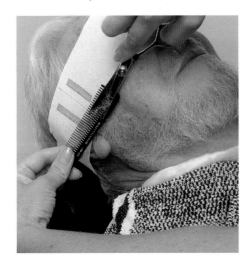
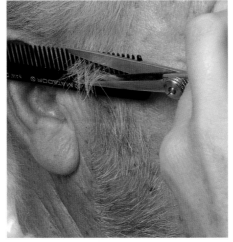

Scissor-over-comb technique to remove length from the sideburns and blend in with the beard

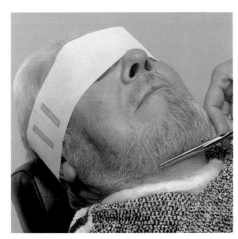

Scissors can be used to neaten off and shape the outside beardline before clippering to remove unwanted hair outside of the neckline shape

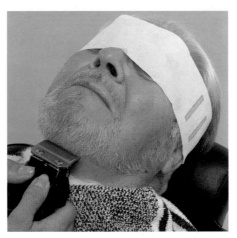

The edge of the clippers are used to give an even, blunt edge to the neckline shape

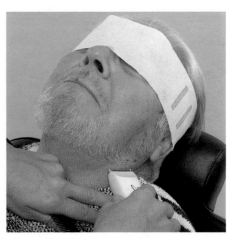

The small rechargeable clippers will help to get into the more difficult-to-reach areas to finish off the neckline shape

Using the clippers with attachments will give an even look to the whole beard trim. Clippers are ideal for cutting thick, coarse hair.

The combs that you use are very important. When cutting a beard you will need to use a rigid cutting comb. When tapering in closely to the neck or carrying out a moustache trim, you should use a flexible comb that will allow you to work in hard-to-reach areas. The fine teeth on a comb allow the hair to be controlled and closely cut; the coarser teeth allow for repeated combing and positioning of the hair.

Cutting techniques

When you are carrying out any cutting service, it is important that you work in a methodical manner; one that allows you to see where you are going next in a haircut and where you have already cut. When you are cutting beards and moustaches using either a scissor-over-comb technique or with clippers, you will find it easier if you work in channels. You could start in the middle or at either side and by working in this way you will be able to see the areas of hair that you have cut and where you are working to next.

Scissor-over-comb

Refer to page 305–6 for cutting equipment.

This method of cutting is ideal for beard and moustache trimming as you can work closely to the head. The hair is lifted with the comb and the protruding hair is clipped off. Care must be taken when using this method to ensure that you do not leave a hard line or step in the hair. This is overcome by the correct use of the comb with the points of the teeth directed away from the skin and working in a flowing movement. If you feel the flow is lapsing, stop and move your scissors and comb away from the head, then go back to it again. Cutting while the comb is stationary will create a hard line in the hair. The hair must be held at a 90 degree angle with the comb.

Step-by-step scissor-over-comb technique

Remember

- Sterilise all equipment after each client.
- Ensure the client is protected from hair cuttings entering the eyes or other uncomfortable areas.

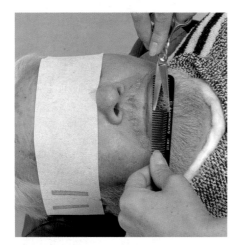

Comb all of the hair into style and place your scissors into the hair to pick up a mesh of hair for cutting. Replace the scissors with your comb to support the section of hair you are going to cut.

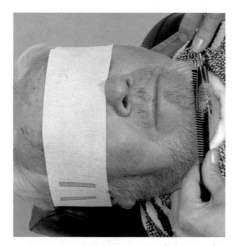

Holding the hair out at 90° to the head, remove the desired length.

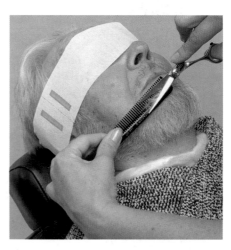

Work your way around the client's beard in small, neat channels.

Clippers with attachment

Refer to page 283 for more information on clipper attachments.

When using the clippers with an attachment, check that you have chosen the right grade to remove the length of hair required by the client. You will need to make sure that you fix the attachment firmly onto the clippers so that it does not fall off during the service.

When you put the clippers into the beard, they should be in contact with the skin. This will help you to maintain an even length throughout the beard trim.

Clipper-over-comb technique

This cutting technique is similar to the scissor-over-comb technique; the difference is that you will be using clippers rather than scissors to cut off the hair that is protruding from your comb. The same principles apply to clipper-over-comb as for scissor-over-comb – you need to cut the hair at a 90-degree angle to ensure you do not put any hard lines into the hair.

Freehand technique

This technique is mainly used for cutting the perimeter shape when trimming moustaches. As the name of the technique suggests, you do not hold the hair with tension but comb the hair into place and cut free hand. The free-hand technique gives you a truer indication of where the hair will sit because you will not have used tension by pulling the hair down.

Step-by-step moustache cutting

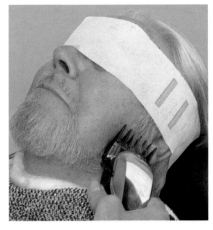

Clippers with attachment

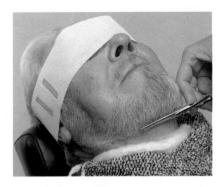

Freehand technique

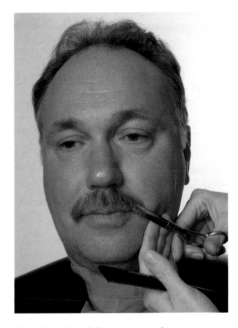

The length of the moustache is decided and perimeter removed accordingly. Use a freehand technique supporting your scissors as you work.

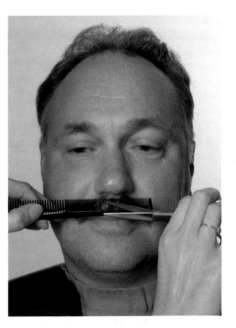

The bulk of the moustache is removed using a scissor-over-comb technique.

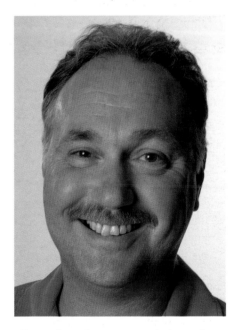

The end result is an even, balanced moustache. Confirm the result with your client.

Critical influencing factors

Head and face shapes

During the consultation with your client you will have looked at the client's head and face shape. If you have a client with a long face shape and you leave the neck outline long, you will emphasise the length of the face. Similarly, if the client has a very round face and you make the neckline very round, you will be emphasising the roundness of the face.

When cutting moustaches, the size of the moustache should correspond to the size of the facial features. Heavy facial features will require a large design, while small, fine, smooth features would suit a small design.

Critical influencing factors you should look out for are:

- length of the mouth
- size of the nose
- size of upper lip area.

Facial features and shape of moustache

Here are a few guidelines to get you started.

- Large coarse facial features – heavy moustache.
- Prominent nose – large moustache.
- Long, narrow nose – narrow, thin moustache.
- Extra large mouth – pyramid-shaped moustache.
- Extra small mouth – narrow, short, thin moustache.
- Smallish regular features – small, triangular-shaped moustache.
- Wide mouth with prominent upper lip – heavy handlebar moustache or large divided moustache.
- Round face with regular features – semi-squarish moustache.
- Square face with prominent features – heavy linear moustache with ends curling slightly downwards.

Hair growth patterns

Not all hair grows in the same direction. You will need to take this into account when you are trimming beards or moustaches. Some beards may have swirls in them; some moustaches may grow unevenly. When cutting facial hair, you may need to change the angle or the length of the cut to take these factors into account.

If the neck hair grows in a specific way, for example, round or square, you will need to follow the natural growth patterns of the hair. If you try to alter the natural shape of the neckline, the client may have difficulty in maintaining the shape at home or the shape may grow out quickly and look untidy.

Reality check!

Always double check that the grade is properly attached before you begin to use the clippers.

You will also need to take care not to push the clipper grade too firmly into the client's neck. Some clients may have more sensitive skin than others and you will cause the skin to go pink or red and look sore.

Check it out

Working in pairs, suggest the best shapes to cut a beard to suit each of the face shapes (round, square, long and oval).

Hair styles

The way in which the client is wearing his hair will need to be taken into account when deciding on the length, shape or thickness of the beard or moustache. If your client has a grade one crew cut and you leave his beard thick and bushy, would that look right? In this instance, what do you think a better look for the client's beard would be?

Hair density

When you talk about the hair's density, you are looking at the amount of hair that the client has on his face. An individual hair might be quite fine but altogether there may be a lot of them. This is when you will refer to the density of the hair. It is the amount of hair the client has per square inch. How would this influence your choice of method or cutting technique when carrying out a beard or moustache trim?

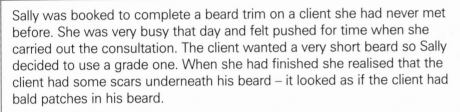

In the salon

Sally was booked to complete a beard trim on a client she had never met before. She was very busy that day and felt pushed for time when she carried out the consultation. The client wanted a very short beard so Sally decided to use a grade one. When she had finished she realised that the client had some scars underneath his beard – it looked as if the client had bald patches in his beard.

- What should Sally have done?

Adverse skin conditions

When you are carrying out a consultation on a client, you are not only looking at the hair growth patterns and hair texture, you are also looking to see if the client has any infestations or infections that might not allow you to carry out the service. You will need to do this in a discreet and professional way, so that you don't make the client feel uncomfortable.

If you come across anything that you are unable to identify but feel will not enable you to carry out the service, you must inform your tutor or salon manager quietly and get them to give you a second opinion.

If you fail to carry out a proper consultation, you could end up passing on infections or infestations to other clients.

In the salon

Tom often forgot to sterilise his tools and, as a result, had a complaint from a customer who had developed a skin condition since coming to the salon for a moustache trim.

- What two things did Tom fail to do correctly before beginning the service?

Check it out

Gather together some style books and cut out some pictures of men's haircuts. Look at the different hairstyles and discuss what shape and thickness, would best suit the different hairstyles you are looking at. If allowed, draw in the the type of beard or moustache that best suits the hairstyle in the picture.

Remember

It is important to take your time on the consultation so get it right!

Adjusting your position to ensure an even, accurate, balanced cut

As you are progressing through your trim, you will need to adjust the position in which you work so that you cover the whole area in a methodical manner. You should ensure that you have not missed any area and that you have achieved an even, balanced result.

If you stand 'square' on to the client and try to cut the hair in one position, you will not achieve a balanced shape since people tend not to have balanced, symmetrical heads and faces. You will need to move around the head as you work so that you are covering all angles of the haircut. This will help you to achieve an accurate cut, ensuring that you have an even distribution of weight and balance throughout the beard and moustache trim.

Your mirror is a good tool to use to check the shape, weight and balance of your cut. If you sit your client up in the chair and stand directly behind him, you will be able to use the mirror to confirm that you have achieved the same length and have achieved a balanced result.

By using your mirror to check the beard or moustache trim, you are giving yourself and your client the opportunity to make any changes to the cut that may be required. It is important to check with your client that he is happy with what you have done and feels that you have achieved the desired result.

Removing unwanted hair outside the desired outline

As part of the complete look you need to make sure that you 'clean up' any hair that is outside of the outline shape of the cut.

You will need to confirm with the client the neck shape that you are going to cut and do that first. You can do this by turning your clippers upside down and using the edge of the blade to gently make a definite line. Once you have put the shape in you require, you then turn your clippers so that the flat side of the clippers are sitting against the client's neck and can continue to remove the unwanted excess hair.

Check it out

In your groups, discuss the types of questions that you can use to confirm with the client that they are happy with the desired look.

Remember to think about using open questions rather than closed questions, which will help you to gain more of a response from your client.

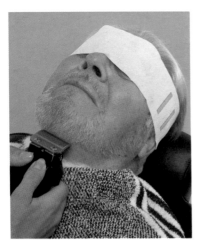

Turn the clippers upside down and use the edge of the blade to create a definite line

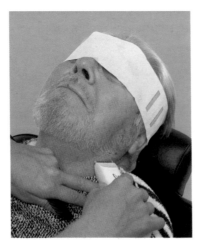

Turn the clippers so the flat side is against the client's neck

Meeting client expectations and ensuring comfort

When you are showing the client the end result you should:

- ensure he is sitting upright
- remove the towel and tissue from his neck so he can see the result
- give him a hand mirror so he can look closely at what you have done
- show him all angles using a hand mirror (if appropriate).

If any hair is sticking to the client, you can use a small amount of talcum powder to absorb the moisture and help to remove the hair cuttings.

You should also be able to give your client the correct after-care advice on home maintenance and discuss a suitable time for him to come back for a trim.

Types of information to give your client

- How often he will require regular trims to maintain the cut.
- Explain how much hair grows on average.
- How you have cut the neck shape and explain to him how to carry out the same process at home.

Your questions answered

What do I do if I cut a client's beard and it appears thinner or shorter on one side?

You could do one of two things. You could use either a scissor-over-comb technique to match up both sides, or use a different clipper attachment on the thicker/longer side.

How would I know how short to cut a moustache?

You need to be guided by your client to a certain degree and it is also important to carry out a thorough consultation. Usually, the length of the moustache sits at the edge of the top lip. It is important to carry out your consultation while the client is sat upright to enable you to see a clear picture.

I have a client who always wants me to shave his neck clean, but I do not like doing this. What should I suggest?

You can use the small rechargeable clippers as these will give a fairly clean, close cut. You would then have to advise the client that he can use his normal shaving technique at home to get a really close shave.

I find it really hard to use the flexible cutting comb for beard trims as it bends too much. Do I have to?

No, you do not have to use this comb. Everyone has preferences for the tools they use. If you can achieve the same result using your rigid cutting comb, continue to do so.

Our salon only has barbicide for us to sterilise our tools in – is this adequate?

Barbicide solution is a good method of sterilisation for the majority of barbering equipment, providing you are following the manufacturer's instructions on how to use it correctly. You will need to use a sterilising spray for electrical clippers as these cannot be immersed in the solution.

The full service

Ensure your client is protected for the service.

Establish and follow the correct cutting guidelines.

Remove any unwanted hair from outside the outline shape.

Confirm the look with the client and give suitable after-care advice.

Test your knowledge

1   What is the correct gowning procedure?

2   What are the legal requirements for the disposal of waste materials?

3   What are your responsibilities under the current Electricity at Work Regulations?

4   Why is it important to avoid cross-infection and infestation?

5   Why is it important to cut to the natural facial hairline?

6   What is the average rate of hair growth?

7   List the methods of sterilisation used in barbershops.

8   What is meant by the term 'critical influencing factor'?

9   List the safety issues that need to be considered when cutting facial hair.

Cut and finish African Caribbean type hair using barbering techniques

Unit H17

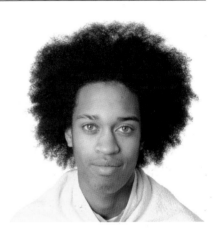

This unit is about using precision cutting skills to achieve a variety of looks that are specifically appropriate for African Caribbean hair. These include club cutting techniques, clipper-over-comb, scissor-over-comb, fading, and freehand techniques. A razor can also be used for cleaner lines and for pattern work. You will also be required to finish the hair using a variety of finishing products specifically created for African Caribbean hair.

What you will learn
• Maintain effective and safe methods of working when cutting and finishing hair H17.1 • Cut hair to achieve a variety of looks H17.2 • Finish hair H17.3

Maintain effective and safe methods of working when cutting and finishing hair

H17.1

Much of the essential knowledge and understanding you need to learn is covered in Unit H7, 'Cut hair using basic barbering techniques', on pages 279–301. However, as this unit is all about cutting and dressing African Caribbean hair, there is specific information you will need to learn and be able to apply.

What you will learn
• Using tools that are safe and fit for their purpose • Minimise the risk of cross-infection to your clients • Factors that may influence the service prior to cutting • Completing the cutting service within a commercially viable time

Many of the topics that you need to know about have been covered previously in Unit H7, such as:

• preparing the client for a cutting service (page 280)
• health and safety issues (page 281)
• safe working methods (page 281).

Using tools that are safe and fit for their purpose

To complete a full service on a client, you may be required to style the hair after the cutting service. In order to do this, you will need a selection of styling tools and equipment. In addition to the tools and equipment outlined in Unit H7, you may need:

- selection of round brushes
- selection of combs
- hairdryer
- wave brush
- afro comb.

In order to maintain your equipment in good working order, you should:

- remove hair and debris from your brushes and combs
- sterilise your tools following the correct procedures and manufacturer's guidelines
- store your tools and equipment in their correct places
- allow electrical equipment to cool down before storing
- not wind flexes or cables tightly around electrical appliances.

By taking good care of your tools you will prolong the life and appearance of all of your equipment.

Make sure that your:
- brushes have straight bristles to avoid tearing hair
- combs have no broken teeth
- scissors are clean and sharp.

Minimise the risk of cross-infection to your clients

To prevent the risk of cross-infection from one client to another, you need to make sure that you carry out a complete and thorough consultation on your client. This is the point where you would be able to identify any infections or infestations that could stop you from being able to carry out a hairdressing service.

Factors that may influence the service prior to cutting

Before cutting the client's hair, you should carry out the consultation. There are a number of important factors to consider before the service can take place and these can be addressed by completing a consultation cutting checklist before you begin. A suggested checklist is given on page 319.

Suspected infections and infestations, particularly ringworm

During your consultation, you should be checking the hair and scalp for any infections or infestations (see the table on pages 287–8).

Ringworm is a highly infectious fungal condition characterised by a bald patch with greyish/white scales and some broken hairs. It is easily spread through skin contact or through contact with equipment. Razor burns on the scalp are very common if clippers aren't cleaned properly before and after use. You must therefore sterilise tools carefully between clients.

Remember

During the consultation, check for any infections or infestations that may not allow you to carry out the service.

Consultation checklist for cutting

Client's name:_____

Address:_____

Tel. no:_____

Stylist:_____

Date:_____

FACTORS TO CONSIDER

Client requirements:

What are your client's wishes? _____

Expectations of the haircut? Dry trim, re-style, neckline shape and sideburns _____

_____

Face shape:

Square ☐   Round ☐   Oval ☐   Oblong ☐

Body proportions:

Hair type/movement: Curly ☐   Wavy ☐   Straight ☐

Extent of wave or curl?_____

Hair texture: Degree of fineness? Very coarse? _____

Abundance of hair: How much hair do you have to work with? _____

Natural growth patterns: Double crown and widow's peak _____

Hair condition: Porosity and elasticity _____

Client personality/dress/lifestyle: _____

Client limitations: Check whether the client will be able to maintain the style at home _____

_____

Suggested style: Use the information gathered above to suggest or guide your client towards a style that you both feel suits his needs _____

_____

Cutting techniques and reason: List the techniques you are going to use and your reasons for using them. Make sure that the chosen cutting techniques, for example, razoring, suit the hair's condition. (This will also act as a record of your consultation and the cut for future reference.) _____

_____

_____

Hair density

When you talk about the hair's density, you are referring to the amount of hair that the client has per square inch of his head. On some clients you can see the scalp through the hair which means that they don't have very dense hair. Other clients may have lots of hair per square inch resulting in very dense hair.

It is sometimes easy to get density and thickness of the hair confused. You will need to remember that density refers to the amount of hair on a head and thickness refers to the texture of an individual hair not the amount of hair the client has.

African Caribbean hair can appear dense because of the colour. However, this is not necessarily so since at root level it can be quite sparse. When assessing density, it is therefore important to check the roots carefully.

Hair texture

You should examine the hair's texture very carefully during your consultation with the client because this may affect the cutting technique that you choose to use. If you decide on a particular cutting technique because of the hair's texture, you will have identified a 'critical influencing factor'. For example, if the client has really thick curly hair that is quite long and wants a grade number 1, you would have to comb the hair through with an afro comb and decrease the grade gradually from a number 4 to a number 1. This will make it easier to cut and prevents the grades from coming off the clippers.

You can identify the texture of the hair by separating a few strands of hair and placing them across the palm of your hand. The texture of the hair usually falls into three categories: fine, medium, and thick. You will need to look at the hair closely and decide which one of these categories the hair falls into.

Head and face shape

When consulting with the client before deciding on the length of the cut, you should take into consideration the client's head and face shape because these can become 'critical influencing factors' in your choice of length for the cut. For example, if a client wanted a graduated cut, you would need to take into account the client's head shape.

The four most common face shapes are: square, round, oblong and oval. You will need to decide what face shape your client has to determine which style will best suit him. For example, to balance out a square face you will need to style the hair to make the 'squareness' of the face less obvious.

Hair elasticity

We test the elasticity of the hair to determine how good the internal strength of the hair is (remember, porosity testing determines the condition of the outside of the hair shaft). Refer to Unit G7 for hair tests. If the hair is in bad condition, you may not choose to use razoring techniques on it. This is because it may be fragile and unable to withstand this method of cutting which can put extra stress on the hair.

Hair growth patterns

On some heads of hair the growth patterns are very apparent. For example, if the client has a prominent crown you need to make sure that you cut the hair in the direction of growth to prevent a patchy cut.

Presence of male pattern baldness

Where a client's hair recedes at the temples or may be thinning slightly at the crown area, you will need to take this into account as a critical influencing factor. The client may ask you to style his hair in such a way that you would be emphasising the male pattern baldness.

Male pattern baldness is a hereditary factor that can affect male clients at a very young age. Most men can look at their fathers or grandfathers to see how their hair will thin or recede (or not). Some clients may be sensitive to this so you should:

* be tactful
* suggest a variation of the style suggested by the client if you think his idea would emphasise the baldness
* leave the hair slightly longer to compensate for these areas.

Not every client who has male pattern baldness will be concerned about it and you may find that they wish to have a very short haircut.

Piercings

If your client has any body piercing to the face you will need to take care. If the piercing is in the eye area cover it with a plaster before carrying out the service.

Completing the cutting service within a commercially viable time

You have looked at making the best use of your working time by ensuring that you are prepared for your client by having all of the relevant tools and equipment to hand and having the client's record card out. What you also need to be aware of is how long your salon allows for each of the services that it offers.

Cut hair to achieve a variety of looks

H17.2

In this element you will be looking at how to complete a thorough consultation to determine any critical influencing factors, the type of haircut your clients' want, and what are the most suitable methods and techniques to achieve the required result. You will be looking at outline and neckline shapes and consulting with the client throughout the service.

What you will learn	

- Preparing the client's hair prior to cutting
- Confirming the desired look with your client prior to cutting
- Accurately establishing and following cutting guidelines
- Cutting techniques
- Critical influencing factors
- Cross checking to establish weight and balance of the cut
- Neckline shapes
- Outline shapes and sideburns
- Confirming the desired look with your client during and after cutting

Preparing the client's hair prior to cutting

Once you have completed the consultation, you will know whether you are going to be carrying out the service on wet or dry hair. You will need to gown the client appropriately, ensuring you maintain good client care throughout.

It is more usual for men to have their hair cut dry and shampooed afterwards. This is because the hair is more manageable in a dry state. However, if the hair is softer and therefore less manageable in its dry state, it is most likely that you will wash it first. You, as the stylist, will have to make the decision.

Confirming the desired look with your client prior to cutting

You would have already discussed how the client wants his hair cut during the consultation and should have him gowned and the hair prepared ready to begin the cut. This is now a good time to confirm what you discussed during your consultation. You can do this by running back through the conversation to check that he is happy for you to continue with the haircut you both discussed.

Some ways of helping you to confirm the desired result with the client would be to:

- ask him to confirm that your suggestions are acceptable
- ask him to repeat or explain himself more, if you do not understand something he is telling you. Then repeat it back to him so that you are sure you have understood correctly.

Accurately establishing and following cutting guidelines

When you are ready to begin your cut on the client, you need to make sure that you work in a methodical manner. You will be working through the haircut by dividing the hair into small workable sections.

The type of haircut you are going to be carrying out will determine how the hair is sectioned throughout the cut.

By following the guidelines below you will be able to work around the head, using your time to the maximum benefit to ensure you achieve the result required.

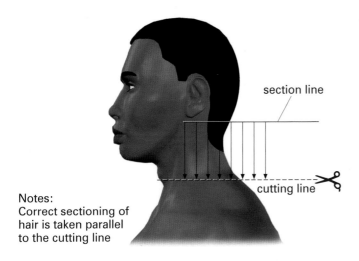

section line

cutting line

Notes:
Correct sectioning of hair is taken parallel to the cutting line

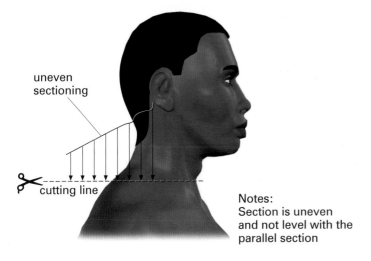

uneven sectioning

cutting line

Notes:
Section is uneven and not level with the parallel section

Cutting techniques

Some of the techniques that you will be using are:

- club cutting
- scissor-over-comb
- clipper-over-comb
- freehand
- fading.

Club cutting

This method leaves the ends of the hair blunt and level. It is sometimes called the blunt cut. The technique is most commonly used for removing length from the hair and is ideal for fine hair, as it gives the appearance of increasing bulk. It can also help to reduce the tendency of the hair to curl.

Club cutting is very suitable for curly hair because the sections are combed through and held with tension, ensuring that the ends of the hair are blunt and level.

Freehand cutting

Freehand techniques are ideal for use on African Caribbean hair. As the name of the technique suggests, you do not hold the hair with tension – the hair is combed into place and cut free hand. The freehand technique gives you a truer indication of how the hair will sit when dried because you will not have used tension by pulling the hair down. This is an ideal method to use on fringes, as they have a tendency to 'jump up' when dried and it is also better suited to one-length looks that are cut above the collar.

Freehand techniques can also be used on hair that has been styled and finished to remove any unwanted stray hairs. When you have styled the hair, you can go back over the cut using a 'topiary' technique to make sure that the perimeter shape is level and even.

Fading

A style is created so that a harsh or bold hairline is not visible. Cutting techniques used in fading include clipper-over-comb, scissor-over-comb, freehand or using clippers with clipper grades.

Scissor-over-comb

This technique is used to cut hair very short following the natural contours of the head. It is most frequently used in the nape area or around the ears and is often used in men's hairdressing to taper the hair into the hairline. The technique can be used on wet or dry hair, although you will achieve a better result on dry hair, as the cutting line is clearer.

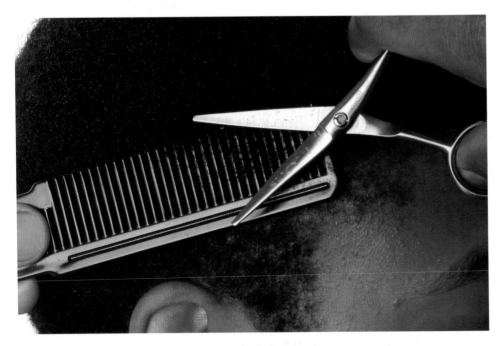

Scissor-over-comb technique used to remove bulk from the hair

Reality check!

When club cutting, sections taken must be combed through so that the hair is smooth and held with even tension to ensure an even result.

Clipper-over-comb

With this technique, the clippers are used instead of scissors to give a similar effect to scissor-over-comb. Both techniques allow you to cut the hair shorter than if you were holding the hair between your fingers. Clipper-over-comb must be carried out on dry hair.

Critical influencing factors

By looking at the cutting consultation checklist, you can see how the hair's texture, density and amount of natural curl will have an influence on your haircut.

Other factors that will have an influence on your haircut are strong hair growth patterns, such as nape whirls, widow's peak, double crowns, and the tightness of the curl in the hair.

Look at the list below to see the explanation of each of the growth patterns.

- Widow's peak – found at the very front of the hairline. The hair comes to a sharp exaggerated point.
- Nape whorls – found in the lower nape area. The hair grows in a strong circular movement each side of the hairline, often pushing up and away from the head.
- Double crown – found on the crown or crown area. There are two circular movements that may encourage the hair to lift or split.
- Cowlick – found in the fringe area. Strong movement will push the hair strongly to one side or up in an arc.

You will need to move around the head as you work so that you are covering all angles of the haircut. Moving around the head will help you to achieve an accurate cut, ensuring that you have even distribution of weight and balance throughout the style.

You may also need to move your client's head during the haircut so that you can reach more awkward areas such as the nape area. You may need to gently guide the client's head in the direction you want them to be in.

Crosschecking to establish weight and balance of the cut

As you are moving around your client, you should be looking at the hair from all angles to check that you have achieved even balance and weight throughout the haircut. It is also important to use your mirror, as this will allow you to see what the client is seeing. Stand behind your client with his head in a normal position, either pull the hair out from each side of the haircut or run your fingers through the hair, and use your mirror to check that you have achieved hair of the same length on both sides.

If you have used thinning methods during the haircut, you can do the same to check that you have an even distribution of weight throughout the cut.

It is important to make sure you have looked at the haircut from every angle, as when the client has left the salon this is what other people will see.

Neckline shapes

Cutting an accurate neckline shape in men's barbering is very important. Everyone's hairline grows differently and you will need to take this into account. It is always best to follow the natural growth pattern of the hairline. Any hair that is outside of the neckline shape will need to be removed by using your clippers to get a clean and accurate finished result.

Remember

Only use clippers on dry hair.

Reality check!

You should sterilise and oil your clippers after every client to maintain their effectiveness.

Check it out

In your groups, discuss how you would have to adapt your cutting methods and techniques to take critical influencing factors into consideration.

Check it out

In pairs, use your mirrors, front on, to look at each other's ears and see if your partner's ears are at the same height.

If they were at very different heights, would you suggest a style that showed the ears? How would you adapt your haircut?

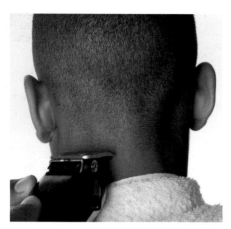

Natural outline

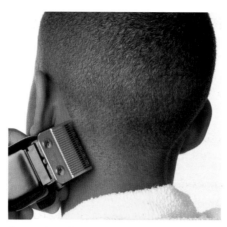

Created outline

Outline shapes and sideburns

Natural and created

When cutting men's hair, you will also be required to shape and balance the client's sideburns. You can use:

- scissor-over-comb techniques
- clipper-over-comb techniques
- freehand techniques
- club cutting techniques.

Scissor- and clipper-over-comb techniques will reduce the bulk from the sideburns, while club cutting and freehand cutting will remove length.

It is not always a good idea to judge the length of the hair by looking at where the hair sits in relation to the client's ears, as they can be uneven! It is best to look at your client straight on in the mirror with a finger at the bottom of each sideburn to determine the correct balance and length.

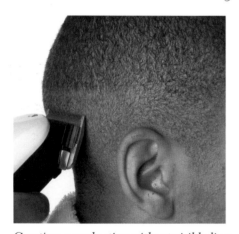

Creating a graduation without visible lines

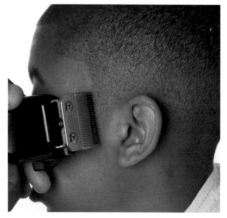

Defining the sideburns to give a finished look

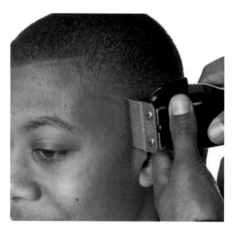

Pattern applied to hairline and sideburn border created

Confirming the desired look with your client during and after cutting

During the treatment you should confirm with the client that he is happy with the way the service is progressing. These are the types of questions you could ask.

- Are you comfortable?
- Have I removed enough length? (Only cut one section of hair before asking this question!)
- Are you happy with the sideburn length?
- How does the whole cut feel? (Let the client run his fingers through his hair.)

It is also important to use the back mirror to show the client the profile and back of his hair, again reaffirming that he is happy with the cut that you have completed.

When using the back mirror:

- hold it at the height of the client's head
- spend time letting the client see all angles of the haircut
- do not stand too far back.

Check it out

Think back to your last visit to the hairdressers. How did the stylist check that you were happy and comfortable during your treatment? Did this make you feel more reassured during your visit?

If the stylist did not ask you any questions, how did this make you feel?

Finish hair

H17.3

In this element you will be looking at how to finish the look by dressing the hair with the appropriate styling and finishing products, and how to control the hair by choosing the correct tools to take into account the relevant influencing factors.

What you will learn

- Consulting with your client
- Styling and finishing products
- Effectively controlling the client's hair
- Styling tools
- Ensuring the look takes into account critical influencing factors

Consulting with your client

You will have already consulted with your client (refer to consultation cutting checklist, page 319) to establish how you are going to cut his hair. It is equally important to consult with the client to find out how you are going to finish and dress the hair into the finished look.

From your cutting consultation you will already have a good idea of how you are going to be finishing the style. It is important however to double-check and confirm with the client the desired effect that you want to achieve as an end result.

Styling and finishing products

To be able to style your client's hair it is essential that you have a knowledge of the types of styling and finishing products that your salon stocks. Products that can be used include gels, activators, dressing creams and sprays. The products are effective in moisturising hair and enhancing the style. Hair and scalp conditioners, are used on African Caribbean hair, in particular, to give the hair a sheen and moisturise the hair and scalp. Follow manufacturer's instructions when applying, using and storing products.

Check it out

In your groups, discuss what types of questions you would ask your client to help you to confirm what the end result will be.

Reality check!

Always follow the manufacturer's instructions. These give you all the information you need to use the product correctly.

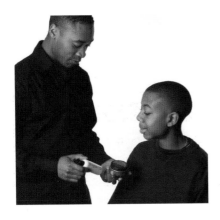

Advise your client on the correct products to use to maintain the style

Effectively controlling the client's hair

From the following chart, you will notice that different products will produce varying holds on the hair. When styling the hair it is important to be aware of what each product will do, as this will affect your choice of product when taking into account any critical influencing factors.

By researching your products you should find that:

- for hair that has a strong growth pattern, a product with a strong/firm hold is be required
- all products will help you to produce totally different effects
- products are applied to the hair in different amounts
- some products can only be applied to wet or dry hair
- you will be able to explain in detail the benefits of the product to the client if you have read the manufacturer's instructions.

Check it out

In your groups, list some of the critical influencing factors that you have already discussed. You can refer back to page 325. Looking at each of these factors in turn, decide which product would be the most suitable to use to give you effective control for the type of hair you would be working on.

Product	Application	Suitability	Comments
Gel (wet or dry look)	Apply to wet or dry hair at the roots and spread through	Firm hold – enhances curls	Ideal for short, textured styles
Glaze	Apply evenly to towel dried hair	Firm hold – dries hardand adds body to hair	Ideal for slicking back unruly hair
Dressing cream	Apply small amount evenly with hands	Light hold – large amounts will produce a slicked back look	Effectively moisturises the hair
Hair gloss	Apply small amounts on wet hair to mid-length and ends of hair	Reduces frizz and increases shine	Ideal for African Caribbean hair
Moisturiser	Apply to hair before styling	Makes hair soft and shiny; loosens tangles	Useful for conditioning African Caribbean hair
Activators	Apply to wet or dry hair	Used to maintain curl or replace moisture in permanent or naturally curly hair	Defines curl; adds moisture and shine to hair

Some styling, dressing and finishing products

Styling tools

As well as understanding the way in which styling products affect the hair, you need to know about the effects different types of equipment can help you to achieve.

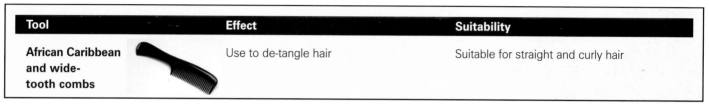

Tool	Effect	Suitability
African Caribbean and wide-tooth combs	Use to de-tangle hair	Suitable for straight and curly hair

Styling tools for African Caribbean hair

Controlling your styling tools

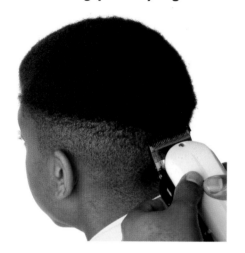 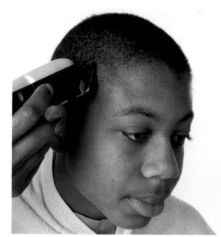 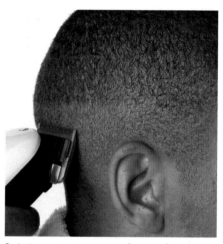

It is important to control your clippers to produce the desired result

You need to be able to control your equipment and the hair as you style it. The way in which you manage the hair is very important, as this will affect the finished result. Here are some tips to help you.

- If your clippers have a guard, make sure it is placed securely.
- You will need to make sure your hands are steady so that they can glide along the hair easily.
- Make sure that your hands are not greasy or wet otherwise the clippers will slip.
- Many barbers use two pairs of clippers and swap over when they get too hot or sticky.
- You need to make sure that your client is sitting comfortably without fidgeting.

Clipper grades

The most commonly used clipper grades for African Caribbean hair are:

Grade 0 – bald effect

Grade 0.1 – skinhead effect

Grade 1 – half an inch

Grade 2 – nearly an inch

Grade 3 – at least an inch

Grade 4 – longer than an inch.

Ensuring the look takes into account critical influencing factors

When you have completed the cut and have styled the hair, you will need to look at the finished result, checking that you:

- have achieved the look requested by the client
- are happy with the balance and weight distribution of the haircut
- have styled the hair to reflect the haircut
- have taken into account any critical influencing factors.

If the client had a widow's peak, double crown or strong growth patterns, have you worked with the hair in such a way that any of these factors are not obvious? Have you used the correct styling and finishing products to dress the hair so that a double crown is less apparent? Have you made an incorrect choice and highlighted a critical influencing factor?

You need to make sure that you make allowances for any factor that may have an effect on your end result from your choice of style to the method of styling, and the products that you decide to use. You may be happy with the end result, but is the client? You will need to check that your client is happy to leave the salon with the finished result.

Another important part of any hairdressing service is to make sure you give your client adequate and correct after-care advice. You will need to discuss with your client a suitable time span for him to come back to the salon for regular trims, for example. You will need to explain about the amount that hair grows every two weeks so that the client understands how frequently he should have his hair cut.

The hair grows on average about half an inch per month, some peoples' hair may grow slightly slower or faster than this and the client should be able to give you an indication of how quickly he thinks his hair grows.

It is also important to explain to your client how to use the styling tools and products so that he can re-create the same result at home. You can talk about what equipment you are using, why and how to use it as you are styling his hair. You can also do the same with styling and finishing products.

Types of information suitable to give a client could include:

- type of comb to use for his length or style of hair
- what products you have used and why you have used them
- where the client can purchase the products
- how much product he should use
- how much the products cost.

All of this information can be given during the service so it will not add any extra time onto the appointment and you will have given the client a complete service by providing advice and recommendations.

Check it out

In your groups, discuss the types of questions you would like to be asked as a client to see if you are happy with the finished result.

Your questions answered

I have heard that African Caribbean and very curly hair can really spring up after it has been cut. What can I do to make sure I do not cut the hair too short?
This is why a thorough consultation is very important. You will need to look at the hair in its dry state first to make sure you know how much hair requires cutting and to make sure that you have a mental guide of the amount to work to. When the hair is wet it will stretch, so it is important that you do not cut off any more hair than was discussed at the initial consultation. If in doubt, cut the hair when it is dry.

How will I be able to tell the difference between alopecia and ringworm?
With ringworm you will find that the skin, where the hair is missing, may not look like the rest of the scalp. It begins with pink patches on the scalp developing into grey scaly areas with broken hairs around the outside.

With alopecia the hair has fallen out. The exposed skin should look like the rest of the scalp and the hairs at the edges of the circle will not be broken.

Whose responsibility is it to have electrical equipment checked under the Electricity at Work Act?
It is the responsibility of the employer to have equipment checked at regular intervals under this Act, but you still have a responsibility under the Health and Safety at Work Act to make sure that you report any faulty or damaged equipment to a senior member of staff.

What could happen if you did not have electrical equipment checked and did not have safety stickers on it?
You may find that if there was an incident and a client or member of staff was injured and wanted to claim compensation that the salon's insurance would not be valid. Depending on the severity of the injury this could be very costly for the salon and end up as a potential court case!

I do not understand the term 'distribution of weight' what does this mean?
Distribution of weight basically means the haircut level. Ask yourself: 'When I look in the mirror, does one side look the same as the other?' If you have left more length or bulk on one side of the hair, you will not have an even distribution of weight.

What would I do if a client asked for a neckline shape that was not suitable for the way his nape hair growth pattern allowed?
You would need to advise and explain to the client why the neckline shape that he wanted wasn't suitable for his particular hair growth pattern. You could use your mirror to show the client why and outline what your recommendations would be. You will always find that if you explain to clients the reasons why something cannot be achieved, they will be understanding and open to your suggestions. If you have a client who still insists on his first request then you have no option but to carry out his wishes having explained the potential outcome.

Would it be more suitable to use clipper-over-comb techniques rather than scissor-over-comb techniques on African Caribbean hair?
It may well be more practical in some instances to use clipper-over-comb techniques as opposed to scissor-over-comb. Clipper-over-comb techniques allow you to cut the hair using a freehand technique to create a precise exterior shape.

Test your knowledge

1   What is the correct gowning procedure for a wet and dry haircut?

2   Why is it important to make sure that your client is seated in the correct position before you carry out the haircut?

3   List three sterilising methods that can be used for your tools and equipment.

4   Where do you dispose of used sharps?

5   Why is it important to follow cutting guidelines?

6   What is meant by the term 'critical influencing factors'?

7   List three critical influencing factors.

8   Why is it important to use the correct degree of tension when cutting?

9   What effect can be achieved by the club cutting technique?

Key Skills Level 1 and NVQ Level 2 Customer Service

When completing tasks for your NVQ Level 2 Hairdressing portfolio you will also be creating evidence that is suitable for your Key Skills portfolio and, if you take it, NVQ Level 2 Customer service.

The following is a guide to which evidence is most suitable for each and what is expected of that evidence. The Key Skills evidence is listed first, and the related Customer Service evidence follows.

Key Skills Level 1 Communication

C1.1 One-to-one discussion

This needs to be about different, straightforward subjects. Any of the following can be used as evidence.

- Practical units H6, H9, H10, H12, H13, H15, H16 – a treatment consultation with the client or G7 (Advise and consult with clients).

The assessor who has observed your client interaction should sign the consultation sheet. The form must be neat and tidy, with clear writing, and no spelling mistakes. (See pages 83–6 for advice on analysing clients' needs)

- Unit G8 – one-to-one discussion for any tutorial interview with a subject or personal tutor

You and your tutor will decide on a clear pathway for your personal progression through the unit you are currently working on and you should both sign this. Any resulting action plan can contribute to Unit G8 (Develop and maintain your effectiveness at work). (See Unit G8, pages 99–105 – self-appraisal.)

- Units G4, G5 and G8 – one-to-one discussion within your role as salon manager

If a discussion arises regarding the treatment page/treatments to do or jobs to be allocated, the discussion should be logged on your duty report form and signed by both parties. Your tutor will supply you with the appropriate paperwork.

- Units G4, G5 and G8 – student discussion between two colleagues

Use a salon situation to discuss any practical issues that arise, and log it on the salon report sheet, or present the solution to a problem to your salon manager/assessor i.e. 'Shelley and I are going to cover the clients for Ramona, who is off sick – I will do XYZ and Shelley will do ABC" (See Unit G4 pages 55–7.)

C1.1 Group discussion

- Units G4, G5 and G8 - class discussion between all class members

Suggestions on how to improve the salon/client set-up – salon organisation, client rota or similar topic.

Class discussion on a straightforward subject linked to Hairdressing e.g. why you have chosen hairdressing as a career, new and interesting products on the market, animal testing on hairdressing products, the importance of keeping up to date with new treatments, styles and products or a similar topic.

Complete an evaluation sheet on the results of your discussion and remember to get signatures. You tutor will provide the marking sheets.

NVQ Level 2 Customer Service

If you complete the evidence for Key Skills Communication C1.1 One-to-one discussion, you have also achieved the following elements and units for NVQ Level 2 Customer Service.

Element 1.1

Find out which products the client has been using or which treatments have been a success.

Element 5.3

Produce evidence that you have worked with clients or colleagues to provide a more reliable service.

C1.2 Read two documents including an image

- Units G1, H6, H9, H10, H12, H13, H15, H16

Working as a salon manager and dealing with any health and safety instructions or manufacturer's instructions for anything relating to practical units H6, H9, H10, H12, H13, H15, H16.

- How to use a steamer. (See Unit G6, page 128.)
- Fire evacuation procedures. (See Unit G1, page 36.)
- Client booking-in sheet – allocation of jobs. (See Unit G4, page 56.)
- Salon rules and regulations for professional attire and safe footwear. (See Unit G1, pages 42–3.)
- Also use information from Unit G1, health and safety for safe practices within the salon and spillage procedures. (See Unit G1, pages 25–6.)

NVQ Level 2 Customer Service

If you complete the evidence for Key Skills Communication C1.2 Read two documents including an image, you have also achieved the following elements and units in NVQ Level 2 Customer Service.

Element 1.1

Using products and services.
Following manufacturer's instructions.
Awareness of legal rights of customers.

C1.3 Write two documents including an image
- Units G1, H6, H9, H10, H12, H13, H15, H16 or G7

Design a safety poster, which could then be presented to the group, and a memo inviting students to attend the briefing. Also, a memo, inviting students to attend a salon manager meeting could be sent. (See Unit G1, pages 22–6.)

Design an after-care leaflet for any practical unit, H12, H13, H15, H16 e.g. perming, relaxing and colouring (pages 194–273).

NVQ Level 2 Customer service

If you complete the evidence for Key Skills Communication C1.3 Write two documents including an image, you have also achieved the following elements and units in NVQ Level 2 Customer Service.

Element 2.1

Design a client record card bearing security of information in mind.

Element 5.3

Work with others to improve reliably of service.

Design a short questionnaire on the back of the record of evidence sheet, for customer evaluation of the service or treatment, or for sales to improve delivery of services.

Key Skills Application of Number Level 1

N1.1 Interpret information from two sources
- Facts about hair and skin

  - Refer to the pH scale in Facts about hair and skin, both the chart and text. Identify five different products you use in your salon. Using the pH scale, decide what you think the pH values for each of the products are and write them down. Design a data collection sheet to record the pH values of the products that you have chosen. Fill it out with your estimated values. Using litmus paper, test the products you have chosen and note down the actual results on your data collection sheet. (See Facts about hair and skin page 19.)

N1.2 Carry out calculations to do with amounts and sizes, scales and proportions, handling statistics
- Unit H9

  - Work out how many re-growth treatments you would realistically get from one tube of tint, using the volume and division of number of tint used each time.
  - Calculate the cost of the tint to purchase, and the cost per treatment, remembering overheads. You should now be able to calculate the profit margin, per tube.

N1.3 Interpret results of calculations and present findings – must include one chart and one diagram

The above calculations lend themselves very nicely to a bar chart, pie chart and/or line graph, to show profit margins and overhead costs. Your lecturer will help you and provide the paperwork. This can also be used for the Key Skills Level 1 IT.

NVQ Level 2 Customer Service

If you complete the evidence for Key Skills Application of Number N1.1 Interpret information from two sources, you have also achieved the following elements and units for NVQ Level 2 Customer Service.

Element 5.2 Using client feed back to improve service reliability

Design and conduct a short questionnaire on client preferences for salon opening times. Using your results, give feedback to colleagues on the most popular choices and why.

Key Skills Level 1 Information and Computer Technology

You may need the help of your IT co-ordinator as this key skill requires you to use ICT resources.

IT1.1 Find, explore and develop information for two different purposes; IT1.2 Present two pieces of information for different purposes – including: x1 text, x1 images and x1 numbers
- Unit H13, page 238

If you are creating client information sheets on, for example, perming or colouring treatments you need to remember the following:

- Don't forget to check the spelling, punctuation and grammar.
- Keep a log detailing: how you found the information you required; the filenames you used to save your work; your reasons for choosing or rejecting information.
- Keep **draft copies** of your work, and note on them why you decided to make changes.

NVQ Level 2 Customer Service

Unit 4 Solve problems for customers

Using a computer, design a short questionnaire to gather information on customer problems – it could be related to grumbles or praise the client has for hygiene procedures.

Or, you could relate your questionnaire to: Availability of stock, quality of products or services, Use of products or services, organisation of systems, booking in etc

Element 4.2

Analyse the results and discuss in a staff meeting with colleagues, the best way to solve the problem.

Design a poster explaining the new method of addressing the clients' problems. Include text, images and numbers.

It could be a timed booking-in system, with a fixed penalty for late clients or non-arrivals.

NB All the above are suggested tasks only, with references to the book to help you identify where you may find evidence. Your lecturer may use other tasks, and give you guidance through your Key Skills and Customer Service activities.

Index

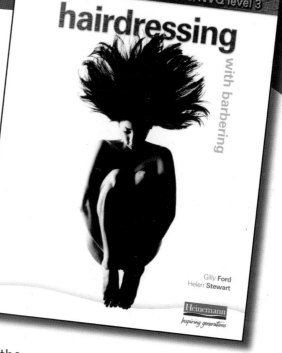
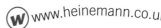
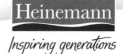
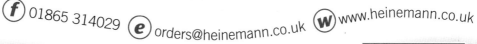